Hoekelman,
Principles of Pediatrics

Hoekelman,
Principles of Pediatrics:
PreTest® Self-Assessment and Review

Edited by
Robert A. Hoekelman

Professor and Associate Chairman, Department of Pediatrics,
University of Rochester School of Medicine and Dentistry
Rochester, New York

McGraw-Hill Book Company
Health Professions Division
PreTest Series

New York   St. Louis   San Francisco
Auckland   Bogotá   Hamburg   Johannesburg
London   Madrid   Mexico   Montreal
New Delhi   Panama   Paris   São Paulo
Singapore   Sydney   Tokyo   Toronto

Library of Congress Cataloging in Publication Data
Main entry under title:

Principles of pediatrics.

  Bibliography: p.
  1. Pediatrics—Examinations, questions, etc.
I. Hoekelman, Robert A. [DNLM: 1. Pediatrics—
Examination questions. WS18 P957]
RJ48.2.P74   618.92′00076   80-19358
ISBN 0-07-051648-0

Editorial Supervisor: *Jane Edwards*
Project Editor: *Aaron E. Klein*
Editorial Assistant: *Donna Altieri*
Production Supervisor: *Susan A. Hillinski*
Production Assistants: *Rosemary J. Pascale*
Judith M. Raccio
Designer: *Robert Tutsky*
Printer: *Hull Printing Company*

1 2 3 4 5 6 7 8 9 HUHU 8 7 6 5 4 3 2 1

Table of Contents

List of Contributors

Margaret T. Colgan, M.D.
Associate Professor of Pediatrics
University of Rochester School of
  Medicine and Dentistry
Rochester, New York

Philip W. Davidson, Ph.D.
Associate Professor of Pediatrics and
  Psychiatry (Psychology)
University of Rochester School of
  Medicine and Dentistry
Rochester, New York

John C. Ellis, M.D.
Instructor and General Pediatrics
  Academic Fellow
University of Rochester School of
  Medicine and Dentistry
Rochester, New York

Charles R. Fikar, M.D.
Preceptor, Department of Pediatrics
Rochester General Hospital
Rochester, New York

Harry L. Gewanter, M.D.
Instructor and General Pediatrics
  Academic Fellow
University of Rochester School of
  Medicine and Dentistry
Rochester, New York

Donald E. Greydanus, M.D.
Assistant Professor of Pediatrics
University of Rochester School of
  Medicine and Dentistry
Rochester, New York

Lisa Beth Handwerker, M.D.
Instructor and General Pediatrics
  Academic Fellow
University of Rochester School of
  Medicine and Dentistry
Rochester, New York

J. Peter Harris, M.D.
Assistant Professor of Pediatrics
University of Rochester School of
  Medicine and Dentistry
Rochester, New York

Richard A. Insel, M.D.
Assistant Professor of Pediatrics
University of Rochester School of
  Medicine and Dentistry
Rochester, New York

Bruce M. Kleene, M.D.
Instructor and Fellow in
  Developmental Pediatrics
University of Rochester School of
  Medicine and Dentistry
Rochester, New York

Richard E. Kreipe, M.D.
Instructor and General Pediatrics
  Academic Fellow
University of Rochester School of
  Medicine and Dentistry
Rochester, New York

Richard A. Lawrence, M.D.
Instructor and Fellow in Pediatric
  Gastroenterology and Nutrition
University of Rochester School of
  Medicine and Dentistry
Rochester, New York

Gregory S. Liptak, M.D.
Assistant Professor of Pediatrics
University of Rochester School of
  Medicine and Dentistry
Rochester, New York

James B. MacWhinney, Jr., M.D.
Clinical Assistant Professor of Pediatrics
University of Rochester School of
  Medicine and Dentistry
Rochester, New York

Kenneth M. McConnochie, M.D.
Assistant Professor of Pediatrics
University of Rochester School of
  Medicine and Dentistry
Rochester, New York

T. Allen Merritt, M.D.
Assistant Professor of Pediatrics and
  Obstetrics and Gynecology
University of Rochester School of
  Medicine and Dentistry
Rochester, New York

Michael E. Pichichero, M.D.
Instructor and Fellow in Pediatric
  Infectious Diseases
University of Rochester School of
  Medicine and Dentistry
Rochester, New York

Olle Jane Z. Sahler, M.D.
Assistant Professor of Pediatrics and
  Psychiatry
University of Rochester School of
  Medicine and Dentistry
Rochester, New York

A. Elisabeth Sommerfelt, M.D.
Instructor in Pediatrics
University of Rochester School of
  Medicine and Dentistry
Rochester, New York

Mark C. Steinhoff, M.D.
Instructor in Pediatrics
University of Rochester School of
  Medicine and Dentistry
Rochester, New York

Scott B. Valet, M.D.
Instructor and Cystic Fibrosis
  Foundation Clinical Fellow
University of Rochester School of
  Medicine and Dentistry
Rochester, New York

E.W. van der Jagt, M.D.
Instructor in Pediatrics
University of Rochester School of
  Medicine and Dentistry
Chief Resident, Strong Memorial
  Hospital Medical Center
Rochester, New York

Introduction

Hoekelman, Principles of Pediatrics: PreTest Self-Assessment and Review has been designed to provide physicians with a comprehensive, relevant, and convenient instrument for self-evaluation and review within the broad area of pediatrics. Although it should be particularly helpful for residents preparing for the American Board of Pediatrics certification examination and for board-certified pediatricians preparing for recertification, it should also be useful for pediatricians, family practitioners, and other physicians in practice who are simply interested in maintaining a high level of competence in pediatrics. Study of this self-assessment and review book should help our readers to (1) identify their areas of relative weakness; (2) confirm their areas of expertise; (3) assess their knowledge of the sciences fundamental to pediatrics; (4) assess their clinical judgment and problem-solving skills; and (5) review recent developments in general pediatrics.

This book consists of 615 multiple-choice questions that (1) are representative of the major pediatric subspecialties and (2) parallel the format and degree of difficulty of the questions on the above-mentioned board exams. Each question is accompanied by an answer, a paragraph-length explanation, and a reference to a major textbook in the field (including *Principles of Pediatrics* by Hoekelman et al., *Nelson Textbook of Pediatrics* by Vaughan et al., and *Pediatrics* by Rudolph et al.) as well as references to more specialized textbooks and current journal articles. A list of normal values used in the laboratory studies in this book can be found in the Appendix, after which follows a Bibliography listing all the sources used for the questions. All of this material was prepared by physicians representing the major subspecialties in pediatrics.

We have assumed that the time available to the reader is limited; as a result, the book can be used profitably a chapter at a time. By allowing no more than two and a half minutes to answer each question, you can simulate the time constraints of the actual board exams. When you finish answering all of the questions in a chapter, spend as much time as necessary verifying answers and carefully reading the accompanying explanations. If after reading the explanations for a given chapter, you feel a need for a more extensive and definitive discussion, consult the references listed with each question.

Based on our testing experience, on most medical examinations, examinees who answer half the questions correctly would score around the 50th or 60th percentile. A score of 65 percent would place the examinee above the 80th percentile, while a score of 30 percent would rank him below the 15th percentile. In other words, if you answer fewer than 30 percent of the questions correctly, you are relatively weak in that area. A score of 50 percent would be approximately average, and 70 percent or higher would probably be honors.

We have used three basic question types in accordance with the format of the American Board of Pediatrics certification and recertification examinations. Considerable editorial time has been spent trying to ensure that each question is clearly stated and discriminates between those physicians who are well-prepared in the subject and those who are less knowledgeable.

This book is a teaching device that provides readers with the opportunity to evaluate and update their clinical expertise, their ability to interpret data, and their ability to diagnose and manage clinical problems. If any of the examinations for which you are preparing use the programmed patient management problem technique, you will also find the companion book, *Hoekelman, Principles of Pediatrics Patient Management Problems: PreTest Self-Assessment and Review*, most helpful.

We hope that you will find this book interesting, relevant, and challenging. The editor and authors, as well as the PreTest staff, would be very happy to receive your comments and suggestions.

Preface

The authors of the 615 questions and answers in this book were commissioned to provide our readers with a review of the most important information needed for the practice of pediatrics. I believe they have succeeded and that those who are familiar with this information will be able to use it to improve the care they provide to their patients. This book also provides its readers with a means for assessing their own knowledge of pediatric subjects and an opportunity to prepare themselves to score well on a variety of tests of pediatric knowledge.

I wish to thank the authors, my colleagues in the Department of Pediatrics at the University of Rochester School of Medicine and Dentistry, for the enthusiasm and expertise they exhibited in the construction of these questions and answers. They made my job as editor both easy and pleasant. Finally, this book could not have been published without the editorial and technical assistance of Sydney A. Sutherland and the support provided by Kathy Schafer in the preparation of the manuscript.

Robert A. Hoekelman
Editor

Reproduction

DIRECTIONS: Each question below contains five suggested answers. Choose the **one best** response to each question.

1. All of the following statements concerning the susceptibility of fetuses to malformations are correct EXCEPT that

(A) the effects of maternal vitamin and iron deficiencies are limited by the ability of the placenta to transport these substances to the fetus
(B) during the first two postconception weeks, the fetus is relatively unsusceptible to teratogens
(C) major malformations of the ear generally result from exposure to teratogens during the fourth to the twelfth postconception weeks
(D) major malformations of the cardiovascular system generally result from exposure to teratogens during the sixth to eighth postconception weeks
(E) major malformations of the central nervous system generally result from exposure to teratogens during the third to sixth postconception weeks

2. The mode of inheritance of all the following diseases is autosomal dominant EXCEPT for

(A) neurofibromatosis
(B) achondroplasia
(C) Hurler's syndrome
(D) Marfan's syndrome
(E) Waardenburg's syndrome

3. In which of the following pregnancies would fetal risk be the LEAST likely?

(A) Uterine bleeding in a 24-year-old woman at 38 weeks gestation
(B) Class D diabetes in a 30-year-old woman at 36 weeks gestation
(C) Previous Rh sensitization in a 20-year-old woman at 34 weeks gestation
(D) A 40 lb weight gain in an 18-year-old woman at 36 weeks gestation
(E) Cigarette smoking and a 12 lb weight gain in a 28-year-old woman at 40 weeks gestation

4. To determine the need for therapeutic intervention, amniocentesis is recommended when

(A) both parents carry the β-thalassemia gene
(B) both parents carry the Tay-Sachs gene
(C) both parents have sickle cell trait
(D) the mother is Rh sensitized
(E) the mother is over 40 years old

5. All of the following statements concerning infant and maternal mortality are correct EXCEPT

(A) the risk of pregnancy-related maternal death is higher than the risk related to oral contraception
(B) the risk of maternal death related to mechanical contraception (diaphragm, condom, or foam) is equal to that of oral contraception
(C) the maternal death rate for pregnancy is 12 per 100,000 pregnancies
(D) the perinatal death rate for spontaneous vertex vaginal deliveries is about four times as high for nonwhites as compared to whites
(E) the perinatal death rate for repeat caesarean section is slightly higher for whites as compared to nonwhites

6. All of the following would be performed during a suction curettage abortion EXCEPT

(A) a measurement of the uterus with uterine sounding
(B) an exploration of the uterine cavity with a sharp curette
(C) the administration of Rh immunoglobulin to an Rh-negative woman
(D) the administration of nitrous oxide anesthesia
(E) the insertion of an IUD at the time of the procedure

7. All of the following syndromes may be a result of chromosomal nondisjunction EXCEPT

(A) Down's syndrome
(B) trisomy 13
(C) Klinefelter's syndrome
(D) cri du chat (cat cry) syndrome
(E) Turner's syndrome

8.   The percentage of unmarried women who report that they were sexually active by age 19 is

(A) 25 percent
(B) 35 percent
(C) 45 percent
(D) 55 percent
(E) 65 percent

9.   Of the one million adolescent pregnancies reported in 1977, approximately how many were terminated by abortion?

(A) 250,000
(B) 350,000
(C) 450,000
(D) 550,000
(E) One million

10. All of the following statements about the human leukocyte antigen (HLA) system are correct EXCEPT

(A) they are histocompatibility antigens
(B) HLA antigens are coded on chromosome no. 6 in humans
(C) HLA antigens are present on red blood cells
(D) juvenile rheumatoid arthritis (JRA) is related to HLA B27
(E) juvenile onset diabetes mellitus is identified with certain HLA types

11. When an adolescent's menstrual period is two weeks late, the most accurate method of determining pregnancy is

(A) a serum pregnancy test
(B) a urine pregnancy test
(C) a sexual history
(D) a pelvic examination
(E) an ultrasound examination

12. All of the following statements about adolescent pregnancy are true EXCEPT that

(A) adolescent mothers eventually complete their education, although pregnancy temporarily interrupts their studies
(B) adolescents often are ambivalent about the responsibilities of motherhood, wanting to be mothers but also wanting to engage in normal adolescent activities
(C) adolescent pregnancy is a medical and psychosocial high risk condition, especially for those 15 years of age or less
(D) pregnancy rates for adolescents in general are decreasing, except for black and white girls under age 15 and for white girls 15 to 17 years of age
(E) a greater percentage of infants weighing less than 2500 g are born to adolescents 15 years of age or less than those born to women aged 25-29

13. Which of the following most closely approximates the current average age range of menarche in the United States?

(A) 11.2 - 11.4
(B) 12.0 - 12.2
(C) 12.6 - 12.9
(D) 13.0 - 13.2
(E) 13.6 - 13.9

14. The most effective form of contraception for adolescents is

(A) the progesterone-only pill (mini-pill)
(B) the intrauterine device
(C) depo-medroxyprogesterone acetate
(D) the condom
(E) the diaphragm

15. According to the American College of Obstetrics and Gynecology, all of the following conditions are **absolute** contraindications for combined oral contraceptive use EXCEPT

(A) a history of thromboembolism
(B) active liver disease
(C) undiagnosed uterine bleeding
(D) diabetes mellitus
(E) pregnancy

DIRECTIONS: Each question below contains four suggested answers of which **one** or **more** is correct. Choose the answer

A	if	1, 2, and 3	are correct
B	if	1 and 3	are correct
C	if	2 and 4	are correct
D	if	4	is correct
E	if	1, 2, 3, and 4	are correct

16. Correct statements concerning the effects of anesthetics on the fetus include which of the following?

(1) Meperidine given during the delivery may not exert its maximum effect on the fetus for 20 or 30 minutes
(2) Barbiturates, which may interfere with infant feeding and bonding for extended periods, have no effective antagonist
(3) Inhaled agents may achieve higher levels in the fetus than in the mother
(4) Epidural anesthesia may result in decreased placental perfusion and prolonged labor

17. To determine if an infant who weighs 2,436 g (5 lb, 6 oz) at birth has maintained normal intrauterine growth according to the Colorado Intrauterine Growth Charts, which of the following factors must be considered?

(1) Length
(2) Race
(3) Head circumference
(4) Sex

18. Correct statements regarding caesarean section include which of the following?

(1) Uterine dysfunction, fetal distress, diabetes mellitus, and carcinoma of the cervix are all valid indications for caesarean section
(2) Prior caesarean section is an absolute contraindication to vaginal delivery
(3) Amniocentesis is indicated prior to repeat caesarean section
(4) The prognosis for fetal survival after caesarean section is better than that following vaginal delivery

19. A 37-year-old woman, gravida 5, para 2 (2 abortions), with blood type B, Rh-negative (cde), presents for ultrasound evaluation and amniocentesis at 36 weeks gestation because of rising titers suggestive of rhesus isoimmunization. Which of the following ultrasound findings or amniotic fluid chemistries would indicate immediate delivery of the fetus?

(1) Ultrasound evidence of placental edema
(2) Spectrophotometric absorption with an optical density at 450 mμ of 0.02 on the chloroform extracted amniotic fluid
(3) Biparietal diameter of 8.5 cm by ultrasound
(4) Lecithin/sphingomyelin (L/S) ratio of 3.1

20. Middle adolescent pregnancy is often the result of which of the following factors?

(1) A means of competing with the mother for the father
(2) A means of manipulating the environment
(3) An attempt to acquire autonomy
(4) A means of proving physiological maturity

21. Correct statements regarding infants of mothers addicted to narcotics include which of the following?

(1) They are frequently hyperactive, irritable, and subject to sleep disorders
(2) They may show more severe withdrawal symptoms if their mothers are on methadone maintenance rather than heroin
(3) They have a high-pitched, shrill cry and cry excessively
(4) The mortality rates and incidence of congenital anomalies in these infants are higher than those in the normal population

SUMMARY OF DIRECTIONS				
A	B	C	D	E
1, 2, 3 only	1, 3 only	2, 4 only	4 only	All are correct

22. Which of the following individuals would have no Barr bodies in their cells?

(1) A phenotypic female with Down's syndrome
(2) A phenotypic female with Turner's syndrome
(3) A phenotypic male with Kleinfelter's syndrome
(4) A phenotypic male with trisomy 18

23. Correct statements about dysmenorrhea include which of the following?

(1) It is the largest single cause of absenteeism for high school girls
(2) It appears to be related to prostaglandin metabolism
(3) It can be relieved completely by combined estrogen-progesterone therapy
(4) It can be modified by diuretic therapy

24. Correct statements about mucocolpos in infancy include which of the following?

(1) It is characterized by a bulging vaginal membrane
(2) It is treated by surgical removal of the mass
(3) It is an obstructive lesion
(4) It is associated with absent ovaries

DIRECTIONS: The groups of questions below consist of lettered choices followed by several numbered items. For each numbered item select the **one** lettered choice with which it is **most** closely associated. Each lettered choice may be used once, more than once, or not at all.

Questions 25-28

For each of the hereditary conditions listed below, select the mode of inheritance with which it is most likely to be associated.

    (A) Autosomal dominant trait
    (B) Autosomal recessive trait
    (C) Sex-linked recessive trait
    (D) Multifactorial or mode of inheritance unknown
    (E) None of the above

25. Fanconi's syndrome

26. Oculocerebrorenal syndrome of Lowe

27. Cystinuria

28. Alport's syndrome

Questions 29-33

The conditions listed below have been associated with alterations in fetal growth. Select the growth parameters most severely affected in each of these.

    (A) Weight, length, and head circumference
    (B) Head circumference and upper segment-lower segment disproportion
    (C) Weight
    (D) Length and head circumference
    (E) Ponderal index (weight/length^3)

29. Congenital pancreatic agenesis

30. Achondroplasia

31. Maternal cigarette smoking

32. Fetal alcohol syndrome

33. Infant of a diabetic mother

Questions 34-37

The agents listed below are thought to produce **irreversible** changes in the fetus. For each condition listed below, select the agent that is most likely to be responsible.

    (A) Ethanol
    (B) Diethylstilbestrol
    (C) Glucocorticoids
    (D) Lead
    (E) Diphenylhydantoin

34. Abnormal epithelialization of vagina and cervix

35. Central nervous system damage

36. Cleft palate

37. Intrauterine growth retardation and microcephaly

Questions 38-40

For each statement that follows, select the venereal disease which it best describes.

    (A) Gonorrhea
    (B) Syphilis
    (C) Lymphogranuloma venereum
    (D) Granuloma inguinale
    (E) Chancroid

38. It is characterized by ulceration of the genitals with regional adenopathy and abscess formation. Diagnosis is confirmed by skin biopsy showing gram-negative plump bipolar rods

39. It is characterized by urethral discharge in males. Diagnosis is confirmed by Gram stain showing gram-negative intracellular diplococci

40. It is characterized by ulceration of the genitals with regional adenopathy. Diagnosis is confirmed by serologic testing

Reproduction

Answers

1. **The answer is D**. *(Hoekelman, pp 364, 366.)* The first trimester represents the period of highest vulnerability to teratogenic agents. Different anatomic systems have different times of greatest susceptibility: the ear is most susceptible from four to twelve weeks and the central nervous and cardiovascular systems are most susceptible from three to six weeks postconception. The central nervous system and the ear retain their susceptibility longer than the first trimester but at a lesser level. Interestingly, during the first two weeks postconception, the fetus is relatively safe from teratogenic effects. Other problems, such as maternal deficiencies of iron, vitamins, minerals, and many other substances, are corrected to some extent by the placenta at the expense of the maternal stores.

2. **The answer is C**. *(Hoekelman, pp 334-335. Smith, 1976. pp 264-265.)* Hurler's syndrome, also classified as mucopolysaccharidosis type I-H, is an autosomal recessive disease. Autosomal recessive diseases are caused by single gene mutations and are expressed only in homozygotes. Symptoms are not evident in heterozygotes (carriers) of most autosomal recessive diseases. Rare autosomal recessive diseases generally occur with greater frequency among offspring of consanguineous parents (who are not affected) than among the general population. Autosomal dominant traits are also single gene mutations but are expressed in homozygotes or heterozygotes. At least one of the parents is affected, and the risk among children and siblings of acquiring the disease of the affected individual is 50 percent.

3. **The answer is D**. *(Hoekelman, pp 383-387.)* There are numerous contributors to fetal risk, including placenta and membrane disorders, such as placenta previa, villamentous insertion of the cord, abruptio placentae, and premature rupture of the membranes with infection. Uterine bleeding in the third trimester of pregnancy is always an ominous sign, since it may indicate a placental dysfunction with possible fetal exsanguination. Diabetes is also a major risk factor in pregnancy, with possible complications, including stillbirth, congenital anomalies, hypoglycemia, renal vein thrombosis, and others. Previous Rh sensitization can lead to problems in the Rh-positive fetus with a risk of stillbirth, hydrops fetalis, and hyperbilirubinemia plus anemia. Cigarette smoking has been associated with small-for-gestational age infants, and a high incidence of prematurity, perinatal mortality, and sudden infant death syndrome. Poor weight gain also has been associated with small-for-gestational age children and perinatal abnormalities. Although, in the past, weight gain of more than 20 lb per pregnancy was felt to be a significant risk factor for the infant, leading to a restrictive diet for the mother, it has been shown recently that weight gains within reasonable limits have no adverse effect on the infant. When the weight gain is associated with toxemia, there are complications. However, in most mothers, weight gain in excess of 20 lb during pregnancy is simply associated with increased food intake rather than edema. Again, although young maternal age had been thought to be a risk factor in and of itself, it appears that this is not the case and that a maternal age greater than 30 is a more significant risk factor than an age less than 20.

4. The answer is D. *(Hoekelman, p 188.)* Amniocentesis performed during the second and third trimester will demonstrate whether an infant of an Rh-sensitized mother has erythroblastosis fetalis. Severely affected fetuses can receive intrauterine transfusions. If Tay-Sachs disease, sickle cell disease, or chromosomal disorders (more frequently seen if the mother is over 40 years old) are detected, termination of pregnancy can be considered. No treatment is available for the affected fetus. Prenatal detection of β-thalassemia is possible by sampling fetal blood, although the safety and accuracy of this technique have not yet been resolved. Again, no treatment is available for the affected fetus.

5. The answer is D. *(Hoekelman, pp 318, 357, 436.)* The perinatal death rate for white and nonwhite infants following spontaneous vertex vaginal delivery is approximately equal. The mortality rate following repeat caesarean section is slightly higher for white as compared to nonwhite infants. Studies have indicated that the risks associated with pregnancy are considerably higher than those associated with oral contraceptives. The use of oral contraception appears to be as safe as that of mechanical contraceptives, if the consequences of their failures (pregnancy and abortion) are taken into consideration. The maternal mortality rate for pregnancy is 12 per 100,000 pregnancies.

6. The answer is D. *(Hoekelman, pp 356-358.)* Suction curettage abortion, the method of choice for early first trimester abortion, is the most commonly used method in the United States. After determining uterine size, the cervix is cleansed, a paracervical block is administered, and the uterus sounded. In most cases, general anesthesia such as nitrous oxide is not used. The cervix is dilated and the uterine contents aspirated. The cavity is explored with a sharp curette, and, finally, an additional suction curettage is performed to remove any remaining products of conception. Rh immunoglobulin is administered to Rh-negative women. An IUD can be put in place at this time in those women who have chosen to use this form of contraception. Women who choose to use oral contraceptives should be advised to start using them at any point during the first week following the abortion procedure. Fitting for diaphragms is done during a postoperative checkup.

7. The answer is D. *(Hoekelman, pp 329, 332, 352-354.)* Down's syndrome, trisomy 13, Klinefelter's syndrome, and Turner's syndrome are all aneuploidic situations resulting from chromosomal nondisjunction in early postzygotic divisions. The cri du chat (cat cry) syndrome results from an autosomal deletion. Nondisjunction is a phenomenon of cell division during which duplicated chromosomal parts (chromatids) fail to separate normally during meiotic cell divisions (spermatogenesis or oogenesis). Such a failure results in daughter cells with an extra or absent chromosome or chromosomal parts. To the extent that this situation is compatible with survival, the defect may be expressed in a variety of ways. If the nondisjunction occurs in early meiotic divisions, all the cells in the organism may be affected. If not, a mosaic results, with two or more cell types being expressed.

8. The answer is D. *(Zelnick, Fam Plann Perspect 10:135-142, 1978.)* Recent data indicate that 55 percent of unmarried women report that they were sexually active by age 19. This percentage is based on the well-known studies of Zelnick and Kantner, who noted an increase of 30 percent in sexual activity by unwed adolescent girls between 1971 and 1976. Perhaps as many as 70 percent or more American adolescents have had coitus at least once by age 19. The more "open" society in which adolescents live today, as well as their earlier maturation, may be contributing factors to this marked increase in sexual activity. Thus, the physician should always consider initiating the discussion of contraceptive use with adolescent patients.

9. The answer is B. *(McAnarney, Am J Dis Child 132:125-126, 1978.)* Of the one million adolescent pregnancies reported in 1977, approximately 350,000 were terminated by abortion. Although the number of adolescent pregnancies is not increasing at this time, it still represents a major problem. Physicians should encourage their sexually active adolescent patients to use effective contraceptive methods. A major difficulty in the prevention of these pregnancies is that so many are based on the adolescent girl's conscious (or unconscious) motivation to become pregnant.

10. The answer is C. *(Hoekelman, pp 1061-1062. Rosenberg, N Engl J Med 297:1060-1062, 1977.)* The human leukocyte antigen (HLA) system is a chromosomal region in man that controls histocompatibility or transplantation antigens and in some way influences the immune process. The gene complex is found in the short arm of chromosome no. 6. Four highly polymorphic loci have been identified, and various combinations of genes are found in increased frequency in association with a variety of chronic diseases including juvenile rheumatoid arthritis (B27), juvenile onset diabetes mellitus, psoriasis, multiple sclerosis, and chronic aggressive hepatitis. HLA antigens are not present on erythrocytes.

11. The answer is A. *(Hoekelman, pp 660-661. Emans, p 18.)* The most accurate method of pregnancy detection if the adolescent patient is two weeks late for her expected menstrual period is the serum pregnancy test. This test measures the very low levels of human chorionic gonadotropin, which are present within several days or less of conception. Urine pregnancy tests may be inaccurate until six weeks after conception. Sexual histories are often inaccurate, and determination of uterine size by pelvic examination is not accurate at this time. Ultrasound examination is not done routinely to determine pregnancy.

12. The answer is A. *(Hoekelman, pp 655-662. McAnarney, Pediatr Rev 1:123-126, 1979.)* Adolescent pregnancy is a recognized medical and psychosocial high risk condition, especially for girls 15 years of age and younger. In 1975, the prematurity rate of infants born to girls in this younger group was double that for women 25-29 years old (13 percent vs. 6 percent, respectively). Unfortunately, the pregnancy rate for these younger adolescents (15 years of age and younger) seems to be increasing. The psychological reaction of adolescents to their pregnancy is varied and often ambivalent. For example, the young mother might want the baby but will also want the freedom to engage in normal adolescent activity. A major tragedy of pregnant adolescents is that many never complete their educational or vocational training.

13. The answer is C. *(Hoekelman, pp 642-643. Barnes, Med Clin North Am 59:1315-1316, 1975.)* Current data indicate that the **average** age of menarche in the United States is 12.6-12.9 years of age and in Europe is 13.0-13.5. The actual age range of menarche in the United States is from 11.5 to 16 years of age; it should begin within 2-5 years of the onset of thelarche (breast development). During the past century a downward trend in the age at which biologic maturity is reached has been observed in children in the United States and Europe; however, recent data indicate that this downward trend has stopped in middle-class American girls. The average age of menarche for this group is approximately the same as it was during the late 1940s. Menstrual periods, though irregular at first, usually become regular within one to two years after menarche. The average age of thelarche is 11.2 years (with a range of 8 to 15 years), while the average age of the growth spurt in females is 12.2 years. Adult-type pubertal development (Tanner V) is often achieved by 14-16 years (with a range of 12.5 to 18).

14. The answer is C. *(Hoekelman, pp 315-322. Greydanus, Pediatrics 65:1-12, 1980. Jaffe, N Engl J Med 297:612-614, 1977.)* The two most effective forms of contraception are the combined estrogen-progesterone birth control pill taken orally and depo-medroxyprogesterone acetate given by injection. Both methods have pregnancy rates under 1 per 100 woman years of use. The mini-pill (progesterone-only), intrauterine device, condom, and diaphragm are acceptable but are not as effective as combined estrogen-progesterone and depo-medroxyprogesterone. The Federal Drug Administration does not approve the use of the injectable depo-medroxyprogesterone acetate for most individuals.

15. The answer is D. *(Hoekelman, pp 315-322. Mishell, Am J Dis Child 132:912-920, 1978. Wiese, Acta Endocrinol [Suppl] 182:87-94, 1974.)* The six absolute contraindications to combined oral contraceptive use are (1) estrogen-dependent neoplasia, (2) breast cancer, (3) history of thromboembolism, (4) active acute or chronic liver disease, (5) pregnancy, and (6) undiagnosed uterine bleeding. Diabetes mellitus is considered a relative (not absolute) contraindication. An impaired glucose tolerance curve is noted in many women who are on the pill, although there is no increased risk of developing diabetes mellitus in these women. Insulin requirements may increase for diabetic females on the pill, but metabolic control is possible. The mini-pill, with minimal carbohydrate effects, may be a better alternative for diabetic women who wish to use a contraceptive pill.

16. The answer is E (all). *(Hoekelman, pp 437-440.)* The maximum effect on the fetus of meperidine given during the delivery may occur 20 to 30 minutes later and last for up to an hour, causing significant respiratory depression. Barbiturates, on the other hand, may be present in measurable amounts in the newborn for up to several days following their use at delivery; they thereby sedate the infant and prevent normal feeding and bonding. There is no antagonist for barbiturates comparable to naloxone, which is used to counteract the effects of meperidine and morphine. All inhalation anesthetics traverse the placenta readily and thus affect the infant. Some are preferentially transported and result in higher infant levels compared to maternal levels. Epidural anesthesia may result in peripheral vasodilatation below the level of the block and decrease placental perfusion. Abdominal muscle incoordination after the block can result in prolonged labor or in the necessity for the use of forceps.

17. The answer is B (1, 3). *(Hoekelman, pp 375-376, 452.)* In the past newborns were classified as full-term or premature solely on the basis of birth weight. Those who weighed more than 2500 g at birth were considered to be full-term, while those less than that weight were considered to be premature. It is now known that a birth weight less than 2500 g is not necessarily a sign of prematurity. Many factors such as smoking, nutrition, and disease states can affect intrauterine growth. The Colorado Intrauterine Growth Charts are now widely used criteria for determining if normal intrauterine growth was maintained during gestation. The growth curves in the Colorado charts are plottings of gestational age against birth weight, length, and head circumference. Sex and race are not included as determinants. Small for gestational age (SGA) intrauterine growth is classified as ≤ 10th percentile on the charts; appropriate for gestational age (AGA) is 10th to 90th percentile, and large for gestational age (LGA) is ≥ 90th percentile.

18. The answer is B (1, 3). *(Hoekelman, p 436. Danforth, ed 3. pp 691-694. Vaughan, ed 11. p 388.)* The incidence of caesarean section has increased dramatically over the past 20 years; it is recognized that, in a variety of circumstances, it is safer for both mother and child than the alternatives of prolonged labor or difficult delivery. Current indications for caesarean section include fetal distress, uterine dysfunction, diabetes mellitus, and carcinoma of the cervix. However, because of its high risk, the overall survival rate following caesarean section is worse than that of vaginal delivery. The belief, "once a casearean, always a cae- sarean," is not strictly held in all cases. In the following circumstances, a vaginal delivery may be attempted: (1) absence of the original indication; (2) successful prior vaginal delivery; (3) low, transverse incision; (4) no apparent incisional weakness; (5) excellent monitoring ca- pacity; and (6) informed consent. However, if an elective repeat section is deemed neces- sary, it is imperative to have accurate information regarding length of gestation before pro- ceeding, as an error of two to four weeks increases perinatal morbidity and mortality sig- nificantly. Amniocentesis is an accurate method of making this assessment in most cases.

19. The answer is D (4). *(Hoekelman, pp 406-407, 412-415. Avery, pp 389-390.)* Ante- natal management of the fetus of an Rh-negative, sensitized mother is based upon previous pregnancy history of isoimmunization as well as that of a previously affected infant. In addition, rising Coombs' titers, amniotic fluid bilirubin pigments measured spectrophoto- metrically from 350 mμ to 700 mμ, and ultrasound findings of fetal congestive heart failure and edema are indicators of the presence of erythroblastosis fetalis, hydrops fetalis, or both in this fetus. When hydrops fetalis is suspected, induction of labor or caesarean section is indicated, but only when the gestational age is at least 32 to 34 weeks, or pulmonary maturity is evident, as determined by an L/S ratio > 2. In this case, pulmonary maturity, as indicated by an L/S ratio of 3.1, would prompt delivery prior to term to prevent worsen- ing of the fetal condition (as evidenced by ultrasound and amniocentesis results) and intra- uterine death. A biparietal diameter of 8.5 cm corresponds to the 50th percentile for 34 weeks. These data of fetal growth do not assist in the decision as to whether pulmonary maturity or progressive hydrops is occurring. Fetal ultrasound, however, can provide evidence of fetal edema, placental edema, and analysis of fetal activity in utero.

20. The answer is A (1, 2, 3). *(Hoekelman, pp 659-660. McAnarney, Pediatr Rev 1:123-126, 1979.)* The reasons for adolescent pregnancies are many. The **early** adolescent often be- comes pregnant to discover if her changing body is mature enough to become pregnant or to become closer to her own mother by becoming a mother herself. The **middle** adolescent often uses the pregnancy to compete with the mother for the father's attention or uses the preg- nancy to acquire new autonomy in her life – to acquire something of her own without the help of her parents. The middle adolescent also wants to manipulate her environment. **Late** adolescents may use the pregnancy to force a marriage commitment from a boyfriend. As expected, of the three stages of adolescence, the older adolescent seems to be the most aware of her reasons for becoming pregnant.

21. The answer is A (1, 2, 3). *(Hoekelman, pp 403-406.)* Infants of mothers addicted to narcotics present a challenging problem to the physician. Although they may be asympto- matic, infants of mothers addicted to heroin, cocaine, meperidine, and propoxyphene fre- quently are irritable, hyperactive, and subject to sleep disorders. High pitched, shrill, exces- sive crying has been observed in many infants of addict mothers. Methadone does not pro- vide a ready solution, as the child of a mother on methadone maintenance therapy occa- sionally shows a more severe withdrawal than that of a mother on heroin. A higher inci- dence of congenital anomalies and neonatal deaths in the addicted compared to the non- addicted population has not been demonstrated.

22. The answer is C (2, 4). *(Hoekelman, p 332.)* The Barr body, generally located just within the nuclear membrane of the cell, appears to be the inactive X chromatin in individuals who have more than one X chromosome. Cells of girls with Turner's syndrome (XO) have no Barr body, whereas cells of boys with Kleinfelter's syndrome (XXY) have Barr bodies, despite their phenotypic appearances. Trisomy 18 and Down's syndrome (trisomy 21) are not associated with sex chromosome aberrations; therefore, cells of a phenotypic female with Down's syndrome would have a Barr body, and cells of a phenotypic male with trisomy 18 would not.

23. The answer is A (1, 2, 3). *(Hoekelman, pp 1327-1328.)* Dysmenorrhea outranks respiratory infections as the leading cause of absenteeism among high school girls. There appears to be an association between levels of prostaglandins and dysmenorrhea. Drugs that inhibit or antagonize prostaglandins are effective in relieving dysmenorrhea. Also effective in treatment of severe primary dysmenorrhea is combined estrogen-progesterone therapy, which provides relief by suppressing ovulation. Diuretics have no role in the treatment of this disorder.

24. The answer is B (1, 3). *(Hoekelman, p 1318.)* Mucocolpos describes a bulging cystic mass at the introitus. It is caused by the accumulation of mucoid secretions behind a vaginal membrane. This obstructive lesion is treated by surgical drainage. Surgical removal of the mass by the abdominal route is contraindicated because the mass will contain the reproductive tract of the female. It is best not to treat asymptomatic obstructions during infancy. The ovaries are normally present in this syndrome.

25-28. The answers are: 25-B, 26-C, 27-B, 28-D. *(Hoekelman, pp 1589-1593.)* Fanconi's syndrome is an autosomal-recessive disease state that usually manifests by age two with symptoms of failure to thrive, anorexia, vomiting, and dehydration. The main features are aminoaciduria, renal tubular acidosis, hyperuricemia, glucosuria, hypophosphatemic rickets, and nephrogenic diabetes insipidus. Treatment regimens may include bicarbonate, phosphate, and vitamin D supplementation.

The oculocerebrorenal syndrome of Lowe is inherited as a sex-linked recessive trait, occurring only in males. The main features are striking physical stigmata (atypical facies, congenital cataracts, and buphthalmos), varying degrees of mental retardation and hypotonia, and a type of hyperaminoaciduria that affects all the amino acids. Vitamin D supplementation and alkalinization therapy should be given to those with tubular acidosis.

Cystinurea is a defect in amino acid transport inherited as an autosomal-recessive trait that usually presents with urinary lithiasis. There are no systemic abnormalities. Treatment consists of urine alkalinization, frequently with sodium or potassium citrate, or the use of d-penicillamine.

Alport's syndrome or hereditary nephritis is characterized by renal disease, sensorineural hearing loss, and ocular abnormalities. Males are more severely affected than females, but the mode of inheritance is unclear. There is no specific treatment.

29-33. The answers are: 29-A, 30-B, 31-C, 32-D, 33-A. *(Avery, p 695. Miller and Merritt, pp 9-24, 103-109. Smith, 1976. pp 336-337.)* Infants with pancreatic agenesis are short, microcephalic, and small for gestational age. The syndrome is characterized by low or absent levels of fetal insulin levels critical for normal fetal growth. These infants manifest overt signs of clinical diabetes and remain short and underweight during postnatal life.

The upper segment to lower segment ratio is disturbed in infants with achondroplasia. Major manifestations include short stature with the proximal segments of the limbs being more involved than the distal segments. The hands are short with stubby fingers. The head is also enlarged, which may be due to either macrocephaly or hydrocephalus. The trunk is normal in length. Achondroplasia is an autosomal-dominant disorder.

Maternal cigarette smoking reduces both the length of gestation and birth weight. Studies demonstrate conclusively that the infant of a mother who smokes as few as five cigarettes per day during pregnancy will weigh less than expected for gestational age at birth. This decrease in birth weight may be related to alterations in uterine blood flow induced by nicotine and to the adverse effects of carboxyhemoglobin on placental transfer of oxygen to the fetus.

Infants born to women known to have been severe alcoholics prior to or during gestation have substantial alterations in all parameters of fetal growth. Pre- and postnatal growth deficiency in this, the fetal alcohol syndrome, is characterized by the presence of microcephaly and by birth length being affected more severely than birth weight. Postnatal linear growth and rate of weight gain are lower than normal despite adequate caloric intake.

Infants of diabetic mothers are larger than expected for their gestational age (> 90th percentile) in weight, length, and head circumference. These infants have an excess of body fat. Morphologic evaluation has demonstrated organ hypertrophy with increases in cell size and cell nuclei. Infants who are born to mothers with diabetes classes D, E, and F tend to be of normal weight; approximately 10 percent may even be small for gestational age.

34-37. The answers are: 34-B, 35-D, 36-C, 37-A. *(Hoekelman, pp 356, 395, 397.)* Some agents produce severe, irreversible changes in the fetus. Among these are diethylstilbestrol, which results in abnormal epithelialization of the vagina and cervix, hence an increased risk of malignancy; lead, which yields central nervous system damage; and glucocorticoids, which are believed to yield an increased incidence of cleft palate. Intrauterine growth retardation, microcephaly, and mental retardation have been documented to occur with maternal ethanol abuse. Although not definitely demonstrated, diphenylhydantoin (Dilantin) is suspected of producing irreversible changes of the face, central nervous system, and circulatory system.

38-40. The answers are: 38-E, 39-A, 40-B. *(Hoekelman, pp 293, 1310-1311.)* Chancroid, caused by *Hemophilus ducreyi*, is characterized by ulceration and adenopathy. It is diagnosed by the identification of gram-negative plump bipolar rods on skin biopsy. Treatment with sulfisoxazole or tetracycline usually is effective. Chancroid is very rare in adolescents in the United States.

Gram-negative intracellular diplococci found on gram-stained smears of urethral discharge are diagnostic of gonorrhea. The diagnosis is confirmed by culture, but treatment with penicillin should be given if organisms are seen on Gram stain.

Syphilis is characterized by genital ulceration, inguinal adenopathy, and a positive serological blood test.

Lymphogranuloma venereum rarely occurs in adolescents in the United States. It is caused by an organism of the Chlamydia group, closely related to those organisms that cause psittacosis *(Chlamydia psittaci)* and trachoma *(Chlamydia trachomatis)*.

Granuloma inguinale, also rare among adolescents in the United States, is characterized by genital ulcers and can be diagnosed by demonstrating Donovan bodies (gram-negative bacilli) in infected material. Treatment is with chloramphenicol or tetracycline.

Neonatology

DIRECTIONS: Each question below contains five suggested answers. Choose the **one best** response to each question.

41. A nasogastric tube cannot be passed in a newborn who has air within the gastrointestinal tract. Which figure below represents the most likely anatomic configuration of the trachea and esophagus in this infant?

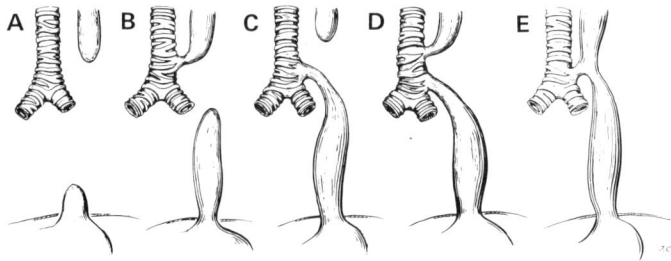

Used with permission of McGraw-Hill Book Company, from *Principles of Pediatrics: Health Care of the Young* (pp 750, 752), by Hoekelman RA et al, © 1978 McGraw-Hill Inc.

(A)   Figure A
(B)   Figure B
(C)   Figure C
(D)   Figure D
(E)   Figure E

42. Which of the following statements regarding the TORCHES diseases is NOT true?

(A) They represent forms of transplacental chorioamnionitis
(B) The prognosis for congenital cytomegalovirus infections is quite good
(C) The degree of intrauterine growth retardation in congenital rubella correlates well with future neurologic development
(D) Toxoplasmosis in pregnant women is acquired by eating undercooked meat
(E) Congenital syphilis frequently is suspected from the appearance of the long bones on x-ray

43. Physiologic hyperbilirubinemia is characterized by which of the following statements?

F (A) Clinical jaundice appears within the first 24 hours of life
F (B) Jaundice persists for 10 days in an infant of at least 37 weeks gestation
T (C) Kernicterus is not a complication in term infants
F (D) ~~Phototherapy is the best treatment~~ common in formula-fed infants
T (E) Direct reacting bilirubin fraction is less than 2 mg/100 ml

40 micromol/L

44. The best method of reducing temperature in a neonate is to

(A) administer salicylates orally
(B) administer acetaminophen orally
(C) administer acetaminophen rectally
(D) sponge with alcohol and water
(E) sponge with tepid water

45. All of the following are manifestations of congenital syphilis EXCEPT

(A) osteochondritis
(B) cerebrospinal fluid pleocytosis
(C) pseudoparalysis
(D) conjunctivitis
(E) maculopapular rash

46. Over a six hour period a two-week-old preterm infant being fed mother's breast milk by nasogastric tube develops abdominal distension, apnea, and gastric residuals of 7 ml following 25 ml feedings. The suspected diagnosis of necrotizing enterocolitis can best be established by

(A) a loss of bowel sounds
(B) guaiac positive stools
(C) an elevated white blood count and thrombocytopenia
(D) free air within the peritoneum detected by abdominal x-ray
(E) pneumatosis intestinalis detected on abdominal x-ray

47. Mechanical ventilation of infants with respiratory distress syndrome is indicated when

(A) the F_IO_2 cannot be lowered to $\leqslant 0.5$ within the first 24 hours of age with the administration of oxygen
(B) there is evidence of a pneumothorax or pneumomediastinum
(C) there is evidence of hypercarbia ($\geqslant 60$ torr), hypoxemia ($\leqslant 50$ torr in a $F_IO_2 \geqslant 0.6$), or apnea
(D) the continuous positive airway pressure cannot be maintained at arterial $P_{O_2} \geqslant 90$ torr
(E) the infant has a respiratory rate of $\geqslant 80$/min

13

48. All of the following statements about neonatal sepsis are true EXCEPT that

(A) the most common causative organisms are group B beta-hemolytic streptococcus and *Escherichia coli*
(B) the complete blood count and differential are not useful diagnostically
(C) important clinical signs include hyperthermia, jaundice, and lethargy
(D) prolonged rupture of the maternal amniotic membranes (≥ 24 hours) predisposes to the disease
(E) initial therapy should include ampicillin and an aminoglycoside parenterally

49. Pictured below is a three-month-old infant who weighs 2980 g (6 lb, 9 oz) and has a pattern of malformations consistent with

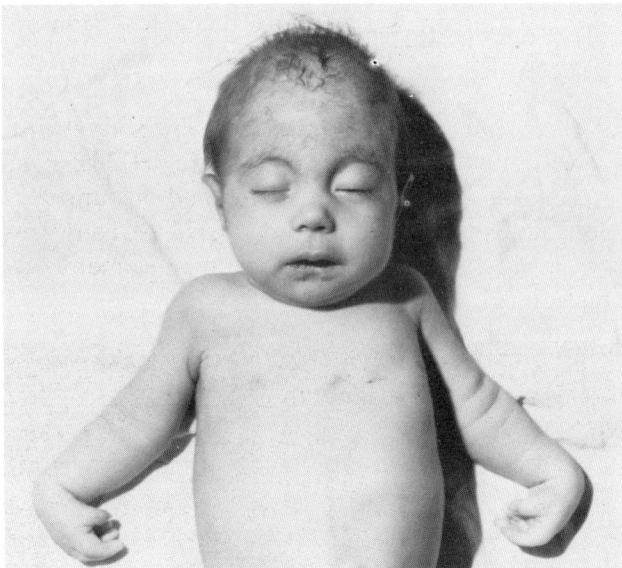

(A) maternal mercury exposure during pregnancy
(B) maternal ionizing radiation exposure during the second trimester of pregnancy
(C) maternal hydantonin exposure during pregnancy
(D) a chromosomal disorder
(E) none of the above

50. All of the following conditions may be associated with a history of meconium ileus in the newborn period EXCEPT

(A) systemic hypertension
(B) nasal polyposis
(C) decreased fertility in adulthood
(D) biliary cirrhosis
(E) failure to thrive

51. A four-day-old 1480 g (3 lb, 4 oz) preterm infant is recovering from respiratory distress syndrome treated by continuous positive airway pressure and elevated ambient oxygen. Over a period of 12-18 hours, the infant develops a rising P_{CO_2} and requires mechanical ventilation for both the hypercarbia and increasing apnea. The ambient oxygen requirement rises from an F_IO_2 of 0.25 to an F_IO_2 of 0.50. The chest x-ray shows increased pulmonary vascularity, air bronchograms, a mildly enlarged cardiothoracic ratio, and a small thymus. On physical examination, the infant is found to have a heart rate of 158/min, a blood pressure of 52/23 mm Hg, and brisk femoral pulses. This change in the infant's clinical state is consistent with

(A) worsening respiratory distress syndrome secondary to surfactant deficiency
(B) patency of the ductus arteriosus
(C) intraventricular hemorrhage and associated central pulmonary edema
(D) a large atrial septal defect
(E) arteriovenous malformation in the right iliofemoral region

52. A three-week-old girl is brought to a physician's office for her first routine health maintenance visit. It is noted that a positive phenylketonuria screening test was obtained previously; on follow-up, her serum phenylalanine was elevated while her serum tyrosine was normal. All of the following statements about this infant are correct EXCEPT that

(A) her feeding history probably reveals recurrent vomiting
(B) untreated, her major problem would be seizures
(C) she is probably blond and blue-eyed
(D) her children may have a greater risk of mental retardation than she has
(E) if she had an elevated tyrosine, it would probably be unnecessary to treat her

DIRECTIONS: Each question below contains four suggested answers of which **one** or **more** is correct. Choose the answer

A	if	1, 2, and 3	are correct
B	if	1 and 3	are correct
C	if	2 and 4	are correct
D	if	4	is correct
E	if	1, 2, 3, and 4	are correct

53. The full-term neonate has normal levels and function of

(1) the primary antibody response
(2) polymorphonuclear white blood cell chemotaxis and phagocytosis
(3) complement components
(4) IgG antibody

54. The mother of a full-term, one-day-old girl (pictured below) asks that her baby be checked because of a "crooked cry." There is no history of birth trauma. Which of the following would be helpful in evaluating this child's problem?

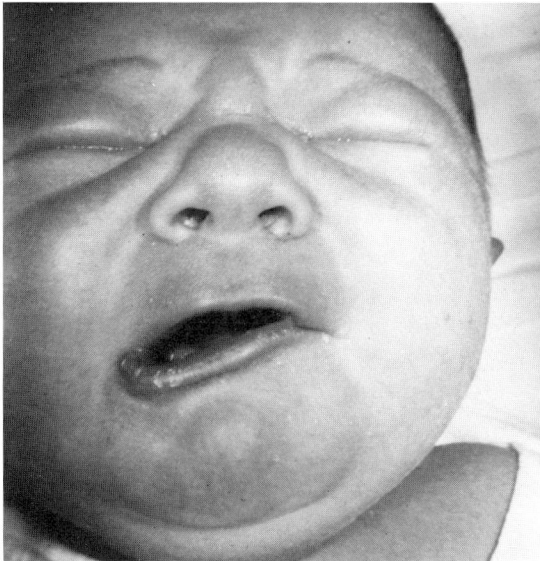

(1) Family history for asymmetric facies
(2) Evaluation of corneal reflex
(3) Cardiac examination, electrocardiogram, and chest x-ray
(4) Barium swallow for gastroesophageal reflux

55. Correct statements concerning single umbilical artery include which of the following?

(1) Single umbilical artery is believied to be associated with an increased incidence of congenital anomalies
(2) The second umbilical artery is believed to have been present but atrophied
(3) Twenty-five percent of infants with single umbilical artery die in the perinatal period
(4) Single umbilical artery is most often found with a marginal or velamentous insertion of the cord

56. A 1900 g (4 lb, 3 oz) infant who shared the placenta pictured below is plethoric, lethargic, and tachypneic. A hematocrit performed on venous blood drawn from this infant was 71 percent. Immediate steps to be taken in the management of this condition include the

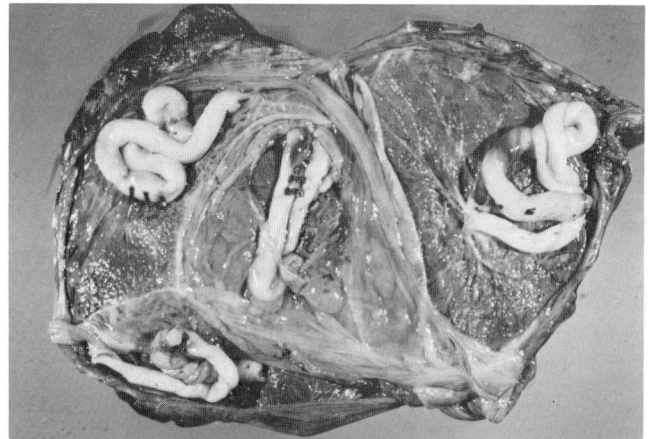

(1) examination of the placenta for bridging vessels
(2) performance of a hematocrit on the infant's siblings
(3) partial exchange transfusion with fresh frozen plasma
(4) prompt feeding and blood volume expansion with a solution of 10 percent dextrose in water

SUMMARY OF DIRECTIONS				
A	B	C	D	E
1, 2, 3 only	1, 3 only	2, 4 only	4 only	All are correct

57. True statements relating to umbilical artery catheterization in preterm infants include which of the following?

(1) A high incidence of umbilical artery thrombosis has been associated with its catheterization
(2) Blanching and cyanosis of the legs occur frequently but rarely result in loss of the femoral pulse
(3) The occurrence of serious complications is reduced when the tip of the catheter is placed in the thoracic portion of the aorta as opposed to the lower lumbar portion
(4) In double volume exchange transfusion, it is preferable to use an umbilical artery catheter interchangeably with an umbilical vein catheter

58. Prophylactic instillation of 1 percent silver nitrate into the neonatal conjunctivae

(1) prevents gonorrhea ophthalmia
(2) must be followed with a normal saline solution rinse to prevent chemical conjunctivitis
(3) must be administered soon after birth to ensure protection
(4) has been associated with inclusion conjunctivitis

59. Asphyxia neonatorum frequently accompanies which of the following conditions?

(1) Cord prolapse
(2) Late and variable decelerations of fetal heart rate
(3) Preterm births
(4) Infants of diabetic mothers

60. Exchange transfusions are associated with severe life-threatening complications infrequently. Metabolic complications associated with exchange transfusions include

(1) hyperkalemia
(2) hypernatremia
(3) hypocalcemia
(4) hypoglycemia

61. Factors associated with an increased incidence of the respiratory distress syndrome include

(1) a negative foam stability test
(2) maternal diabetes
(3) an amniotic fluid lecithin/sphingomyelin ratio (L/S ratio) of < 1.0
(4) rupture of the chorion and amnion in premature infants 24 hours or more prior to delivery

62. The neonatal hyperviscosity syndrome is characterized by which of the following statements?

(1) It is found most frequently in term infants who are either small or large for gestational age
(2) It is associated with central hematocrits $\geqslant 65$ percent
(3) It is manifested by tachypnea, seizures, oliguria, and abdominal distension
(4) It is treated effectively by a partial transfusion of 20 percent of an infant's blood volume and replacement by a solution of 5 percent dextrose in water and 0.5 normal saline

63. Correct statements concerning ABO hemolytic disease include which of the following?

(1) The mother is usually blood type O
(2) The isoimmune antibodies responsible for this problem are of the IgG class of immunoglobulins
(3) First pregnancies may be affected
(4) Successive affected pregnancies usually result in more severe disease

64. Correct statements concerning meconium aspiration syndrome include which of the following?

(1) It occurs frequently in infants $\geqslant 34$ weeks
(2) It is found in 10-20 percent of deliveries with meconium-stained amniotic fluid
(3) It may result in pulmonary hypertension
(4) It frequently is associated with pneumothorax

65. Transient neonatal hypoglycemia can be anticipated if the prenatal history and the birth weight are known. It is also more likely to occur in

(1) infants of diabetic mothers
(2) association with erythroblastosis fetalis
(3) infants who are small for gestational age
(4) association with the respiratory distress syndrome

66. True statements about hemorrhagic disease of the newborn include which of the following?

(1) The onset of bleeding occurs at three to five days of age in term infants
(2) It is due to a functional defect in coagulation factors III, VI, IX, and X
(3) It can be prevented by a single 1 mg parenteral dose of vitamin K
(4) It occurs more frequently in infants of diabetic mothers

67. Fluid replacement in an infant with necrotizing enterocolitis should be administered by

(1) subcutaneous fluid clysis
(2) peripheral vein
(3) nasogastric tube
(4) central venous line

68. The Brazleton Neonatal Behavioral Assessment Scale is an evaluation of the

(1) degree of variability of the infant's state of consciousness
(2) ability of the infant to calm himself after aversive stimuli
(3) degree of responsiveness of the infant to inanimate and animate stimuli
(4) infant's neurologic status

69. A five-day-old infant is brought to the pediatrician only 48 hours after discharge from the hospital because of a 3 cm area of periumbilical erythema, induration of the abdominal wall, a temperature of 38.0° (100.4°F), and jaundice. This infant's condition is described by which of the following statements?

(1) Hepatic abscesses are a frequent complication of this condition
(2) Cellulitis of the abdominal wall frequently results in peritonitis
(3) Even with systemic antibiotic therapy and debridement, many infants die from this condition
(4) *Escherichia coli* is the organism isolated most frequently in this disorder

DIRECTIONS: The groups of questions below consist of lettered choices followed by several numbered items. For each numbered item select the **one** lettered choice with which it is **most** closely associated. Each lettered choice may be used once, more than once, or not at all.

Questions 70-72

For each upper extremity deficit, select the presentation at delivery with which it is most commonly associated.

(A) Forcible vertex with traction
(B) Forcible breech with difficult shoulder delivery
(C) Persistent transverse lie
(D) Persistent occipitoposterior position with forceps rotation to an anterior position
(E) None of the above

70. Volkmann's contracture

71. Erb's palsy

72. Klumpke's palsy

Questions 73-76

The four conditions listed below may produce biliary obstruction in the first month of life. For each condition, select the statement which most closely applies.

(A) It presents as conjugated hyperbilirubinemia following severe erythroblastosis
(B) It is diagnosed by the finding of giant cell transformation on liver biopsy
(C) It is excluded as a diagnosis by a rose bengal test in which excretion of injected radioactive iodine from the liver into the intestine exceeds 10 percent
(D) It may present with jaundice in the neonate or with cholangitis in older patients
(E) It has a relatively good prognosis, but may result in liver failure or cirrhosis

E 73. Idiopathic neonatal hepatitis

C 74. Extrahepatic biliary atresia

A 75. Inspissated bile syndrome

D 76. A choledochal cyst

Questions 77-79

For each of the clinical presentations listed below, select the anorectal anomaly most likely to be associated with it.

(A) Anal stenosis
(B) Imperforate anal membrane
(C) Anal agenesis (low pouch imperforate anus)
(D) Rectal agenesis (high pouch imperforate anus)
(E) Rectal atresia

77. A newborn presents with abdominal distension and a normal-appearing anus, which easily admits the examiner's finger

78. An anal dimple is present and an abdominal x-ray (with the infant in an upside down position) shows air below the pubococcygeal line

79. Air above the pubococcygeal line is shown on x-ray, and there is a dark vaginal discharge in the absence of an anus

Neonatology

Answers

41. The answer is C. *(Hoekelman, p 750.)* The most common form of esophageal atresia (90 percent of cases) in a child with abdominal air consists of a blind upper esophageal pouch and a distal tracheoesophageal fistula (**C**). Infants with this type of atresia drool because of their inability to swallow saliva. Initial feedings result in choking, coughing, and regurgitation. The second most common defect (9 percent) is esophageal atresia without a fistula (**A**), but these infants have an airless abdomen as do those with a proximal tracheoesophageal fistula (**B**). This latter type, the K-type (**D**), and the H-type (**E**) each occur in less than 1 percent of cases and present with cough and complications of tracheal aspiration, rather than with regurgitation. Failure to pass a nasogastric tube into the stomach is a feature of all except the H-type tracheoesophageal anomaly (**E**).

42. The answer is B. *(Hoekelman, pp 389-390, 461-463. Brumback, p 916.)* Congenital infections produce a broad spectrum of clinical pathology primarily on the basis of transplacental chorioamnionitis. The TORCHES acronym represents a diffuse set of diseases which may demand attention during the neonatal period. The acronym is derived from **to**xoplasmosis, **r**ubella, **c**ytomegalovirus disease, **he**rpes simplex infection, and **s**yphilis—all congenital infections. Toxoplasmosis, a parasitic disease, usually results from eating inadequately-cooked meat. It can also be obtained from contact with contaminated cat feces or handling raw, infected meat with open cuts or scratches on the hands. Hepatosplenomegaly, jaundice, anemia, thrombocytopenia, chorioretinitis, intracranial calcifications, and hydrocephaly commonly occur in congenital toxoplasmosis. Viral infection in the form of rubella yields intrauterine growth retardation, which parallels central nervous system damage and predicts future development. Congenital cytomegalovirus is known to produce devastating results, including chorioretinitis, mental retardation, and neonatal death. Transplacental transmission of the herpes simplex virus (usually type 2) can result in a disseminated infection of the fetus and fetal death. If the infant is born alive, a serious disseminated infection occurs characterized by mucocutaneous lesions, hepatomegaly, anemia, thrombocytopenia, and meningoencephalitis. Mortality and morbidity are extremely high. Syphilis, caused by a spirochete, frequently results in periostitis of the long bones (demonstrable on x-ray), a serosanguineous nasal discharge, maculopapular skin rash, pneumonitis, hepatosplenomegaly, and meningoencephalitis. The prognosis is good if the condition is recognized and treated promptly after birth.

43. The answer is E. *(Hoekelman, pp 478, 737. Avery, pp 339-340.)* Physiologic jaundice is defined as an elevation of the serum indirect bilirubin for which no clear-cut pathology can be defined. The elevation in bilirubin can be termed "physiologic" only after a careful review of the maternal and infant history, a thorough examination of the infant, and assessment of laboratory values that clearly eliminate infection, metabolic disorders, hemolysis (regardless of etiology), liver and gastrointestinal disease, and fetal exposure to toxins. Specific criteria that rule out a diagnosis of "physiologic" jaundice include: (1) clinical jaundice occurring within the first 24 hours of life; (2) a total serum bilirubin concentration which increases more than 5 mg/100 ml every 24 hours; (3) total serum bilirubin $\geq$ 12 mg/100 ml in term infants or $\geq$ 15 mg/100 ml in preterm infants; (4) direct reacting bilirubin $\geq$ 2 mg/100 ml; and (5) clinical hyperbilirubinemia persisting for more than one week in term infants or more than two weeks in preterm infants. Physiologic jaundice does not carry a risk for kernicterus in the term infant; therefore, no treatment is required. However, premature, low birth weight infants are at risk for kernicterus. Phototherapy and, at times, exchange transfusion may be required to prevent this complication in these infants.

44. The answer is E. *(Hoekelman, pp 275-279.)* The safest and best way to reduce temperature in a neonate is tepid-water sponging. The addition of alcohol to the sponge water does not increase appreciably the temperature-reducing effectiveness of the process and may produce severe chilling as well as burning of irritated areas of the skin. Because there is a decreased ability of the neonate to excrete salicylates and acetaminophen because of immature liver and kidneys, serum levels may become toxic quite readily. The absorption of drugs from the rectum may be very erratic, especially when there is severe gastroenteritis. Therefore, administration of any drug in suppository form ordinarily is not advisable in infants and children.

45. The answer is D. *(Hoekelman, p 391. Vaughan, ed 11. p 846.)* In recent years prenatal screening and treatment with antibiotics have reduced the incidence of congenital syphilis. There appears, however, to be a resurgence of this disease. Since the sequelae may be severe, early diagnosis and treatment are imperative. Many infected infants have no symptoms; however, the following are common in symptomatic newborns: rashes, rhinitis, meningitis, chorioretinitis, periostitis, osteochondritis, and pseudoparalysis. Conjunctivitis is not one of the protean manifestations of this infection.

46. The answer is E. *(Hoekelman, pp 472-473, 843-845. Avery, pp 645-646.)* Although the etiology, pathogenesis, and pathophysiology of necrotizing enterocolitis (NEC) remain controversial, the clinical presentation of abdominal distension and apnea with gastric residuals strongly suggests this diagnosis. Progression to florid NEC is often gradual and insidious. Early signs include gastric distension often associated with a tender abdomen and erythema of the abdominal wall. Edema of the bowel wall and peritonitis may result. Ileus (loss of bowel sounds), intestinal bleeding (positive guaiac), and signs of infection, such as elevated white blood cell count and thrombocytopenia, are found in a variety of gastrointestinal disorders in infancy and are not diagnostic of NEC. Pneumatosis intestinalis (the presence of air bubbles in the walls of the small intestine caused by invading gas-forming organisms) is the radiographic hallmark of NEC. Free peritoneal air visualized on abdominal radiographs indicates intestinal perforation, a late complication of NEC. Several reports have established that necrotizing enterocolitis may occur in infants fed only breast milk; however, it has also been suggested that the overall incidence is decreased in infants who are fed breast milk.

47. The answer is C. *(Thibeault, pp 272-274.)* Ventilatory failure is defined as the inability to maintain blood oxygen and carbon dioxide concentrations at the levels needed to maintain aerobic metabolism and to overcome respiratory acidosis. Failure to breathe (apnea) is also an indication for mechanical ventilation when it is clearly associated with a rising arterial P_{CO_2} and a falling arterial P_{O_2}. (Generally accepted as indications of ventilatory failure are a $P_{CO_2} \geq 60$ torr and $P_{O_2} \leq 50$ torr in an $F_IO_2 \geq 0.6$.) Failure of continuous positive airway pressure to maintain a $P_{O_2} \geq 50$-60 torr would indicate that this treatment is ineffective, and alternate treatment modalities must be employed.

48. The answer is B. *(Hoekelman, p 464. Wientzen, Curr Probl Pediatr VIII:3-54, 1977.)* Predisposing factors to neonatal sepsis include prolonged rupture of maternal amniotic membranes, infant prematurity, fetal hypoxia, and virulent organism exposure of the immunologically immature newborn in intensive care nursery units. The most common causative bacterium is group B beta-hemolytic streptococcus, followed by *Escherichia coli*. There are many clinical signs of sepsis in the newborn, including hyper- and hypothermia, respiratory distress, jaundice, lethargy, irritability, and feeding difficulties. Differentiating laboratory tests that indicate the presence of infection include a white blood cell count of less than 5,000 cells/mm³, a platelet count of less than 100,000/mm³, and a buffy coat smear if organisms are seen. After appropriate cultures have been obtained, empiric treatment with ampicillin and an aminoglycoside is appropriate.

49. The answer is D. *(Hoekelman, pp 353, 923. Smith, 1976. pp 10-11.)* The infant in the figure that accompanies this question has a pattern of malformations most consistent with trisomy 18 (the presence of an extra chromosome 18 in diploid cells). Chromosomal analysis substantiated the diagnosis based upon the clinical appearance of dysmorphic features, including those readily seen in this photograph—growth failure, a narrowed bifrontal distance, ptosis of the eyelids, low-set ears, short palpebral fissures, micrognathia, a shortened sternum, and clenched hands with radial deviation secondary to radial aplasia—as well as other features characteristic of trisomy 18—nail hypoplasia, low arch dermal ridge patterns on a majority of fingertips, overlapping of the index finger over the third finger and of the fourth over the fifth finger, inguinal hernia, a small pelvis with limited hip adduction, ventricular septal defects, and patent ductus arteriosus. This infant's pattern of malformations usually is not seen with maternal mercury exposure during pregnancy, ionizing radiation during the second trimester of pregnancy, or maternal hydantonin exposure during pregnancy. Parental chromosomal analyses were normal. The mother was 26 years old; future risk of recurrence is less than one percent.

50. The answer is A. *(Hoekelman, pp 795, 1848.)* In the vast majority of cases, the presence of meconium ileus in the newborn period is associated with cystic fibrosis (CF). A decrease in fertility is a manifestation of CF in both males and females. Males are almost invariably sterile, secondary to aspermia; females have thick cervical mucus, which makes fertilization more difficult. Nasal polyposis is also common in cystic fibrosis, with an incidence of over 10 percent in CF patients greater than five years of age. Although systemic hypertension is not usually seen in patients with CF, portal and pulmonary hypertension may be associated findings. Biliary cirrhosis is the liver complication usually associated with CF, and microscopic changes can be found in livers of all patients with this disease. Failure to thrive is extremely common and is the result of both pulmonary and gastrointestinal abnormalities.

51. The answer is B. *(Thibeault, pp 261-276.)* The clinical presentation of the infant described in the question is very typical of patency of the ductus arteriosus, a condition often recognized between four and seven days of life. In these infants, ductal patency persists after birth but because of superimposed respiratory distress syndrome, is not manifested clinically until the respiratory distress begins to improve. With a decline in pulmonary artery pressures and normalization of oxygenation as evidenced by a normal P_{CO_2}, a balanced shunt through the ductus arteriosus changes to one that moves from left-to-right. Injudicious parenteral fluid management may also contribute to the magnitude of the shunt. Physical signs and symptoms of this phenomenon include (1) a rising P_{CO_2}, (2) increasing ventilatory and oxygen requirements, (3) apnea, (4) late or holosystolic cardiac murmur, (5) bounding peripheral pulses, (6) a hyperkinetic precordium, and (7) a widened pulse pressure. Radiographic clues to patency of the ductus arteriosus include: (1) pulmonary plethora [because of increased pulmonary blood flow], (2) mild cardiac dilatation, and (3) later, frank pulmonary "white-out" associated with severe pulmonary edema. Respiratory distress syndrome improves by day four in most infants. Although some may develop acute worsening of ventilatory status and pulmonary edema, the physical and radiographic findings presented in this infant are not seen in those infants or in infants with intraventricular hemorrhage and associated central nervous system-mediated pulmonary edema. Defects of the atrial septum do not cause signs of congestive heart failure in the newborn period. Large arteriovenous malformations may result in severe congestive heart failure in the neonate, but other signs localized to the affected region, including bruits, color changes, and diminutive pulses peripheral to this site, usually are observed.

52. The answer is B. *(Hoekelman, pp 349-350. Buist, Clin Endocrinol Metab 5:265-288, 1976. Mamunes, Clin Perinatol 3:231-250, 1976.)* Although phenylketonuria (PKU) has no clinical signs in the neonatal period, these predominantly fair-haired, blue-eyed patients most often are diagnosed by routine newborn screening. An elevated serum phenylalanine usually is diagnostic if it does not result from hypertyrosinemia. Recurrent vomiting is an outstanding feature of the untreated child who, almost without exception, goes on to develop severe mental retardation. Seizure disorders occur in approximately one-fourth of the untreated patients. If expeditiously started on a reduced phenylalanine diet and monitored closely, development proceeds well. The female PKU patient of childbearing age presents a severe threat to her unborn child, as she frequently is no longer on a controlled diet. The result is a very high incidence of severe mental retardation in the offspring, even though they are not phenylalanine hydroxylase deficient and even though the parent is of relatively normal intelligence. Current practice is to restrict maternal phenylalanine intake during pregnancy.

53. The answer is D (4). *(Hoekelman, pp 1062-1063. Stiehm, pp 168-180.)* The full-term newborn has levels of maternal IgG equal to those of the mother. The majority of IgG crosses the placenta during the third trimester. The normal newborn may be deficient in several immune defenses. The primary response to antigens is delayed; there is no mucosal IgA nor is there IgM in the blood. Maternal IgG may suppress some antibody responses, and there is a decreased C5 level. The polymorphonuclear white blood cells show abnormal chemotactic responses and suboptimal phagocytosis.

54. The answer is A (1, 2, 3). *(Miller, Am J Dis Child 133:743-746, 1979.)* Asymmetric crying facies in the newborn can result from facial nerve dysfunction secondary to birth trauma or to hypoplasia of the anguli oris depressor muscle. The latter cause has been found to occur in families and has also been associated with congenital anomalies in the cardiovascular system (ventricular septal defect, coarctation of the aorta, tetralogy of Fallot), genitourinary, skeletal, and respiratory systems. When evaluating a child with a crooked cry, one should first try to differentiate seventh cranial nerve (facial) dysfunction from hypoplastic muscle. Since birth trauma commonly produces peripheral seventh nerve involvement, the presence of normal muscles of the upper face (including the corneal reflex) makes it more likely that the cause is muscle hypoplasia. Definitive differentiation can be made with electromyelogram. Because cardiovascular defects are the ones most likely to be associated with muscle dysfunction, they should be investigated most thoroughly. There is no correlation between asymmetric facies and gastroesophageal reflux.

55. The answer is E (all). *(Hoekelman, p 372.)* Most often associated with a marginal or velamentous insertion of the umbilical cord, the single umbilical artery (SUA) remains controversial; most investigators, however, believe it is linked to an increased incidence of congenital anomalies. One current belief is that two vessels were present but that one atrophied. It has been suggested that up to 25 percent of the affected newborns will die during the perinatal period. Because SUA is associated with congenital anomalies, those infants who survive the perinatal period should be carefully examined for the presence of these anomalies.

56. The answer is A (1, 2, 3). *(Hoekelman, pp 368-369. Benirschke, Curr Probl Pediatr II: 10-11, 1971.)* Twin-to-twin transfusion occurs in monochorionic twin pairs or in monochorionic multiple births. This often results in polycythemia in one member and anemia in the other. Careful observation or injection of the placental vessels with contrast media will reveal an artery-to-vein, an artery-to-artery, or a vein-to-vein anastomosis. Thus, placental examination is mandatory in multiple births in whom markedly different hematocrits are observed. In addition, differences in twin size occur frequently—the plethoric member is macrosomic and the anemic counterpart is much smaller. Management includes transfusion of the anemic twin and phlebotomy of the polycythemic member, with a partial exchange of fresh frozen plasma to lower the central hematocrit, should it exceed 65-70 percent.

57. The answer is A (1, 2, 3). *(Mokohisky, N Engl J Med 299:561-563, 1978.)* Umbilical artery catheterization is a part of routine high-risk newborn care when serial sampling of arterial blood gases or continuous blood pressure recordings are required. Blanching or cyanosis of the lower extremities is more frequent in catheters positioned in the lower lumbar region; loss of pulse, which fortunately is a rare occurrence, is the criterion for removal of the catheter. Whether this blanching is due to vascular spasm, thromboembolization, or air embolization has not been determined adequately. Overall, the occurrence of thrombosis of the umbilical artery has been reported to be in excess of 90 percent; however, often no clinical evidence of occlusion can be detected. Use of arterial catheters for double volume exchange transfusions is not warranted because of the potential for microthrombi, air emboli, and dramatic drops in arterial perfusion pressure. Overall, the complication rate for umbilical artery catheters is reduced when the tip is placed at the 7th to 8th thoracic vertebrae.

58. The answer is B (1, 3). *(Hoekelman, pp 450-451.)* One percent silver nitrate ($AgNO_3$) dispensed in single-dose containers is recommended by the American Academy of Pediatrics for prophylaxis of gonococcal ophthalmia neonatorum. It should be instilled soon after birth (preferably within the first hour of life) and should reach all parts of the conjunctival sac. The eyes should not be irrigated with saline or distilled water after $AgNO_3$ instillation. Chemical conjunctivitis occurs in 30-40 percent of infants receiving 1 percent $AgNO_3$ and is self-limited and not associated with later inclusion conjunctivitis or blennorrhea.

59.   The answer is A (1, 2, 3). *(Hoekelman, pp 440-443. Thibeault, pp 199-200.)* The incidence of neonatal asphyxia as measured by low Apgar scores $\leqslant 4$ at 5 minutes and cord blood acidosis (pH < 7.10) is directly related to the degree of prematurity and events within the fetomaternal unit prior to birth. Fetal monitoring patterns reflecting uteroplacental insufficiency are found frequently in fetuses asphyxiated at birth. Prolapse of the umbilical cord through the dilated os often results in compression of the umbilical venous circulation and later the umbilical arterial circulation. Cord prolapse frequently is accompanied by severe variable decelerations of the fetal heart rate, fetal tachycardia and, finally, fetal bradycardia. Usual obstetric management would include an emergency caesarean section in hopes of delivering the infant promptly and averting the progressive effects of asphyxia. Asphyxia neonatorum, in the absence of other factors, is not a common occurrence in infants of diabetic mothers.

60.   The answer is E (all). *(Hoekelman, pp 283, 1964-1965. Avery, p 391.)* Exchange transfusions have a host of potential metabolic complications, including hyperkalemia, hypernatremia, hypocalcemia, and hypoglycemia. Hypomagnesia and acidemia are also found occasionally. These disturbances are related to the acid-citrate-dextrose anticoagulant-preservative present in the transfused blood and hemolysis of red cells secondary to improper warming of the blood. Prolonged storage, injudicious admixture of the blood with hypotonic solutions, and mechanical injury that occurs during the exchange transfusion process are also factors contributing to the metabolic problems.

61.   The answer is A (1, 2, 3). *(Hoekelman, pp 466-468. Farrell, Am Rev Respir Dis 111: 657, 1975. Sell, Obstet Gynecol 49:167, 1977.)* Respiratory distress syndrome (RDS), also called hyaline membrane disease (HMD), is the most common respiratory disorder of the newborn. RDS involves an inability to synthesize, store, and release the surface active material (surfactant) into the lining of the alveoli. The resultant high surface tension in the alveoli causes them to collapse during expiration. The foam stability test (FST) or "shake test" is a semiquantitative way of assessing surface active material in the amniotic fluid. A negative FST indicates a 95 percent risk for RDS, while a positive FST indicates a risk of less than 20 percent. Infants of mothers with diabetes have a five-fold greater risk of RDS than infants born to nondiabetic mothers. Using the method of Gluck and his associates, an L/S > 2.0 reflects lung maturity and freedom from RDS. The lecithin/sphingomyelin ratio in amniotic fluid is an indication of lung maturity and the chances for the development of RDS. A ratio of < 1.0 is an indication of lung immaturity and high potential for RDS. Several studies have demonstrated a decreased incidence of RDS associated with prolonged rupture of the fetal membranes in infants of less than 32 weeks gestation. There is a higher incidence of RDS among monozygotic twins than among dizygotic twins, a circumstance that suggests a genetic predisposition to RDS.

62.   The answer is A (1, 2, 3). *(Oski, p 81. Wirth, Pediatrics 63:833-836, 1979.)* In a recent study only 4 of 790 infants (0.5 percent), studied four hours after birth, were found to have polycythemia (central hematocrits $\geqslant 65$ percent). However, because hyperviscosity occurs for reasons other than an elevated hematocrit (Hct), the incidence of hyperviscosity in this group of infants was found to be five percent. All infants with central venous hematocrits $\geqslant 65$ percent were hyperviscous when measured on the viscometer. The highest incidence of polycythemia was found in term and post-term infants who were either small or large for gestational age. Clinical manifestations accompanying polycythemia include respiratory distress, abnormal renal function (oliguria and hematuria), central nervous system disorders, and abdominal distension. Reduction in the hematocrit is necessary and is performed by replacing a fraction of the infant's blood with fresh frozen plasma. This fraction can be calculated by the following formula:

$$\text{Volume of partial exchange (ml)} = \frac{(\text{baby's weight} \times .8) \times (\text{baby's Hct} - \text{desired Hct})}{\text{baby's Hct}}$$

63. The answer is A (1, 2, 3). *(Hoekelman, pp 412-414, 475-477.)* Isoimmune hemolytic disease of the newborn resulting from ABO incompatibility is primarily a disease of type A or B infants born to type O mothers. Isoimmune antibodies are primarily of the IgM class of immunoglobulins. However, only IgG antibodies can cross the placenta and involve the infant's hematopoietic system. Occasionally, despite a negative history for blood transfusion, a first pregnancy is affected as a result of an earlier unrecognized spontaneous abortion. In contrast with Rh hemolytic disease, the clinical severity of ABO incompatibility usually declines with successive pregnancies.

64. The answer is E (all). *(Hoekelman, pp 440, 457, 470.)* Meconium aspiration at birth occurs in infants close to term. A recent survey found meconium-stained amniotic fluid and meconium-stained infants exclusively among infants of 34 or more weeks gestation. Approximately 10-20 percent of babies born at deliveries in which the amniotic fluid contains meconium will develop signs and symptoms of meconium aspiration syndrome. Prominent clinical features include frequent pneumothoraxes, difficulty in oxygenation, and acidosis resulting from pulmonary hypertension. The syndrome may be prevented or its severity reduced significantly by endotracheal intubation and removal of meconium within the airways. Tracheobronchial lavage has not been shown to reduce the severity of the disorder.

65. The answer is E (all). *(Hoekelman, pp 1268-1269.)* Transient neonatal hypoglycemia may be seen when there is (1) low birth weight, (2) transient hyperinsulinism, and (3) neonatal stress. Undernourished infants who are small for gestational age are especially at risk for hypoglycemia and must be monitored closely. Hypoglycemia secondary to hyperinsulinism and associated with beta cell hyperplasia is seen in infants of diabetic mothers and when there is erythroblastosis fetalis. Different forms of stress, including the respiratory distress syndrome, sepsis, and maternal toxemia, may produce transient hypoglycemia, especially in premature infants.

66. The answer is B (1, 3). *(Schaffer, ed 4. pp 573-574.)* Hemorrhagic disease of the newborn is due to vitamin K deficiency and the decreased activity of vitamin K-dependent coagulation factors II, VII, IX, and X. These clotting factors are synthesized and stored in the liver until activated by vitamin K. Newborn infants are capable of normal factor synthesis, but because of slow gastrointestinal colonization with organisms that synthesize vitamin K, they are relatively deficient in this vitamin. Bleeding due to vitamin K deficiency characteristically occurs in a thriving infant between three and five days of age and frequently is localized in the gastrointestinal tract or the skin where it manifests as diffuse ecchymoses. The platelet count is normal, but the partial thromboplastin time (PTT) and prothrombin time (PT) are prolonged. Within four hours after vitamin K administration, the PTT and PT begin to normalize. Vitamin K deficiency is no more frequent in infants of diabetic mothers than in those of nondiabetic mothers. In most centers, prophylactic vitamin K is given intramuscularly at the time of delivery. A single dose of 1 mg of vitamin K oxide prevents the disorder.

67.   The answer is C (2, 4). *(Hoekelman, p 261.)* In a child with necrotizing enterocolitis, nasogastric fluid administration would cause increased distension of the bowel because of lack of absorption. Subcutaneous fluid clysis has no place in fluid therapy of any kind, since the fluids are absorbed slowly and thus can cause significant fluid and electrolyte shifts. Intravenous administration of fluids is the only reliable and safe method, that is, via peripheral vein or central line.

68.   The answer is E (all). *(Brazleton, pp 1-8.)* The Brazleton Neonatal Behavioral Assessment Scale is a measurement of how an infant interacts with his or her environment. An important part of the Brazleton Scale is observation of changes in an infant's state of consciousness as it is presented with the various tests and maneuvers. Other parts include assessment of the infant's ability to calm down after aversive stimuli and to attend to both animate stimuli (such as the examiner's voice and face) and inanimate stimuli (such as a rattle or a ball). A neurologic examination is done as well.

69.   The answer is A (1, 2, 3). *(Avery, pp 960-962.)* Omphalitis or infection of the umbilicus is a serious infection in neonates. Formerly associated with home deliveries and unskilled perinatal care in the United States, omphalitis remains a common cause of neonatal morbidity in developing areas of the world. Cellulitis of the umbilicus and surrounding abdominal wall may lead to direct extension to the peritoneal cavity. Ascending infection through the umbilical vein may result in hepatic abscesses and portal vein thrombosis. Staphylococci and group B streptococci organisms are isolated more frequently than are gram-negative organisms. *Clostridium tetani* often is the offending organism in unattended deliveries in countries where surgical asepsis is not practiced in cutting the umbilical cord after delivery. Even with systemic antibiotics, local wound care, and surgical debridement, many of these infants die.

70-72.   The answers are: 70-E, 71-A, 72-B. *(Hoekelman, pp 460, 954, 1643-1644.)* Erb's palsy, with the resultant "waiter asking for the tip" attitude of wrist flexion and pronation of the forearm, follows brachial plexus injuries to C5 and C6, usually from traction on the head. The injury can occur in cephalic presentations during delivery of the head and shoulder. On the other hand, Klumpke's palsy results from injury to C8 and T1, usually from hyperabduction during breech presentation with difficult shoulder delivery. Persistent occipitoposterior presentations that require forceps version maneuvers do not predispose the infant to any upper extremity deficit. Volkmann's contracture is secondary to ischemia to the muscles of the forearm; it most commonly follows supracondylar fracture of the humerus and is not associated with birth trauma.

73-76.   The answers are: 73-E, 74-C, 75-A, 76-D. *(Hoekelman, pp 773-777. Avery, pp 359-368.)* Neonatal hepatitis and extrahepatic biliary atresia may be indistinguishable by clinical course, laboratory findings, or liver biopsy. However, a rose bengal test, which demonstrates the recoverability of the radioactive isotope of iodine (^{131}I) in the intestine of greater than ten percent of the injected dose, does require patency of the biliary tract and therefore excludes the diagnosis of extrahepatic biliary atresia. Neonatal hepatitis in general has a good prognosis, although some infants do develop hepatic failure or cirrhosis. Conjugated hyperbilirubinemia due to inspissation of bile in the hepatic caniculae can be seen following severe erythroblastosis. The finding of giant cell transformation on biopsy is nonspecific and may be present in hepatitis, intrahepatic biliary obstruction and, to a lesser extent, in extrahepatic biliary obstruction. Eighteen percent of cases of choledochal cyst present as prolonged neonatal jaundice, while the remainder become manifest later with symptoms of cholangitis.

77-79. The answers are: 77-E, 78-C, 79-D. *(Roy, ed 2. pp 73-75.)* Rectal atresia is associated with early intestinal obstruction and a normal-appearing anus, which, unlike anal stenosis, is not narrowed to the examining finger. Difficult to diagnose, it is fortunately a rare condition.

A low pouch imperforate anus of anal agenesis is associated with air below the pubococcygeal line on x-ray, low intestinal obstruction (or the presence of a fistulous tract), and an anal dimple. A high pouch imperforate anus or rectal agenesis is associated with air above the pubococcygeal line, fistula formation (to the vagina or bladder), and the absence of an anal dimple. In general, the lesions below the pubococcygeal line are associated with good prognostic outcome in regard to continence compared with those above the pubococcygeal line. A high incidence of associated congenital anomalies occurs with lesions at both levels.

Anal stenosis may present with obstructive signs and symptoms in the newborn period. The anal opening is present, but the anal canal is quite tight. This usually responds well to dilatations, and surgery is not required. An imperforate anal membrane may present with obstruction, but the contents of the anal canal and rectum usually are visible behind the membrane.

Gastroenterology

DIRECTIONS: Each question below contains five suggested answers. Choose the **one best** response to each question.

80. A newborn infant who presents with signs of intestinal obstruction is given a barium enema (illustrated below). Initial management of this infant should include

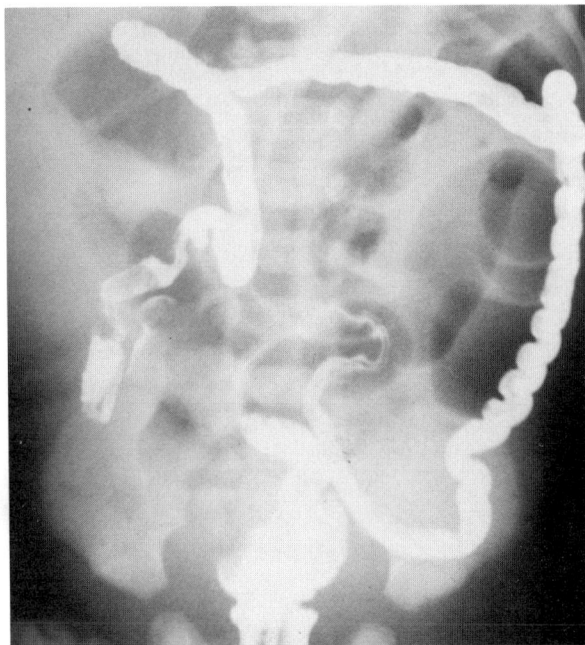

Used with permission of McGraw-Hill Book Company, from *Principles of Pediatrics: Health Care of the Young* (p 796), by Hoekelman RA et al, © 1978 McGraw-Hill Inc.

(A) careful observation and elimination of oral feedings
(B) the administration of thyroid hormone
(C) a Gastrografin enema
(D) surgical intervention
(E) decompression with a Miller-Abbott tube

81. Malrotation of the intestine, which is characterized by abnormal placement and fixation of the cecum, is best demonstrated by

(A) a flat plate of the abdomen
(B) an upper gastrointestinal series
(C) a lateral decubitus view of the abdomen
(D) a barium enema
(E) an intravenous pyelogram

82. The diagnosis of pyloric stenosis is best confirmed by

(A) a family history of pyloric stenosis
(B) a history of projectile vomiting
(C) a history of recurrent vomiting
(D) palpation of a mass in the right upper quadrant
(E) an upper gastrointestinal x-ray series

83. A five-month-old boy is brought to the physician's office because of persistent vomiting and mild jaundice. There are no other symptoms or findings. The mother reports that she breast-fed her child until six weeks ago at which time one type of solid food was introduced. The vomiting began after the ingestion of this solid food, stopped when the solid food was discontinued, but resumed when it was reintroduced. The food most likely to be responsible for this pattern is

(A) fruit
(B) vegetables
(C) cereal
(D) meat
(E) eggs

84. The most likely mechanism for diarrhea in association with *Salmonella* enteritis is

(A) increased intraluminal osmotic pressure
(B) increased secretory activity of intestinal mucosa
(C) malabsorption of intestinal contents
(D) decreased intestinal motility
(E) increased intestinal motility

85. A seven-year-old child presents with a four-month history of recurrent, acute, colicky abdominal pain and associated rectal bleeding. The physical examination is normal. A solitary lesion is seen in the colon on barium enema. The most likely etiology is

(A) Crohn's disease
(B) *Yersinia* enterocolitis
(C) recurrent intussusception
(D) lymphoid nodular hyperplasia
(E) Henoch-Schönlein purpura

86. Which of the following is the best method for diagnosing Wilson's disease?

(A) Slit lamp examination of the cornea
(B) Determination of serum ceruloplasmin levels
(C) Determination of 24-hour urinary copper excretion
(D) Determination of hepatic copper content
(E) Determination of serum copper levels

87. A seven-year-old boy is seen with massive painless hematochezia. Sigmoidoscopy reveals no lesions but shows deep red blood coming from 25 cm above the internal sphincter. Further evaluation is best made by

(A) a barium enema
(B) Meckel's scan
(C) a laparotomy
(D) an arteriogram
(E) a colonoscopy

88. The most common helminth infection in adults and children in the United States is

(A) *Necator americanus* (hookworm)
(B) *Trichinella spiralis* (trichinosis)
(C) *Toxocara canis* (visceral larva migrans)
(D) *Enterobius vermicularis* (pinworm)
(E) *Ascaris lumbricoides* (roundworm)

89. An eight-year-old boy presents with abdominal pain and vomiting. Four days previously he had fallen from his bicycle on his way home from school. As he fell to the ground, the handlebar struck him in the abdomen. He also sustained minor abrasions on the right knee and elbow. The most likely diagnosis is

(A) an intramural hematoma of the duodenum
(B) post-traumatic intussusception
(C) a pseudocyst of the spleen
(D) a posterior subcapsular hematoma of the liver
(E) a pseudocyst of the pancreas

90. A six-month-old child is brought in for a routine checkup, at which time the mother voices some concern about blood-streaked stools. The most likely diagnosis is

(A) a cavernous hemangioma
(B) an anal fissure
(C) a rectal tear
(D) a juvenile polyp
(E) milk intolerance

91. A 16-year-old girl complains of fatigue and appears pale. Menstrual history is normal, and her stool is 2+ guaiac positive. The most likely etiology is

(A) pernicious anemia
(B) peptic ulcer disease
(C) Menetrier's disease
(D) a gastric polyp
(E) Zollinger-Ellison syndrome

92. All the following clinical presentations have been associated with gastrointestinal duplications EXCEPT

(A) an abdominal mass
(B) rectal bleeding
(C) an obstruction
(D) jaundice
(E) colicky pain

93. A 24-month-old white male is admitted to the hospital because of acute onset of colicky abdominal pain, anorexia, bile-stained vomiting, and abdominal distension. X-ray examination reveals dilated air-filled loops in both the large and small bowel. The child had previously been healthy with no history of serious illness, hospitalizations, or allergies. On examination, the patient is in moderate distress. Vital signs are: temperature, 39°C (102.2°F); pulse, 120; and respirations, 40. Which of the following procedures would NOT be useful in the evaluation and management of this child?

(A) An upper gastrointestinal series
(B) Determination of serum electrolyte levels
(C) Examination of stools for occult blood
(D) A barium enema
(E) A urinalysis

94. After the ingestion of strong acid, severe lesions are most likely to appear at which of the following sections of the gastrointestinal tract illustrated below?

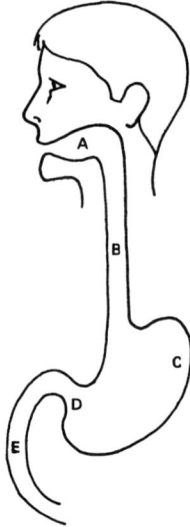

(A) A
(B) B
(C) C
(D) D
(E) E

95. A 12-month-old child with a long history of regurgitating after meals shows a low resting level of the esophageal sphincter pressure, normal peristalsis, and a normal sphincter relaxation time. No anemia is noted, and stools are guaiac negative. These findings can be explained best by

(A) achalasia
(B) chalasia
(C) esophagitis
(D) normal physiologic variation
(E) central core disease

96. A 12-year-old white male is brought to the physician's office by his mother because of blood in his stool for the past two days. The patient has been taking penicillin for group A β-hemolytic streptococcal pharyngitis. He has had anorexia and mid-abdominal pain but no vomiting. Blood pressure is normal both standing and lying, but the pulse increases from 85 to 100 when he stands. A nasogastric tube is passed, and bright red blood is obtained on aspiration. The stool contains red blood with a small amount of feces. The most likely diagnosis is

(A) Peutz-Jeghers syndrome
(B) regional enteritis
(C) acute gastritis
(D) serum sickness
(E) Henoch-Schönlein purpura

97. A six-year-old white male comes in with a chief complaint of continuous stool soiling of six months duration. The child has had no other medical problems nor has he been on any medication. He is doing relatively well in the first grade. On physical examination, the patient is at the 50th percentile for height and weight, with good muscle tone and strength. Neurologic examination is normal, including deep tendon reflexes and an anal wink bilaterally. There are no lesions on the skin. Abdominal examination reveals firm, irregular masses throughout the abdomen. Rectal examination reveals decreased tone in the muscle sphincter with a large rectal ampulla filled with feces. Stool is guaiac negative. This child's history would most probably reveal

(A) a family history of muscular dystrophy
(B) a family history of thyroid dysfunction
(C) a history of back injury
(D) constipation and abdominal distension since birth
(E) difficulties with toilet training

98. A nine-year-old black male presents with recurrent abdominal pain present since age six. The pain is periumbilical and nonradiating and does not awaken him at night. Bowel movements, which are soft, occur once or twice a day; there has been no vomiting. Physical examination is unremarkable. Stool guaiacs have been repeatedly negative. Blood count is normal, and sedimentation rate is 4. Urinalysis reveals 0-1 white cells, no red cells, and no casts. Urine is negative for glucose, protein, and ketones. Which of the following disease entities is the most likely cause of this patient's pain?

(A) Disaccharide intolerance
(B) Inflammatory bowel disease
(C) Chronic appendicitis
(D) Hydronephrosis
(E) Ascariasis

99. An eight-year-old child develops jaundice and malaise with a serum glutamic oxaloacetic transaminase level (SGOT) of 2000. Liver biopsy shows scattered mild ballooning degeneration, periportal mononuclear infiltrates, councilman bodies, and some cholestasis. This clinical picture is most consistent with

(A) cystic fibrosis
(B) acute viral hepatitis
(C) Wilson's disease
(D) chronic active hepatitis
(E) alpha$_1$-antitrypsin deficiency

100. If bacteremia is suspected in a patient who is undergoing parenteral hyperalimentation, the most important **initial** therapeutic measure is to

(A) obtain blood cultures
(B) remove the hyperalimentation catheter
(C) change the fluid to normal saline
(D) start antibiotics
(E) replace the infusion pump

101. A jejunal biopsy is performed on a patient with a history of chronic diarrhea. The histologic findings of the biopsy are shown below. The most likely cause of this patient's symptoms is

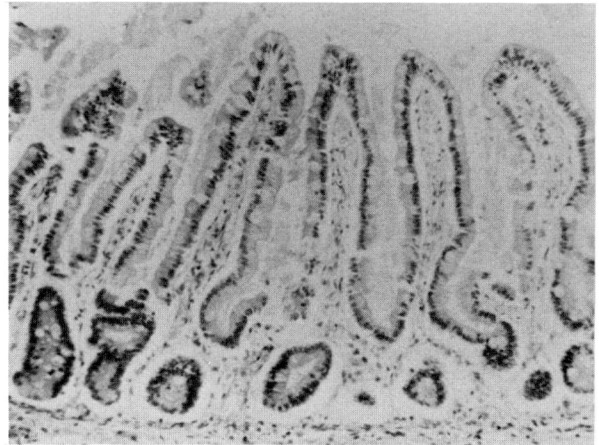

(A) gluten sensitive enteropathy
(B) selective IgA deficiency
(C) cystic fibrosis
(D) eosinophilic gastroenteritis
(E) bacterial overgrowth

DIRECTIONS: Each question below contains four suggested answers of which **one** or **more** is correct. Choose the answer

A	if	**1, 2, and 3**	are correct
B	if	**1 and 3**	are correct
C	if	**2 and 4**	are correct
D	if	**4**	is correct
E	if	**1, 2, 3, and 4**	are correct

102. A neonate who has not passed meconium 24 hours after birth is found on examination to have no anal orifice. The infant can be expected to have which of the following complications?

(1) Coughing and vomiting with feedings
(2) Anomalies of the vertebral column
(3) An abnormal intravenous pyelogram
(4) A severe convulsive disorder

103. Functional and biochemical changes that can occur in association with liver disease include

(1) menstrual irregularities in adolescent girls with cirrhosis
(2) hypoglycemia with Reye's syndrome
(3) deficiencies in fat soluble vitamins with biliary atresia
(4) metabolic acidosis with acute serum hepatitis

104. The clinical picture of tracheoesophageal fistula with esophageal atresia is consistent with

(1) a distended abdomen at three hours of age
(2) an imperforate anus
(3) "aspiration pneumonia"
(4) a cleft palate

105. A five-month-old boy is suspected of having lactose intolerance following an episode of gastroenteritis. The child's mother is instructed to avoid lactose feedings for four weeks. Acceptable feedings would include

(1) cow's milk-based formula
(2) soy formulas
(3) clear liquids
(4) a carbohydrate-free formula with added honey

106. The diagnosis of acute appendicitis in children under two years of age may be aided by which of the following observations?

(1) The presence of a fecalith
(2) An abnormal bowel gas pattern
(3) A normal psoas shadow
(4) A normal urinalysis

107. A ten-year-old white male presents with a four-month history of constant localized right lower quadrant pain, which occasionally awakens him from sleep. The initial approach would be to obtain a history of

(1) previous surgery
(2) familial stress points
(3) urinary tract infections
(4) milk intolerance

108. Diseases that may mimic the clinical presentation of inflammatory bowel disease include

(1) shigellosis
(2) yersinosis
(3) salmonellosis
(4) rotavirus infection

109. Intestinal polyposis syndromes associated with malignant transformation include

(1) Gardner's syndrome
(2) Canada-Cronkhite syndrome
(3) familial polyposis
(4) Peutz-Jeghers syndrome

110. A child is below the third percentile for weight and 25th percentile for height. A 72-hour quantitative stool collection for fat on a measured high fat intake shows elimination of 50 g of fat every 24 hours. A differential diagnosis should include which of the following diseases?

(1) Cystic fibrosis
(2) Giardiasis
(3) Shwachman-Diamond syndrome
(4) Gluten-sensitive enteropathy

111. A 12-year-old child with a recent history of blunt abdominal trauma is found to have back pain and a large epigastric mass. Initial diagnostic studies should include

✓(1) determination of serum amylase levels
(2) an exploratory laparotomy
✓(3) abdominal ultrasonography
(4) transabdominal needle biopsy

112. Which of the following may be found in association with gluten-sensitive enteropathy?

✓(1) Finger clubbing
✓(2) Constipation
✓(3) Anorexia
✓(4) Epistaxis

113. A 13-year-old white male presents with a four-month history of weight loss, stool frequency, and rectal bleeding. The physical examination is remarkable for small stature and pallor. Laboratory findings include an elevated sedimentation rate and iron deficiency anemia. Sigmoidoscopy and mucosal biopsy may reveal

✓(1) friability of the mucosa
✓(2) goblet cell depletion
✓(3) crypt abscesses
✓(4) granulomatous changes

114. Extraintestinal manifestations of chronic ulcerative colitis in children frequently include

✓(1) erythema nodosum
✓(2) fatty infiltration of the liver
✓(3) arthritis
(4) ankylosing spondylitis

115. Correct statements concerning the outpatient management of a child with gastroenteritis include which of the following?

✓(1) Since most gastroenteritis results in isotonic dehydration, replacement fluid approximates maintenance fluid in composition
(2) Although infrequently used today, boiled skim milk is an adequate replacement fluid for most cases of gastroenteritis
✓(3) For mild gastroenteritis, hypotonic liquids such as soda pop and broth are appropriate replacement fluids
(4) A homemade electrolyte solution consisting of ½ teaspoon of salt and ¼ teaspoon of baking soda per quart of water is a good alternative to commercial electrolyte solutions

116. Appropriate antimicrobials shorten the course of acute diarrhea when it is associated with which of the following infections?

✓(1) Giardiasis
✓(2) Cholera
✓(3) Shigellosis
(4) Salmonellosis

117. Which of the following drugs should be avoided in hepatic failure?

(1) Penicillin
(2) Chloramphenicol
(3) Gentamicin
(4) Nafcillin

118. Splenomegaly is noted on a routine physical examination in a ten-year-old girl. Among the subsequent studies that were carried out was the x-ray shown below. A differential diagnosis should include

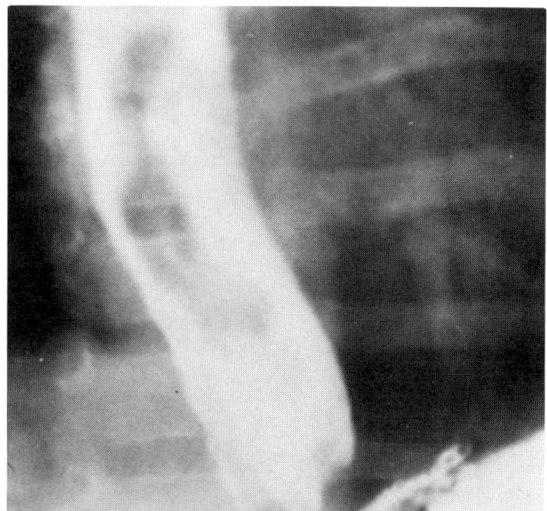

✓(1) alpha₁-antitrypsin deficiency
(2) extrahepatic biliary atresia
✓(3) cavernous transformation of the portal vein
(4) childhood lymphoma

119. The consequences of malabsorption associated with regional enteritis (Crohn's disease) include

(1) megaloblastic anemia
✓(2) zinc deficiency
✓(3) steatorrhea
✓(4) oxalate stones

SUMMARY OF DIRECTIONS				
A	B	C	D	E
1, 2, 3 only	1, 3 only	2, 4 only	4 only	All are correct

120. On examination, an infant is found to have a liver span of 8 cm. Subsequent examination by computerized axial tomography (CAT scan) reveals fatty infiltration. Inherited metabolic diseases likely to produce such a clinical picture include

(1) tyrosinemia
(2) galactosemia
(3) Gaucher's disease
(4) hereditary fructose intolerance

121. In the evaluation of chronic diarrhea, hereditary lactose intolerance is suspected in the presence of which of the following factors?

(1) Non-Caucasian ethnic background
(2) Acid pH of stool
(3) Onset after six years of age
(4) Presence of reducing substances in the stool

122. A previously healthy four-year-old boy is brought to a poison control center with hematemesis. Endoscopy reveals diffuse gastritis. Likely etiologies include

(1) aspirin ingestion
(2) alcohol ingestion
(3) iron intoxication
(4) chronic granulomatous disease

Gastroenterology

Answers

80.   The answer is C. *(Hoekelman, pp 795-796, 1274.)* The barium enema illustrated in the figure accompanying the question demonstrates dilatation of loops of small bowel (secondary to thick meconium, which fails to pass normally and results in ileal obstruction) and microcolon (secondary to disuse) typical of meconium ileus. Under closely controlled conditions, meglumine diatrizoate (a Gastrografin enema) may relieve the obstruction without surgery and should be tried first. Hypothyroidism would not be associated with a narrow colon, and while hypothyroidism may cause constipation in the newborn period, intestinal obstruction is highly unlikely. No newborn with intestinal obstruction should merely be observed with supportive therapy; for the infant's safety, the etiology must be discerned as soon as possible. Palliative procedures, such as decompression of the distended upper gastrointestinal tract, have no place in the management of intestinal obstruction in the newborn.

81.   The answer is D. *(Hoekelman, pp 471-472.)* In malrotation of the intestine, there is failure, embryologically, of the intestine to rotate counterclockwise, so that normal placement and fixation of the cecum in the right lower quadrant does not occur. The usual clinical presentation is that of duodenal obstruction during the first year of life due to compression of the duodenum by the band of tissue that normally anchors the cecum in the right lower quadrant. A barium enema demonstrates the abnormal position of the cecum. A flat plate of the abdomen or an upper gastrointestinal series may show duodenal obstruction but will not establish its etiology. No specific findings on intravenous pyelogram or on a lateral decubitus view of the abdomen are found in this condition.

82.   The answer is D. *(Hoekelman, p 754.)* The diagnosis of pyloric stenosis is best made by direct palpation of the pyloric tumor after emesis. An upper gastrointestinal x-ray series also may be used, but pyloric stenosis may be difficult to distinguish from pylorospasm by this means. X-ray criteria for the diagnosis of pyloric stenosis include delayed emptying, persistent narrowing of the barium column, and persistent elongation of the pyloric channel. Often the double-track, or so-called "railroad-track" sign—that is, two or more parallel linear streaks of barium extending through the pyloric canal—is seen in the x-ray. Projectile or recurrent vomiting is not pathognomonic of pyloric stenosis. A family history is present in only about 15 percent of cases.

83.   The answer is A. *(Hoekelman, pp 336, 889.)* Children with hereditary fructose intolerance present with vomiting following the introduction of fruits into their diet. Jaundice may be present on initial presentation. Fructose should be eliminated from their diet to prevent liver damage and renal tubular acidosis. The introduction of vegetables, cereal, meat, or eggs to the diet of a four-month-old infant is not associated with the pattern of vomiting described or with jaundice. Fructose intolerance is inherited as an autosomal recessive trait.

84. The answer is B. *(Hoekelman, pp 722-725.)* The most likely pathophysiologic mechanism for diarrhea in *Salmonella* enteritis is stimulation of intestinal secretion by an enterotoxin. Other organisms associated with secretory toxins include *Escherichia coli, Klebsiella, Staphylococcus aureus,* and *Shigella dysenteriae.* Diarrhea also may be caused by: ingestion of osmotically active particles, such as magnesium citrate; malabsorption of carbohydrates and fat, which produces an osmotic or toxic effect in the colon; increased motility with resultant malabsorption of intestinal water; and decreased motility, which in producing intraluminal stasis encourages malabsorption of fats with secondary osmotic effects.

85. The answer is C. *(Hoekelman, pp 744-745, 803, 847-849.)* The most likely etiology for intermittent, acute, colicky abdominal pain with associated rectal bleeding is recurrent intussusception, usually secondary to a polyp or tumor being taken up by the fecal stream. Crohn's disease may be associated with pain and bloody diarrhea, but it is uncommon in this age group and does not produce acute colicky pain. *Yersinia* also may be associated with a chronic enterocolitis-like picture but not with rectal bleeding. Lymphoid nodular hyperplasia, which may be associated with abdominal pain or bleeding, has many 1 to 3 mm ileal or colonic lesions that are evident on x-ray. Henoch-Schönlein purpura is a hypersensitivity angiitis of a more acute nature, which may cause colicky bowel pain and bleeding but usually has associated skin or renal lesions. Rarely, intramural hematomas due to this disorder may act as a leading edge for intussusception.

86. The answer is D. *(Hoekelman, pp 790-791.)* The best method for diagnosing Wilson's disease is the determination of the hepatic copper content on liver biopsy. The earliest stage of the disease is marked by the accumulation of copper in the liver. Acute release of hepatic copper may produce hemolysis. Chronic accumulation may result in hepatitis, neurologic disease, and the development of Kayser-Fleischer rings. The only pathognomonic physical finding in pediatric Wilson's disease is Kayser-Fleischer rings detected on slit-lamp examination of the cornea; however, their absence does not rule out the hepatic form of the disease. Serum copper levels and copper excretion in the urine are usually increased, and serum ceruloplasmin levels are decreased in Wilson's disease, but these findings may also occur in patients with chronic acute hepatitis.

87. The answer is D. *(Hoekelman, pp 735-737.)* The evaluation of massive, painless, ongoing hematochezia in the absence of lower large bowel pathology is best made by arteriography. The possibility of upper gastrointestinal bleeding must first be excluded by nasogastric intubation. Arteriography localizes the lesion best if the blood loss is greater than 0.5 cc/min. Colonoscopy may be difficult with ongoing bleeding. Meckel's scan is indicated if the bleeding has stopped, but the yield may be low due to absence of destruction of gastric mucosa in the diverticulum. Barium enema in the presence of massive painless bleeding may have a low yield in an unprepared bowel. Laparotomy also should be delayed until a bleeding site is located. If the bleeding stops before a bleeding site is determined, surgery is best postponed until future bleeding occurs.

88. The answer is D. *(Hoekelman, pp 846, 1242-1249.)* The most common helminth infestation in the United States is due to *Enterobius vermicularis* (pinworm) in both adults and children. It is followed by *Ascaris* and *Trichuris* (whipworm) in frequency. Hookworm, trichinosis, and visceral larva migrans are relatively uncommon in the United States. Trichinosis is more often a problem in adults than in children. Infants are almost never infected with *Trichinella.*

89.   The answer is A. *(Hoekelman, pp 799-801, 858. Touloukian, pp 403-420.)* This is a classic history for an intramural hematoma of the duodenum. Although symptoms may appear immediately, there is usually a delay of several days before bilious vomiting and pain begin. Conservative treatment with nasogastric decompression and parenteral nutrition are usually sufficient. A subcapsular hematoma of the liver would result in severe pain very soon after injury. While a pseudocyst of the spleen may be entirely asymptomatic, it usually takes several weeks to form. A pseudocyst of the pancreas also would take longer to develop, but otherwise the history is compatible. Post-traumatic intussusception has not been described clinically.

90.   The answer is B. *(Roy, ed 2. p 30.)* The most likely cause of blood-streaked stools in infancy is an anal fissure. Cavernous hemangiomas may produce lower gastrointestinal bleeding, but they are rare. Rectal tears occur most commonly with rectal manipulation, usually by the careless use of thermometers. Juvenile polyps in this age group are uncommon; however, these polyps are the most common cause of painless bleeding in early childhood. Milk intolerance may present with enterocolitis and bloody diarrhea but usually only during the first two months of life.

91.   The answer is B. *(Hoekelman, pp 758-760.)* Pallor and positive guaiac stools in an adolescent should raise the question of peptic ulcer disease. Symptoms, however, may be quite atypical; for example, the disease may simply present as iron deficiency anemia. Also, menstruation abnormalities and inflammatory bowel disease must be ruled out. Because of this pattern, determining the actual incidence of peptic ulcer disease in this age group is difficult. The other entities listed are all rare disorders. Inflammatory gastric polyps are rarely seen in individuals under 30 years of age. Zollinger-Ellison syndrome, which is characterized by gastric hypersecretion and hypergastrinemia, may have multiple associated ulcers, but it is quite rare. Menetrier's disease, or gastric hypertrophy, may present with gastritis and an associated exudative gastropathy, but it is also rare. Pernicious anemia, which has an associated megaloblastic anemia secondary to vitamin B_{12} malabsorption, is quite uncommon at this age.

92.   The answer is D. *(Hoekelman, pp 796-798. Roy, ed 2. pp 78-79.)* Duplication (or "doubling") is a term commonly used to describe enteric cysts and diverticula. Gastrointestinal duplications, which usually occur in the small intestine or esophagus, may (1) present as an abdominal or thoracic mass, (2) produce bleeding or obstruction, or (3) cause colicky pain. Pathologically, they may exhibit mucosa similar to that found in the stomach or small intestine or form a neurenteric cyst with associated vertebral abnormalities. Jaundice is not associated with gastrointestinal duplications.

93.   The answer is A. *(Hoekelman, pp 63, 744-745.)* The presentation of acute abdominal pain, bile-stained vomitus, and abdominal distension in this patient would indicate intestinal obstruction. X-ray examination, which reveals dilated air-filled loops in both the large and small bowel, not only confirms the suspicion of intestinal obstruction, but indicates that the obstruction is low—that is, either in the large intestine or rectum. The differential diagnosis of obstruction in a two-year-old child includes (1) intussusception, (2) incarcerated inguinal hernia, (3) adhesions postsurgery, (4) unrecognized congenital stenoses, (5) midgut volvulus, (6) Hirschsprung's disease, (7) fecal impaction associated with cystic fibrosis, and (8) obstructing duplication cysts. The most common of these in a 24-month-old child is intussusception. Determination of serum electrolyte levels would be useful in managing this patient, since the vomiting and third spacing of fluid may lead to serious disorders of fluids and electrolytes. Examination of stools for occult blood (stool guaiac) would help narrow the differential because intussusception and volvulus may be associated with a positive guaiac. Since a paralytic ileus in a young child may be caused by significant infection such as septicemia, peritonitis, pyelonephritis, or pneumonia, a urinalysis would be useful to rule out a urinary tract infection. The definitive diagnostic test would be a barium enema, since plain x-rays have already indicated that the lesion is low. The least appropriate choice in this case would be an upper gastrointestinal series, since the obstruction is below the small intestine.

94.   The answer is D. *(Hoekelman, p 753.)* Ingestion of strong acid is likely to produce the most severe lesions in the gastric antrum. One postulated mechanism includes relaxation of the esophagus with decreased direct mucosal contact. Oral and esophageal lesions may occur, but they are seldom problematic. Acids pass rapidly to the stomach, causing transmural necrosis in that organ. Strong alkalies, on the other hand, produce the most severe lesions in the esophagus, with a high incidence of secondary strictures.

95.   The answer is B. *(Hoekelman, pp 747-750. Roy, ed 2. pp 150-152.)* Chronic regurgitation coupled with a low resting level of the lower esophageal pressure (LES) and normal sphincter relaxation time best fits the clinical picture of chalasia. Low sphincter pressure represents a defect in the intrinsic mechanism for preventing gastroesophageal reflux. Although sphincter pressure can be low in the early neonatal period, low pressure after three to four weeks of age is abnormal. Additional factors thought to prevent reflux include the esophageal cardiac angle, the amount of intraabdominal esophagus, and the phrenoesophageal ligament. Achalasia is an uncommon disorder characterized by the loss of tertiary peristalsis, failure to relax the LES on swallowing, and a high or normal LES resting pressure. About 10 percent of all achalasia presents in childhood. Esophagitis may occur as a complication of recurrent reflux. Often low LES pressure and abnormal distal peristalsis are present. Significant esophagitis usually is accompanied by blood loss. A low LES resting pressure may be encountered in the first few weeks of life but is abnormal at 12 months of age. Central core disease, a skeletal muscle myopathy, would not affect smooth muscle function in the distal esophagus.

96.   The answer is C. *(Hoekelman, pp 734-737, 758, 838, 851, 1121.)* Blood in bowel movements may occur from a lesion anywhere in the gastrointestinal (GI) tract. Even though this patient's blood pressure does not change with position, an increase of pulse from 85 to 100 indicates a significant loss of blood. The presence of blood in the nasogastric tube indicates that the lesion is proximal to the ligament of Treitz. Red blood in the stool may occur from upper GI lesions and is related to the amount of bacteria in the stool (with antibiotics, one is more likely to find bright red blood in the stool associated with bleeding from high lesions), and the transit time (the more rapid the time, the more likely the blood is to be red). Peutz-Jeghers syndrome produces GI bleeding from polyps located distal to the ligament of Treitz. Regional enteritis and Henoch-Schönlein purpura also produce bleeding from lesions in the lower intestines. Serum sickness is generally not associated with gastrointestinal bleeding, making the most likely diagnosis in this patient acute gastritis (in this case, secondary to aspirin ingestion).

97. The answer is E. *(Hoekelman, pp 719-720.)* Although neurologic diseases (muscular dystrophies, neurofibromatoses, and myotonia), metabolic diseases (hypothyroidism and hypocalcemia), anorectal lesions, and chronic use of cathartics may lead to acquired megacolon with secondary encopresis, the most common etiology is "psychogenic." Very often these children have a history of problematic toilet training and stressful events. For example, painful stooling such as that caused by anal fissure may precipitate an episode of retention followed by encopresis. Distension and pressure build-up in the rectal lumen lead to relaxation of the internal sphincter as constipation continues. Because stooling is painful, the child begins to hold back bowel movements, which leads to enlargement of the rectum with less and less function of the external sphincter. This is ultimately followed by continuous leakage of soft stool around the hard mass. Aganglionic megacolon may present at birth with constipation and abdominal distension, but would not then disappear and reappear at age six. Again, although back injury may lead to neurologic damage and encopresis, this is extremely unlikely and would be associated with abnormal anal reflexes. A normal neurologic examination in a normally developing child (both physically and mentally) makes the diagnosis of psychogenic constipation with encopresis the most likely one.

98. The answer is A. *(Hoekelman, pp 816-820, 1245. Liebman, Pediatrics 64:43-45, 1979.)* Although all the diseases listed can cause recurrent abdominal pain, several recent studies have implicated disaccharide intolerance—especially lactose intolerance—as a significant cause of recurrent abdominal pain, especially in black Americans. In several studies, 25 to 43 percent of children with recurrent abdominal pain have been found to have lactose intolerance. None of the other choices occurs with such high frequency as a cause of recurrent abdominal pain. *Ascaris lumbricoides* infestation is frequently asymptomatic. In addition, the negative stool guaiacs and normal sedimentation rate make inflammatory bowel disease less likely. The normal urinalysis makes hydronephrosis less likely.

99. The answer is B. *(Hoekelman, pp 777-781. Schiff, ed 4. pp 533-540, 594-601, 613-614.)* A high serum transaminase level and jaundice in the presence of mild diffuse hepatocellular damage is consistent with acute viral hepatitis. Etiologic agents frequently are hepatitis A virus (infectious) and hepatitis B virus (serum), with the latter often becoming more chronic or persistent. Other agents include cytomegalovirus, Epstein-Barr virus, non-A and non-B hepatitis virus, and coxsackievirus. Drug-induced hepatitis may resemble acute viral hepatitis both clinically and pathologically and should be considered in the differential diagnosis. Cystic fibrosis may present with portal hypertension and biliary cirrhosis. Serum transaminase levels are generally lower in cystic fibrosis than in viral hepatitis, and jaundice is not evident until liver decompensation occurs. Hepatitis is a common presenting feature of Wilson's disease in childhood. It should be considered in fulminant or chronic active hepatitis and postnecrotic cirrhosis occurring between 8 and 14 years of age. Chronic active hepatitis characteristically has a histologic picture showing (1) periportal inflammation and varying degrees of fibrosis, (2) focal loss of hepatocytes, and (3) spillage of inflammatory cells from the limiting plates into the parenchyma. It often culminates in cirrhosis. Serum transaminases are generally only mildly elevated. Alpha$_1$-antitrypsin deficiency may present with prolonged jaundice in the neonatal period or with cirrhosis in early life.

100. The answer is B. *(Hoekelman, p 272.)* Infection (bacteremia or fungemia) is common with parenteral hyperalimentation. Initial measures should be to remove the venous catheter, culture its tip, and discontinue hyperalimentation altogether. Frequently, the bacteremia disappears as soon as the catheter is removed. Blood cultures should be taken, but unless the patient is clinically septic, antibiotic therapy need not be initiated immediately. However, the tip of the catheter should be cultured.

101. The answer is C. *(Hoekelman, pp 812-813, 815.)* The jejunal biopsy shown in the figure accompanying the question is normal. Chronic diarrhea with a normal jejunal biopsy is compatible with cystic fibrosis. The remaining choices are all associated with varying degrees of villous atrophy on the basis of chronic mucosal destruction. A flat villus lesion is seen with gluten-sensitive enteropathy, acute and chronic diarrhea, giardiasis, and immunodeficiency disorders.

102. The answer is A (1, 2, 3). *(McMillan, vol 2. p 116.)* Imperforate anus may be part of Vater's syndrome. Patients with this syndrome may have associated vertebral, anal, tracheal, esophageal, and renal anomalies as well as those involving the heart and radii. Two-thirds of those children without an anal orifice will have associated spinal and urologic anomalies. Disorders of the central nervous system are not usually part of this syndrome.

103. The answer is A (1, 2, 3). *(Hoekelman, pp 763-766, 781-790.)* The function of the liver in carbohydrate metabolism includes: glycogen storage, gluconeogenesis, glycogenolysis, and conversion of carbohydrate to fat. Fasting hypoglycemia may occur in situations of mild hepatic injury. With significant degeneration of the liver, such as in Reye's syndrome, marked hypoglycemia may result. The liver also plays a role in the absorption of fat soluble vitamins which require bile salts for absorption from the intestines. Vitamins A, D, and K will become deficient with diseases such as biliary atresia in which there is a loss of bile salts. The liver also plays an important role in hormone metabolism and detoxification of corticosteroid hormones. The latter role, however, is diminished with liver disease. Gynecomastia, testicular atrophy, infertility, and menstrual disorders may occur in adolescents with cirrhosis. Although acute serum hepatitis may cause vomiting with acid base disturbances, metabolic acidosis is not found consistently.

104. The answer is A (1, 2, 3). *(Hoekelman, pp 750-752. Roy, ed 2. pp 52-53.)* Tracheoesophageal fistula with esophageal atresia is a congenital anomaly that may not be apparent in the newborn period; it can have numerous clinical presentations. Secretions and feedings with an atretic esophagus are either regurgitated or aspirated into the lungs (aspiration pneumonia). The tracheoesophageal fistula may allow air to pass from the respiratory tract to the gastrointestinal tract (particularly with forceful crying), resulting in early abdominal distension. A number of associated anomalies may actually be more threatening to the infant, including cardiovascular, renal, vertebral, and radial anomalies or an imperforate anus. Cleft palate is not an associated anomaly.

105. The answer is C (2, 4). *(Hoekelman, pp 816-820, 897-898. Diem, p 509.)* As dextrose and levulose are the principal sugars in honey, a carbohydrate-free formula with added honey could be used in a child with lactose intolerance. Sucrose is the carbohydrate in soy formulas, which would also be acceptable for this child. The commonly used formulas based on cow's milk contain lactose. Clear liquids do not contain lactose, but should not be used for prolonged periods since they do not provide adequate nutrition.

106. The answer is C (2, 4). *(Hoekelman, pp 827-830.)* Factors useful in diagnosing acute appendicitis in young children include the presence of an abnormal bowel gas pattern (particularly a paucity of luminal gas in the right lower quadrant) and the absence of urinary tract disease. A high incidence of perforation occurs in this age group. Periumbilical pain followed by vomiting and progressive toxicity should alert the clinician to this possibility. Obscuration of the psoas shadow occurs in over half of the cases of appendicitis in children under two years of age. Although a fecalith is found in approximately one-third of cases, the presence of one in the region of the appendix is not too helpful in the diagnosis of acute appendicitis, since fecaliths also may be present in healthy children.

107. The answer is B (1, 3). *(Hoekelman, pp 713-715.)* A history of constant localized pain, which frequently awakens one from sleep, suggests an underlying organic lesion, rather than dysfunctional disease due to stress, constipation, or lactose deficiency, particularly if the pain is in an area other than the periumbilical region. Etiologies of right lower quadrant (RLQ) pain such as that disturbing this patient include adhesions from previous surgery, inflammatory bowel disease, particularly Crohn's disease, and urinary tract abnormalities.

108. The answer is A (1, 2, 3). *(Hoekelman, pp 802-803.)* Disorders that have been associated with an enterocolitis include shigellosis, salmonellosis, and yersinosis. The organisms that cause these disorders invade intestinal mucosal cells and produce necrosis of the bowel with bloody diarrhea. Shigellosis and salmonellosis are usually self-limited, whereas yersinosis may be acute or chronic with remissions and exacerbations. Rotavirus, which is associated with acute diarrhea and superficial mucosal damage, may present with polymorphonuclear leukocytes in the stool; bleeding, however, is quite rare.

109. The answer is B (1, 3). *(Hoekelman, pp 850-851.)* Malignant transformation is associated with the adenomatous polyps seen in familial (adenomatous) polyposis and Gardner's syndrome (also characterized by bony exostosis, connective tissue tumors, and sebaceous cysts). Syndromes characterized by hamartomatous polyps include Peutz-Jeghers syndrome with its associated mucocutaneous pigmentation and Canada-Cronkhite syndrome with its abnormal pigmentation, nail dystrophy, and alopecia. Care must be taken not to confuse familial polyposis with juvenile polyposis. Juvenile polyposis occurs mostly in children between 2 and 12 years of age. The polyps, which are usually single but can occur in multiples, are thought to arise from chronic inflammation, which leads to obstruction of glands and inspissation of mucus. Juvenile polyps are not premalignant.

110. The answer is B (1, 3). *(Hoekelman, pp 859-860.)* A child with low weight for height and massive steatorrhea (> 6 g of stool fat every 24 hours is abnormal) probably has pancreatic insufficiency. Cystic fibrosis is the most common etiology, but others include Shwachmann-Diamond syndrome with associated neutropenia and chronic pancreatitis. Although giardiasis and gluten-sensitive enteropathy have mild to moderate associated steatorrhea, fat absorption does not fall below 65-70 percent of that ingested.

111. The answer is B (1, 3). *(Hoekelman, p 858. Roy, ed 2. pp 648-649.)* An epigastric mass and a history of blunt abdominal trauma suggest a pancreatic pseudocyst, which may be evaluated further by checking the serum amylase level and delineating the extent and origin of the mass by ultrasonography. Pseudocysts require several weeks for maturation before attempts at internal drainage are made. Early manipulation such as transabdominal needle biopsy and exploratory laparotomy may result in perforation and peritoneal spillage. Elemental diets or parenteral nutrition may be useful temporizing adjuncts in reducing the size of the lesion.

112. The answer is E (all). *(Hoekelman, pp 804-808, 811-816. Roy, ed 2. p 229.)* Gluten-sensitive enteropathy (celiac disease) is believed to be a genetic disease, but the mode of inheritance is not known. Except for cystic fibrosis, it it the most common cause of malabsorption in children. Anorexia, wasting, irritability, and steatorrhea are the cardinal manifestations of gluten-sensitive enteropathy. However, it may also present with finger clubbing, fat soluble vitamin deficiencies (including vitamin K deficiency, which may lead to epistaxis), anemia, rickets, edema, vomiting, and constipation (present in about 10 percent of cases).

113. The answer is E (all). *(Sleisenger, ed 2. pp 1606-1608, 1664-1665.)* Friable mucosa, goblet cell depletion, crypt abscesses, and granulomas are all pathologic manifestations of inflammatory bowel disease (IBD). The first three findings occur most often in ulcerative colitis; granulomas are seen in Crohn's disease (in about 30 percent of biopsies). Sigmoidoscopy in ulcerative colitis may reveal abnormalities of the mucosa of the sigmoid colon varying from slight hyperemia, to granularity with mild bleeding, to pseudopolyp formation, depending on the severity of disease. Similar granularity, punctate bleeding, linear ulcers, and "cobblestone" formation within the mucosa of the large intestine may be seen in Crohn's disease. However, differentiation by sigmoidoscopy and biopsy may be difficult. Occasionally the biopsy will be abnormal despite normal-appearing mucosa. Additional clinical features of IBD in children include failure to thrive and iron deficiency anemia.

114. The answer is A (1, 2, 3). *(Hoekelman, pp 832-837. Roy, ed 2. p 295.)* Extraintestinal manifestations of chronic ulcerative colitis in children include growth failure, erythema nodosum, and arthritis. Although ankylosing spondylitis is often an extraintestinal manifestation of chronic ulcerative colitis in adults, it has not been reported in children. Liver abnormalities (including fatty infiltration, chronic active hepatitis, and occasionally, pericholangitis) and finger clubbing are also observed.

115. The answer is B (1, 3). *(Hoekelman, pp 259-262.)* Approximately 70 percent of children with gastroenteritis have isotonic dehydration—that is, fluid loss in which serum concentrations of electrolytes remain constant. To replace this fluid, liquids approximating maintenance fluid may be used, including sodium and potassium replacements of about 50 to 70 mEq/m^2 each. Commonly used clear liquids, including broth, soda pop, and gelatin solution, are hypotonic and may be used appropriately in the outpatient management of gastroenteritis. Although these liquids are quite hypotonic compared with commercial electrolyte solutions, the kidneys of most children with gastroenteritis are able to conserve sodium. Boiled skim milk, which contains a very high sodium concentration, should not be used because it may lead to hypernatremia. The lactose in the milk may also cause the diarrhea to persist. Homemade electrolyte solutions should also be avoided because of the frequent errors made when parents mix the solutions. These errors often result in hypernatremia.

116. The answer is A (1, 2, 3). *(Hoekelman, pp 725-729, 801-804. Vaughan, ed 11. pp 777, 785, 789, 1017.)* Controlled trials have shown that the course of acute diarrhea caused by *Salmonella* species is not shortened significantly by antibiotic therapy. In fact, the carrier state is prolonged by antibiotic therapy. The acute diarrhea associated with giardiasis, shigellosis, and cholera all are shortened by appropriate antibiotic therapy.

117. The answer is C (2, 4). *(Rudolph, ed 16. pp 402, 406.)* Penicillin and gentamicin are excreted by renal mechanisms and are not affected by hepatic failure. Chloramphenicol is metabolized and nafcillin is excreted by hepatic mechanisms. The half-lives and serum levels of these drugs would be difficult to estimate in hepatic failure, so other drugs should be used when hepatic failure is present.

118. The answer is B (1, 3). *(Hoekelman, pp 788-790, 792.)* Splenomegaly and esophageal varices (seen on x-ray) are signs of portal hypertension, as may be seen in cirrhosis due to alpha$_1$-antitrypsin deficiency or cavernous transformation of the portal vein. Both may present with evidence of advanced portal obstruction on physical examination. Extra-hepatic biliary atresia causes portal hypertension but is manifested early in life. Biliary cirrhosis in cystic fibrosis, however, may present in a manner similar to extrahepatic biliary atresia. Although an enlarged spleen may be the first finding in childhood lymphomas, esophageal varices do not occur with this condition.

119. The answer is E (all). *(Hoekelman, pp 837-841. Sleisenger, ed 2. pp 1676-1677.)* Crohn's disease has been referred to by a variety of terms, including regional enteritis, ileal regional enteritis, right-sided colitis, and granulomatous colitis. It can occur anywhere in the gastrointestinal tract. Malabsorptive consequences of this disease include vitamin B$_{12}$ deficiency, with resultant megaloblastic anemia, and bile salt deficiency, with resultant steatorrhea. Fat malabsorption, in turn, is thought to alter oxalate absorption, resulting in hyperoxaluria. Zinc deficiency has been reported with small intestinal Crohn's disease and may be one reason for delayed sexual maturation in some children.

120. The answer is E (all). *(Hoekelman, pp 771-772, 898-899.)* Hepatomegaly with fatty infiltration has been associated with metabolic diseases, including tyrosinemia, galactosemia, Gaucher's disease, and hereditary fructose intolerance. Most of these present in the first few months of life with vomiting, neurologic impairment, or failure to thrive. Galactosemia also presents with jaundice in about 60 percent of patients. Posterior subcapsular cataracts are sometimes seen in newborns and are found in about 50 percent of infants with this disorder by the age of six months. Tyrosinemia presents with fever, edema, and a peculiar urine odor in about 50 percent of patients. Melena, ascites, and splenomegaly also occur. Hereditary fructose intolerance may present early with hypoglycemia, hepatomegaly, jaundice, or shock following introduction to sucrose or fructose, or later with milder disease manifested by aversion to sweets or fruits.

121. The answer is E (all). *(Hoekelman, pp 816-820, 896-898.)* Acquired lactose intolerance is a relatively frequent finding in Caucasian and non-Caucasian infants with acute or chronic inflammatory diarrhea. Treatment consists of a lactose-free diet for several days or weeks after which normal digestion and absorption of lactose returns. Inherited lactose intolerance is common among members of non-Caucasian groups after five or six years of age, even in industrial societies where milk is a prominent food source well past the time of weaning. Acid pH and reducing substances are formed in individuals with either acquired or inherited lactose intolerance.

122. The answer is A (1, 2, 3). *(Hoekelman, p 758. Gellis, pp 190, 662, 685.)* Ingested agents that produce acute gastritis in a young child include aspirin, alcohol, and iron. Aspirin and alcohol both appear to injure the gastric mucosal barrier and facilitate further damage by gastric acid. Chronic granulomatous disease can present with chronic gastritis and iron deficiency anemia, but this is quite rare.

Neurology and Child Development

DIRECTIONS: Each question below contains five suggested answers. Choose the **one best** response to each question.

123. A previously well three-year-old white girl comes in with a chief complaint of left-sided hemiparesis of acute onset following a left-sided seizure. On examination, it is found that in addition to her flaccid left hemiparesis the left side of her mouth droops. The most likely cause of this disorder is

(A) a lateral sinus thrombosis following mastoiditis
(B) an embolus secondary to cardiac valve vegetations
(C) a sagittal sinus thrombosis secondary to hypernatremic dehydration
(D) lead encephalopathy
(E) a hemiplegic migraine

124. A four-year-old girl is brought to the emergency room at 9 P.M., one hour after falling off her tricycle and bumping her head. There was no loss of consciousness, but she is sleepy and has vomited once. Neurological examination is normal. To help rule out serious intracranial pathology before discharge, the pediatrician should

(A) obtain a series of skull x-rays
(B) obtain a neurosurgical consultation
(C) obtain cerebrospinal fluid by lumbar puncture
(D) monitor vital and neurological signs for four hours
(E) monitor consciousness level for four hours of forced wakefulness

125. Neurotoxicity may occur following the topical absorption of which of the following antiseptics?

(A) Hexachlorophene
(B) Benzalkonium chloride
(C) Bacitracin
(D) Silver sulfadiazine
(E) Providone-iodine

126. A three-year-old child with a brain tumor is most likely to present with which of the following symptoms?

(A) Early morning vomiting without nausea
(B) Blurred vision
(C) Behavioral changes
(D) Diplopia
(E) A petit mal seizure

127. The presence of a chronic subdural hematoma should be strongly suspected in a six-month-old infant presenting with

(A) recent head trauma, transient loss of consciousness, and bilateral abducens nerve palsy
(B) recent head trauma, coma, and hemiplegia
(C) fever, lethargy, and flaccid weakness of one leg
(D) seizures, repeated vomiting, and retinal hemorrhages
(E) failure to thrive, repeated vomiting, and nystagmus

128. A five-year-old child with no previous history of central nervous system problems is reported by her parents to have had numerous episodes of "losing contact for brief periods of time" but no loss of consciousness. They also report lip smacking and some automatisms. After each episode, the child complains, "my head hurts." An electroencephalogram shows no abnormality. The **initial** management of this patient would be to

(A) request a sleep electroencephalogram
(B) start the child on phenobarbital
(C) request a CAT scan
(D) obtain skull x-rays
(E) treat the child with ethosuximide

129. An eight-year-old girl presents with acute emotional depression and lability, severe hypotonia, and mild choreiform movements. The family history is negative for rheumatic fever. Blood tests and a throat culture reveal no evidence of streptococcal infection or liver dysfunction. The most probable diagnosis is

(A) Syndenham's chorea
(B) Wilson's disease
(C) Parkinson's disease
(D) Huntington's chorea
(E) Gilles de la Tourette's syndrome

130. The diagnosis of narcolepsy is based on the presence of

(A) sudden attacks of sleep, cataplexy, and focal seizures
(B) sudden attacks of sleep, sleep paralysis, depression, and an abnormal electroencephalogram
(C) sudden attacks of sleep, sleep paralysis, cataplexy, and hallucinations
(D) sudden attacks of sleep, hallucinations, and an abnormal electroencephalogram
(E) sudden attacks of sleep, sleep paralysis, hypoglycemia, and an abnormal electroencephalogram

131. Cerebral palsy is a developmental disability related to

(A) prematurity
(B) brain damage due to anoxia at birth
(C) perinatal factors primarily
(D) a specific brain lesion
(E) no single pathophysiological process in the central nervous system

132. Which of the following conditions does not cause headaches in children?

(A) Spasm of the distal branches of the cerebral arteries
(B) Vascular edema
(C) Muscle tension
(D) Displacement of dural structures
(E) A seizure disorder

133. A mother reports that her five-month-old infant cries vigorously and has irregular sleep, bowel, and feeding habits. Furthermore, the infant reacts with fury every time she prepares a new food and accepts the new food only after many attempts. Physical examination is unremarkable. This behavior is most likely due to

(A) anaclitic depression
(B) complications during the perinatal period
(C) maternal inexperience
(D) excessive coffee consumption during pregnancy
(E) the "difficult child" temperament

134. The etiology of resistance to feeding in a healthy one-year-old child is likely to include all of the following EXCEPT

(A) the child's interest in the tactile properties of food
(B) the child's interest in the trajectories of dropped objects
(C) the child's growing independence as it grows older
(D) the child's decreasing height-growth velocity and resultant loss of appetite
(E) parental attempts to avoid messes that occur when the child attempts to feed itself

135. At two years of age, the average child can be expected to attain approximately

(A) 50 percent of the expected adult height, 20 percent of the expected adult weight, and 87 percent of the expected adult head circumference
(B) 50 percent of the expected adult height, 40 percent of the expected adult weight, and 97 percent of the expected adult head circumference
(C) 30 percent of the expected adult height, 20 percent of the expected adult weight, and 97 percent of the expected adult head circumference
(D) 30 percent of the expected adult height, 30 percent of the expected adult weight, and 87 percent of the expected adult head circumference
(E) 50 percent of the expected adult height, 20 percent of the expected adult weight, and 97 percent of the expected adult head circumference

136. During a routine well-child visit, a six-year-old boy is found to have the language skills of a five year old. The rest of the evaluation is unremarkable. The best **initial** plan of management would be to

(A) suggest that first grade be postponed for a year
(B) refer him for psychometric evaluation
(C) refer him to an audiologist
(D) recommend that first grade be started as planned
(E) recommend a special education class

137. At her son's two-year well-child visit, a mother complains that she is having difficulty toilet training him because he dislikes sitting on the toilet. Questioning reveals that the child has quite irregular bowel habits. Which of the following suggestions would be most likely to lead to successful toilet training within a reasonable period of time?

(A) Delay further attempts until central nervous system maturation yields more regular habits
(B) Place the child on the toilet for fifteen minutes every two hours during the day
(C) Delay further attempts until the child shows an interest in being toilet trained
(D) Express strong disapproval every time the child has an accident and then make him sit on the toilet
(E) Give the child one tablespoon of mineral oil at bedtime and have him sit on the toilet when he gets up in the morning

138. The virtues of being either a "permissive" or a "strict" parent have always been debated. Most studies have shown that children brought up by authoritarian parents—that is, by parents who demand unquestioning obedience and who enforce their will with physical punishment—when compared with children reared by permissive parents, are

(A) better behaved in the classroom
(B) significantly more inhibited in the classroom
(C) more likely to be aggressive with their school-mates
(D) less likely to be in frequent conflict with their mothers
(E) none of the above

139. In a child being evaluated for school failure, the presence of which of the following factors would be most suggestive of a primary "learning disability"?

(A) An impoverished and disordered home
(B) Significantly delayed motor and language milestones
(C) Frequent but brief episodes of ptosis and eye fluttering
(D) Impulsive and distractable behavior
(E) Recently divorced parents

140. A six-year-old boy makes a drawing like the one shown below during the Goodenough-Harris Drawing Test in a school-readiness evaluation. On the basis of this drawing, the physician should

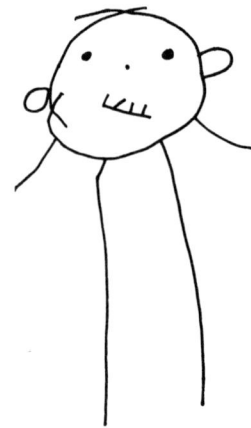

(A) refer the child for psychological evaluation
(B) refer the child for psychiatric evaluation
(C) look for evidence of cerebral palsy
(D) recommend that the child be placed in a special education class
(E) recommend that the child begin school as planned in a regular classroom

141. According to the theories of Freud, Piaget, and Erikson, an eight-year-old child would be in which of the following stages?

(A) Phallic, concrete operations, and initiative versus guilt
(B) Oral, sensorimotor, and trust versus mistrust
(C) Genital, formal operations, and industry versus inferiority
(D) Anal, concrete operations, and initiative versus guilt
(E) Latency, concrete operations, and industry versus inferiority

142. Persons who are mentally retarded can best be described as having a handicapping condition which produces a significant impairment in

(A) intellectual functioning
(B) intellectual and physical functioning
(C) intellectual functioning and adaptive behavior
(D) thinking, language, and perception
(E) development of cognitive skills

143. Although a few prenatally-determined conditions, such as Down's syndrome or the amino-acidurias, are well-known causes of mental retardation, they represent only five to ten percent of all cases. According to currently available data, the most frequent cause of mental retardation is

(A) intrauterine insults, including maternal ingestion of toxic substances
(B) environmental factors of unspecified origin
(C) perinatal complications influencing fetal oxygen supply
(D) maternal deprivation
(E) a mosaic of constitutional and environmental factors

144. All of the following statements concerning adolescents are true EXCEPT that

(A) adolescents with a severe chronic illness often adapt better than those with a milder degree of the same illness
(B) adolescents with a congenital deformity or illness often tolerate it better than those who develop it in early or middle adolescence
(C) early adolescents are often more concerned with the effect of their illness on their appearance than the actual sequelae of the illness
(D) defense mechanisms and other coping methods used in childhood and early adolescence are not often used by late adolescents in dealing with their illnesses
(E) late adolescents often view chronic illness in terms of its effect on their careers or personal relationships

DIRECTIONS: Each question below contains four suggested answers of which **one** or **more** is correct. Choose the answer

A	if	1, 2, and 3	are correct
B	if	1 and 3	are correct
C	if	2 and 4	are correct
D	if	4	is correct
E	if	1, 2, 3, and 4	are correct

145. Appropriate management of a ten-year-old child who has had a generalized tonic-clonic afebrile seizure three hours previously and whose neurological examination is normal includes

(1) determining blood sugar, calcium, and blood urea nitrogen
(2) giving glucose intravenously
(3) obtaining an electroencephalogram
(4) performing a lumbar puncture

146. The infant shown in the figure below was born with spina bifida. Although he had an operative repair in the first day of life, he has a high probability of developing

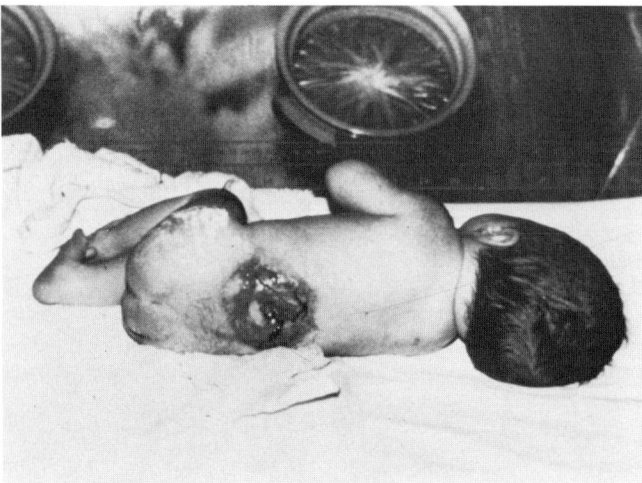

Used with permission of Foundation for Teaching Aids at Low Cost Institute of Child Health, 30 Guilford Street, London WCIN 1EH.

(1) lower extremity paralysis
(2) urinary incontinence
(3) hydrocephalus
(4) mental retardation

147. True statements concerning the current status of treatment for myoclonic epilepsy of infancy include which of the following?

(1) There is no satisfactory treatment
(2) Adrenocorticotropic hormone or steroids typically are administered
(3) Generalized tonic-clonic drugs are used with other medications
(4) Clonazepam is a useful drug

148. A one-year-old child is being evaluated for developmental delay. Physical examination reveals a cherry-red spot on the macula. Diagnostic possibilities include

(1) Canavan's disease
(2) generalized gangliosidosis (G_{M_1})
(3) metachromatic leukodystrophy
(4) Tay-Sachs disease

149. *Pavor nocturnus* is characterized by which of the following statements?

(1) It is rare in children before age five or six
(2) It occurs 90 to 100 minutes after the child has fallen asleep
(3) It is well remembered by the child in the morning
(4) It is not associated with significant psychopathology

150. In treating status epilepticus, which of the following potential complications must be addressed?

(1) Hypotension
(2) Respiratory arrest
(3) Anticonvulsant overdosage
(4) Hyperpyrexia

151. The increase in secular growth in European and American youth over the past 100 years is probably due to

(1) better nutrition
(2) improved living conditions
(3) the control of many serious childhood diseases
(4) improved health habits

152. Early adolescence is characterized by

(1) major arguments and conflicts with parents
(2) rapid pubertal development
(3) the establishment of adolescent sexuality concepts
(4) a preoccupation with physical appearance

153. Late adolescence is characterized by

(1) the maturation of cognitive thinking
(2) the establishment of adult sexuality concepts
(3) maximization of peer group influences
(4) a finalization of the emancipation process

154. Common factors in the etiology of excessive crying in six-week-old infants with normal physical examinations include

(1) the tendency of newborns to cry during the first weeks of life
(2) a "difficult" temperament
(3) over stimulation of the infant
(4) maternal depression or anxiety

155. The average 18-month-old child can be expected to

(1) walk up steps
(2) build a tower of four to eight blocks
(3) point to his eyes or nose on request
(4) copy a circle

156. A mother complains that her two-year-old daughter protests violently when put to bed and then gets up repeatedly. Effective methods for dealing with this situation include

(1) developing a bedtime ritual, such as reading a story to the child
(2) having the child stay up until she is ready to sleep
(3) sitting outside the child's room and insisting that she stay in bed
(4) lying down with the child for a few minutes until she develops a feeling of security

DIRECTIONS: The groups of questions below consist of lettered choices followed by several numbered items. For each numbered item select the **one** lettered choice with which it is **most** closely associated. Each lettered choice may be used once, more than once, or not at all.

Questions 157-161

For each statement that follows, select the type of brain tumor with which it is most likely to be associated.

(A) Medulloblastoma
(B) Cerebellar astrocytoma
(C) Craniopharyngioma
(D) Supratentorial glioma
(E) Meningioma

157. It is rare before adolescence

158. The male to female ratio is approximately 2:1

159. It may produce retarded growth

160. There is a rapid onset of symptoms

161. Approximately 50 percent of all cases are malignant

Questions 162-165

For each statement below, select the cause of abnormal head growth in infancy that it most accurately describes.

(A) Communicating hydrocephalus
(B) Obstructive hydrocephalus
(C) Megalencephaly
(D) Chronic subdural hematoma
(E) None of the above

162. It may be caused by neuronal storage disease

163. It is the most common serious central nervous system manifestation of child abuse

164. It may result from the Arnold-Chiari malformation

165. It may complicate bacterial meningitis

Questions 166-168

For each of the following groups of characteristics, select the age with which they are most likely to be associated.

(A) 2 months
(B) 7 months
(C) 18 months
(D) 3 years
(E) 4 years

166. Stubbornness, temper tantrums, flat feet, and bow legs

167. Crying, sneezing, and straining with bowel movements

168. Talking back, fascination with the processes of elimination, and genital play with other children

Questions 169-172

The primary care physician who manages a developmentally disabled school-age child must relate to various community agencies (this is often mandated by law) for certain aspects of the child's care. For each of the following cases described below, select the appropriate agency which by law must be involved in the patient's care.

(A) Department of Social Services
(B) State Office of Mental Retardation (or equivalent)
(C) Disabled children's program
(D) Family court
(E) Local public school

169. A profoundly mentally retarded 6-year-old child who is in need of an educational program

170. A 20-year-old severely retarded person for whom residential care is desired

171. A 4-year-old nonambulatory child with cerebral palsy left unattended each day for several hours

172. A low-income family of a mentally retarded child that needs financial help

Neurology and Child Development

Answers

123. The answer is B. *(Hoekelman, pp 934, 1524-1525.)* Although a hemiparesis may occur following a seizure (Todd's paralysis), this presentation may also characterize a cerebral vascular accident. Vascular diseases may be either arterial or venous. With arterial occlusion, a previously well child suddenly develops a focal neurologic deficit. There is decreased sensation and weakness in a distribution that corresponds to a single vessel in the cerebral hemisphere or brain stem. Decreased responsiveness in focal seizures is common, and underlying problems such as arteriovenous malformations or aneurysms, vascular disease, emboli, and hemorrhage may also lead to arterial infarctions. Venous obstruction may also occur, but in contrast to children with arterial occlusions, children with venous infarction or hemorrhage are usually ill before the onset of symptoms. The onset of the deficit is slower, and neurologic findings are more diffuse because the venous cerebral circulation overlaps considerably. Lateral and saggital sinus thromboses are venous occlusions. Although lead encephalopathy may have a similar clinical presentation, it would be more likely to present with a generalized rather than focal seizure and would be less likely to be followed by a hemiparesis than would an arterial occlusion. Although a hemiplegic migraine may present as headache with hemiparesis, seizures would be very unlikely. The most likely diagnosis is an embolus secondary to cardiac valve vegetations with occlusion of a cerebral artery, even though prior cardiac disease was not suspected.

124. The answer is D. *(Hoekelman, pp 929-930. Singer, Pediatrics 62:819-821, 1978.)* The history indicates mild trauma without loss of consciousness, and although the child is sleepy, neurological examination is normal. Serious intracranial pathology, therefore, is unlikely. Vomiting several times after minor head trauma is not unusual, nor is it unusual for a child to be sleepy at night. Skull films are rarely useful in the management of minor head trauma. A lumbar puncture will provide no information that will affect therapy and could be dangerous if the injury proved to be serious. Keeping the child awake will make monitoring the consciousness level more difficult than if she is aroused intermittently. Monitoring of vital signs and neurological findings is the procedure most likely to detect significant brain injury. Neurosurgical consultation is not necessary unless signs and symptoms develop that indicate the injury is serious.

125. The answer is A. *(Hoekelman, p 1446.)* The use of hexachlorophene, an effective antistaphylococcal antiseptic, should be limited because of reports of neurotoxicity following topical application, particularly in the neonatal period. Signs of systemic toxicity include increasing irritability, decerebrate rigidity, and seizures. Rarely, topical application of providone-iodine, benzalkonium chloride, and bacitracin is associated with skin sensitization. Silver sulfadiazine may be hazardous in patients with glucose-6-phosphate dehydrogenase deficiency in that it can cause hemolysis, but neurotoxicity has not been reported.

126. The answer is C. *(Nellhaus, Pediatr Ann 3:22-23, 1974.)* The diagnosis of a brain tumor in a young child is difficult because the child often cannot communicate a specific complaint and because signs of increased intracranial pressure (e.g., vomiting) may be minimized by the capacity of cranial sutures to spread. The typical pattern of vomiting seen in adults is not often present in young children. Vomiting in children is generally attributable to other causes. Visual disturbances, such as blurred or double vision, may exist, but the child may not be able to communicate these. Seizures occur in hemispheric tumors but are usually focal, psychomotor, or generalized. In the young child, behavioral changes are relatively common in association with brain tumors, at least in part because more specific symptoms cannot be communicated and thus are expressed in this way.

127. The answer is D. *(Vaughan, ed 11. p 1789.)* Child abuse should be considered in an infant presenting with recent head trauma, but minor, unremembered trauma may also have occurred. A history of head trauma is not obtainable in many infants with subdural hematoma. Symptoms, which develop gradually, include fever, vomiting, lethargy, irritability, failure to thrive, and seizures. Focal neurological findings such as nystagmus, flaccid weakness of a leg, or hemiplegia are unusual. Retinal hemorrhages are present in approximately 50 percent of patients.

128. The answer is A. *(Hoekelman, pp 942-951.)* Although the electroencephalogram (EEG) for many patients with temporal lobe epilepsy will show focality in the temporal lobe, this is not a universal finding and a sleep EEG may be necessary to make a differential diagnosis. Occasionally a sphenoidal or nasopharyngeal recording is needed. Although computerized axial tomography (CAT scan) may be necessary to determine the origin of the seizure disorder, it is not the best course of initial action, as compared to obtaining a sleep EEG. Additional studies, such as plain skull x-rays, may be needed to determine the underlying cause of the seizures. In many instances a CAT scan precludes the necessity of pneumoencephalography and angiography. Obviously, no drug treatment should be started until a definitive diagnosis has been made.

129. The answer is A. *(Hoekelman, pp 937-939.)* Syndenham's chorea, commonly referred to as St. Vitus' dance, usually presents in the first decade of life and is more prevalent in girls than in boys. It is the most common chorea of childhood. Only about 25 percent of these children have a family history of rheumatic fever. It is generally thought to be a delayed complication of a streptococcal infection. However, there may not be an elevated antistreptolysin level, and since the reaction occurs long after the streptococcal infection is over, throat cultures will most likely be negative. Liver dysfunction is present in Wilson's disease but not in Syndenham's chorea. Characteristics of Gilles de la Tourette's syndrome include facial grimacing and tics, as well as coprolalia; this syndrome also occurs more often in boys than girls. Huntington's chorea is more common in adults, although it may present as Parkinson's disease in childhood, with chorea developing later on.

130. The answer is C. *(Hoekelman, pp 951-952.)* The diagnosis of narcolepsy is based on a clinical presentation that includes sudden irresistible attacks of sleep, cataplexy, sleep paralysis, and visual or auditory hallucinations upon falling asleep or awakening. The electroencephalogram (EEG) record of a nonsleeping narcoleptic is normal, but sleep EEG studies do show a rapid eye movement (REM) sleep state coincident with narcoleptic attacks. The differential diagnosis includes hypothyroidism, hypoglycemia, epilepsy, and depression. Narcolepsy rarely begins before the age of ten.

131. The answer is E. *(Drillien, p 259. Hoekelman, pp 962-963, 965.)* Cerebral palsy (CP) results from a heterogeneous group of disorders that are often unknown and imprecisely identified. Cerebral palsy is characterized by fixed motor disabilities that generally follow disorders affecting the immature or developing nervous system. It is clear that a variety of prenatal, postnatal, and perinatal factors may contribute to the development of CP, but the specific pathophysiology of CP is, as yet, ill-defined. Therefore, there is no specific brain lesion in the central nervous system common to all cases of CP. Only 25 percent of children with CP are born prematurely. CP can be related to anoxia at birth, but anoxia does not occur in many newborns who later develop CP.

132. The answer is A. *(Hoekelman, p 916.)* Vascular edema is the main cause of headaches, whether acute or chronic, in children. Headaches that follow a seizure are usually produced by vasodilatation and vascular edema, as are headaches that accompany classic migraine. Intracranial pain-sensitive structures that produce headache are located in the proximal portions of the major cerebral arteries and in the dura. Dilatation of these arteries or displacement of the dural structures, regardless of the cause, will produce headache. Tightening of the muscles of the head and neck may produce headache, due to irritation of the vascular and other intramuscular pain-sensitive structures. The distal branches of the cerebral arteries and the brain parenchyma itself contain no pain receptors; therefore spasm, or even occlusion, of those vessels, per se, is not associated with headache.

133. The answer is E. *(Hoekelman, pp 171-172, 583. Thomas, pp 75-79.)* About 10 percent of infants are irregular in biological functions, are predominantly negative in mood, have strong negative reactions to new situations, and are slow to adapt. This constellation of characteristics has been termed the "difficult child" temperament. Thus, because temperaments are inborn, they can strongly influence the interaction of the infant and its environment. For instance, the mother of a "difficult child" is quite likely to believe she is doing something wrong, and this will affect how she views and handles the child. Maternal experience appears to be unrelated to the child's temperament. The diagnosis of anaclitic depression, a state of profound apathy and unresponsiveness found in infants lacking a consistent mothering figure, is incompatible with the history and physical examination of the child in the question. Insults to the central nervous system during the perinatal period such as hypoxia or a subdural hematoma would be more likely to present with generalized, excessive findings on physical examination. A large caffeine intake during pregnancy has not been associated with long-lasting behavior changes.

134. The answer is D. *(Hoekelman, pp 41, 169, 587.)* Resistance to feeding in a healthy one-year-old infant is usually the result of a difference of opinion between the infant and parent. The infant wants to put his hands into the food, control the spoon, and experiment with dropping his cup. The parents, on the other hand, know that these actions will lead to a mess and therefore try to discourage them. At one year of age, the average infant's height-growth velocity, although decreasing, is still an impressive 14 cm (5.5 inch) per year; thus, it has not decreased significantly enough to account for a loss of appetite.

135. The answer is A. *(Hoekelman, pp 40-41. Schuberth, ed 8. pp 249-257.)* An extra-ordinary capacity for growth is one of the primary features of childhood. Careful, longi-tudinal monitoring of growth provides an early warning system for innumerable diseases. At the age of two years, the average child has attained about half of the expected adult height, 20 percent of the adult weight, and about 87 percent of the head circumference. Thirty per-cent of adult height is attained sometime in the first month of life. Forty percent of adult height is reached at about eight months of age, but this proportion of adult weight is not reached until the child is about eight years old. Ninety-seven percent of adult head circum-ference is generally reached at about 13 years of age.

136. The answer is D. *(Hoekelman, pp 543-546.)* A significant language delay is one of the few conditions that forecasts school problems reliably. Most authorities agree that a "significant delay" is 25 percent or more, which would be a delay of at least one and a half years. However, the child in the question has a language delay of only about 17 percent. If the rest of the school-readiness evaluation is truly unremarkable, including the hearing screen and a search for such conditions as serous otitis media that could produce language delay, there would be no cause for referral, and the child should start first grade as planned. However, the physician should be sure to follow-up carefully on the child's language develop-ment and progress in school.

137. The answer is C. *(Hoekelman, p 169.)* If toilet training is not going well, it is generally best to delay further attempts for a while. Children with irregular bowel habits are often more difficult to toilet train than are other children. Their irregularity is an innate trait and is unrelated to central nervous system maturation. Although these children are unlikely to change their bowel habits, they will usually begin to express interest in toilet training before too long. This interest often takes the form of asking to have their diapers changed or of starting to sit on the toilet in imitation of the others in the family. Attempts to force the issue by scolding and by frequently placing the child on the toilet are likely to create resis-tance in two-year-old children. The use of laxatives has no place in the toilet training of normal children.

138. The answer is E. *(Hoekelman, p 169.)* There does not appear to be any significant difference in school behavior between children raised in an authoritarian manner and chil-dren raised more permissively. The former, however, are more likely to be in frequent con-flict with their parents. In the absence of conclusive evidence of harm arising from the use of a particular childrearing style with a particular child, the physician should probably not interfere with the parents' preference for how they wish to raise their children.

139. The answer is D. *(Hoekelman, pp 539-541.)* The diagnosis of learning disability ap-plies to that child, who, despite having a normal mental age, does poorly in school because of deficiencies in information processing or in the ability to concentrate. A child who is both impulsive and easily distracted—the hallmarks of "hyperactivity"—is most suspect for having a primary learning disability. But before the diagnosis can be made, other causes of school failure must be ruled out. These include social, psychological, and economic factors, mental retardation, and temporal lobe epilepsy.

140. The answer is A. *(Hoekelman, pp 203-208. Schuberth, ed 8. pp 87-88.)* The Good-enough-Harris Drawing Test provides a means for quick screening of general development. The drawing shown would be normal for a four-year-old child. For a six-year-old child, however, the drawing suggests significant developmental delay and indicates the need for formal psychological evaluation. Such evaluation would: confirm the finding of a significant delay, differentiate a global intellectual deficit from a specific one, and provide information about a child's particular strengths and weaknesses. The school placement decision should be delayed until after the psychological evaluation. The test is not used as a screening test for psychiatric illness. The drawing does not show evidences of problems with fine-motor or gross-motor coordination and thus would not suggest the presence of cerebral palsy.

141. The answer is E. *(Gardner, pp 51, 67, 199.)* Freud theorized that the libido is expressed in different parts of the body at different ages. The **oral** stage corresponds to the first year of life; the **anal**, to the second and third years; and the **phallic** (or **Oedipal**), to the fourth through sixth years. **Latency**, a time when the libido is not localized, extends from the seventh year to puberty. The **genital** stage is the stage of adult sexuality. Piaget theorized that a child's way of understanding the world changes sequentially. In the **sensorimotor** stage, which lasts until eighteen months of age, he knows the world by acting upon it. In the **preoperational** stage, which lasts until seven years of age, he becomes skilled in using symbols. In the **concrete operations** stage, which lasts until eleven years of age, the child uses simple logic that is closely tied to the physical world. The final stage is the **formal operations** stage, in which the abstract reasoning of adults takes place. Erikson theorized that there is a series of central life crises that people face. **Trust versus mistrust** occurs during the first year of life; **autonomy versus shame and doubt**, during the second year; **initiative versus guilt**, during the third through fifth years; **industry versus inferiority**, from the sixth year through puberty; and **identity versus identity confusion**, during adolescence. An eight year old, then, would be in the stages of **latency, concrete operations,** and **industry versus inferiority**, according to these theories.

142. The answer is C. *(Hoekelman, p 955. Thompson, pp 25-26.)* The definition of mental retardation adopted by The American Association of Mental Deficiency states that mental retardation is manifested by an impairment in general intellectual functioning that exists concurrently with a deficit in the ability to adapt to the environment. The coincidence of these two disabilities constitutes the definition of mental retardation and distinguishes it from disorders that are either not developmental in nature or that involve deficits other than intellectual and adaptive impairment.

143. The answer is E. *(Johnston, pp 5-7.)* Developmental disorders can be caused by genetic or environmental factors. Genetic factors include chromosome defects and the absence of or increased number of certain genes. Environmental factors include infection, intrauterine insults, perinatal complications, and maternal deprivation. All of these factors are potential causes of developmental problems. There is, however, no identifiable single etiology for most developmental disorders. Very few can be specifically attributed to any one genetic or environmental factor. The most widely accepted hypothesis at the present time is that most developmental disorders are the result of an interaction of any number of genetic and environmental factors.

144. The answer is D. *(Hoekelman, pp 636-642. Leichtman, Med Clin North Am 59:1319-1328, 1975. McAnarney, Pediatrics 53:523-528, 1974.)* The concept of marginality—that is, the concept that individuals who develop a serious chronic illness do better psychologically than an individual with a mild or marginal illness—is applicable to adolescents. This concept has been related to patients with arthritis, epilepsy, hemophilia, and blindness, among others. It is also important to note that early or middle adolescence seems to be a critical time for the development of a chronic illness; thus, this age group often copes poorly with diabetes or epilepsy, as compared to those who developed these illnesses before puberty. Early adolescents are most concerned with how an illness will affect their physical appearance. Late adolescents are more concerned with the effects their illness will have on their careers and relationships with others than they are concerned with the specific sequelae of the disease. Finally, the stress caused by illness **does** lead patients in middle and late adolescence to use defense mechanisms which are used by children and early adolescents. These mechanisms can be positive (intellectualization) or negative (depression or acting out).

145. The answer is B (1, 3). *(Hoekelman, pp 947-949.)* Metabolic abnormalities may present as generalized seizures in a child. While such abnormalities are not a common cause of seizures, if they are present, specific therapy would be indicated. This child now exhibits a normal neurologic examination; therefore, no therapeutic measures for immediate seizure control, including the administration of glucose, are indicated. An electroencephalogram should be performed on any child with an unexplained seizure, but a lumbar puncture is not likely to be helpful unless infection is suspected. Skull films are also of questionable value, and the need for a CAT scan for every child who has had an unexplained seizure is a controversial issue.

146. The answer is A (1, 2, 3). *(Lauder, J Exceptional Child 45:432-436. Scherzer, Pediatrics, 47:426-428, 1971.)* The photograph accompanying the question shows an infant with a lumbar meningomyelocele. This infant can be expected to have significant paralysis of the lower extremities, loss of sensation, and bowel and bladder incontinence. A high proportion of these children develop hydrocephalus. While the average IQ of children with spina bifida is below that of their nonhandicapped siblings, most are not mentally retarded. Poor school performance is often related to their perceptual and cognitive disabilities.

147. The answer is E (all). *(Hoekelman, pp 946-947.)* Although adrenocorticotropic hormone (ACTH) or steroids are used in the treatment of myoclonic epilepsy in infancy, there is no satisfactory treatment available. Phenobarbital, phenytoin, and primidone often are used along with ACTH or steroids. ACTH and steroids are generally used for periods of six to eight weeks. However, these children who show a clearing of the electroencephalogram and a subsidence of seizures after the six to eight weeks of ACTH or steroid treatment (five to ten percent) have a good prognosis. Both diazepam and clonazepam appear to help this condition.

148. The answer is E (all). *(Vaughan, ed 11. pp 558, 560, 1952, 1956.)* All of the conditions listed may present with a cherry-red spot on the macula. In addition, all are associated with a developmental delay. The conditions are distinguishable from each other by biochemical tests of the blood serum. However, it is important to remember the importance of the fundoscopic examination in the evaluation of a child with a developmental lag. A cherry-red spot on the macula may also be seen in Niemann-Pick disease.

149. The answer is C (2, 4). *(Hoekelman, p 601.) Pavor nocturnus,* or night terrors, is a dyssomnia that occurs about 90 to 100 minutes after the child has fallen asleep. The child sits up suddenly and screams and is inconsolable for a while thereafter. It is most common in children three to eight years old, and it is not associated with psychopathology. Unlike nightmares, it is not well remembered in the morning. Quite often attacks of pavor nocturnus occur after a day that has been particularly stressful or fatiguing. An episode of terror that occurs in the latter third of the night is less likely to be pavor nocturnus and more likely to be a nightmare, especially if there is vivid recall of the incident in the morning.

150. The answer is E (all). *(Hoekelman, pp 948-949.)* All of the complications in the question are potential consequences of treatment for status epilepticus. In all probability more deaths are related to the excessive use of medication than to the disease itself. After airway suction and positioning the patient to prevent aspiration of saliva and vomitus are accomplished, the most important step in treating status epilepticus is to establish an intravenous line. This line can be used to: monitor blood chemistries and drug levels, administer glucose and anticonvulsants, and maintain blood volume in the prevention and management of hypotension and shock. Sponging and antipyretic drugs should be used to counteract hyperpyrexia, which may occur even in the absence of an underlying febrile illness. Respiratory arrest and hypotension may occur following the administration of diazepam if phenobarbital or paraldehyde have been given previously. The major cause of death in status epilepticus is anticonvulsant overdosage.

151. The answer is E (all). *(Hoekelman, pp 642-644.)* An increase in height of a half inch per generation from 1840-1950 has been noted in European and American youth. During the same time, there has been a decrease in the age of menarche of 3 to 4 months every 10 to 20 years. There are many factors responsible for this trend in secular pubertal acceleration. Some factors involve improved nutrition, better living conditions, better health habits, and less exposure to serious childhood illnesses. The relative importance of each of these factors in the overall trend is unclear. It is interesting, however, that this trend seems to have stopped in the industrialized countries, but continues in the underdeveloped parts of the world.

152. The answer is C (2, 4). *(Hoekelman, pp 636-640. Daniel, Med Clin North Am 59: 1281-1282, 1975.)* Early adolescence is the psychosocial stage which initiates the whole process of adolescence—that is, the changes converting the child into the adult. The early adolescent stage (usually between 12 and 15 years of age) is the time of rapid pubertal changes and thus the time when most teenagers are concerned with their constantly changing physical appearance. It is not until middle adolescence (approximately between 15 and 17 years of age) that teenagers are at the peak of their emancipation struggles with parents and other authority figures. By this time, their pubertal changes are mostly complete and other issues predominate. Middle adolescence is the time of major arguments with parents, establishment of major sexuality concepts, major drug experimentation, and greatest susceptibility to peer pressures.

153. The answer is C (2, 4). *(Hoekelman, pp 641-642. Hofmann, pp 16-17.)* Late adolescence is the final stage of the adolescent process; it usually occurs between the ages of 17 and 20 years. Prior concerns of early and midadolescence should be resolved by this time, when teenagers turn their attention to two basic tasks: (1) the establishment of an adult sexual role, whether heterosexual, homosexual, or other; and (2) the establishment of an adult vocational role. Sometimes prolonged education or technical training prevents completion of this latter goal until early adulthood. Both of these processes are rooted in successful emancipation from parents, in which the parents and offspring live independently but maintain an adult-to-adult (versus an adult-to-child) relationship. Cognitive thinking matures during early to middle adolescence, while peer group influence is usually greatest during middle adolescence.

154. The answer is A (1, 2, 3). *(Hoekelman, pp 589-590. Thomas, pp 75-80.)* The amount of time an infant spends crying each day reaches a peak at about six weeks of age and then begins to decrease. Infants vary widely in the amount of time they spend crying and in the ease with which they are consoled. Those with the "difficult" temperament are especially prone to excessive crying. This behavior often is aggravated when parents repeatedly attempt to calm the infants, which results in overstimulation. Maternal depression and anxiety in the face of excessive crying are usually an effect rather than a cause of the crying.

155. The answer is B (1, 3). *(Hoekelman, p 957.)* The average 18-month-old child will walk up steps and point to his eyes and nose on request. Most children will not build towers of four to eight cubes until two years of age. Copying a circle is a task not generally mastered until three years of age. Normal motor development is not necessarily an indication of normal intellectual development.

156. The answer is B (1, 3). *(Hoekelman, p 170.)* A bedtime ritual, such as reading a story, and sitting in view of the child outside her room and insisting that she stay in bed, are both effective measures for dealing with the resistance to sleep so common in two-year-old children. The problem seems to have roots both in the increasing independence of children at this age and in a residual separation anxiety. The technique of having one parent sit by a partially open door next to the child's room while engaged in a quiet activity such as reading or knitting is frequently an effective way to handle this problem. The presence of the parent helps to overcome residual separation anxiety, and the parent is present to let the child know that he or she will not be allowed to keep getting up after being put to bed. Lying down with the child is likely to prolong the problem, as is letting the child stay up until exhausted.

157-161. The answers are: 157-E, 158-A, 159-C, 160-A, 161-D. *(Hoekelman, pp 931-933. Ertel, Pediatr Annals 7:90-91, 1978. Isselbacher, ed 9. p 1954.)* The infratentorial tumors, of which medulloblastomas are one, comprise about 50 to 70 percent of brain tumors in children. Medulloblastomas occur most frequently in three- to six-year-old boys (the male to female ratio is 2:1). Usually located near the anterior cerebellar midline, these tumors grow rapidly, and their symptoms are severe. Surgery followed by radiation therapy is the accepted treatment, although radiation does not usually halt recurrence.

The cerebellar astrocytoma is the most common infratentorial tumor. It is a slow-growing cystic tumor that is rarely malignant and is found most commonly in children five to eight years of age. The tumor usually exists in the wall of the cyst; surgical removal is usually effective.

Although supratentorial tumors, of which craniopharyngiomas are one, are more common in adults, they comprise 30 to 40 percent of brain tumors in children. Craniopharyngiomas are benign, but may produce hemianopsia, retarded growth, endocrine dysfunction, or diabetes insipidus. They can also produce hydrocephalus through obstruction of the third ventricle. These tumors are most common in five and six-year-old children, and boys and girls are affected equally. Surgery is often successful; however, treatment outcome with chemotherapy or radiation is controversial.

Supratentorial gliomas account for 10 to 15 percent of all childhood intracranial tumors. Approximately 50 percent of all cases are malignant. Surgery followed by radiation is the treatment of choice, although the prognosis is poor. Males are affected more frequently than females.

Meningiomas are rarely found in children; they are most common in older women. These are benign tumors located on the brain surface or next to the dura. Although they compress or indent brain tissue, these tumors do not invade it.

162-165. The answers are: 162-C, 163-D, 164-A, 165-A. *(Vaughan, ed 11. pp 123, 1754-1756.)* The term megalencephaly describes excessive brain growth. It is often without obvious cause but may be associated with storage diseases. Megalencephaly is most often caused by an overgrowth of glial cells rather than neurons. Subdural hematoma is the most common serious central nervous system (CNS) injury from child abuse and usually results from vigorous shaking of the child. Communicating hydrocephalus occurs when there is interference with the absorption of cerebrospinal fluid (CSF). The Arnold-Chiari malformation involves the downward displacement of the medulla and cerebellum; the result is obstruction of the subarachnoid space surrounding these structures. A similar obstruction may follow CNS infections such as bacterial meningitis. Obstructive hydrocephalus results from obstruction within the ventricular system; aqueductal stenosis or midline brain tumors can also cause this condition. In aqueductal stenosis the aqueduct of Sylvius is narrowed by blind-ended narrow channels.

166-168. The answers are: 166-C, 167-A, 168-E. *(Hoekelman, pp 168-170.)* Crying, sneezing, and straining with bowel movements are all very common characteristics of the young infant. Crying time usually peaks at age 6 weeks and then gradually declines to a lower level at age 2.5 to 3 months when most infants start to sleep through the night. Stubbornness, temper tantrums, flat feet, and bow legs are typical characteristics of the 18-month-old infant. Talking back, repeated use of words such as "poop," and genital play are common behavior patterns in the four year old.

169-172. The answers are: 169-E, 170-B, 171-A, 172-C. *(Arnold, pp 178, 262.)* The school-age child, no matter how disabled, is the responsibility of the local school district for the provision of education, as guaranteed by Public Law 94-142. Each district must maintain a committee for children with special needs, and each child deemed by the committee as one who needs special education must have a written, individualized educational plan designed by the teacher and approved by the parents. If the school district cannot provide for those special needs, it must pay for a suitable program elsewhere.

Residential care for any substantially disabled person is provided either directly or indirectly by state Departments of Mental Retardation (or Developmental Disabilities). In some states, arrangements for residential care are made with the collaboration of the Department of Social Services (DSS), but these arrangements are not their responsibility.

The family in need of help in managing their disabled child at home in a manner beneficial to the child's general welfare is, however, the responsibility of DSS. Any child that shows evidence of either abuse or neglect must be reported by the physician to the DSS's Child Protective Services. This report must be made whether or not the actual neglect was willful. The Protective Services will investigate the case and arrange to provide the identified needs of the family. The identity of the referrer is kept confidential by law.

Low income families in which there is a disabled child are entitled to Supplemental Security Income (SSI) regulated by the state Crippled Children's or Disabled Children's Program.

Hematology and Oncology

DIRECTIONS: Each question below contains five suggested answers. Choose the **one best** response to each question.

173. A peak reticulocyte count should occur how many days after the initiation of iron therapy?

(A) 1-3 days
(B) 4-7 days
✓(C) 7-10 days
(D) 11-14 days
(E) 15-18 days

174. A cryoprecipitate infusion for a spontaneous bleed into the joint of a hemophiliac patient should produce a desired factor VIII serum level of

✓(A) 10-20 percent
(B) 20-30 percent
(C) 30-40 percent
(D) 50-60 percent
(E) 90-100 percent *intra/cranial   bleed/surgery)*

175. A five-year-old white male presents to the emergency room with a recent onset of pallor, easy bruising, and purpura. Physical examination reveals a palpable spleen 3-4 cm below the left costal margin. Hematology studies reveal the following: hemoglobin, 6.6 g/100 ml; hematocrit, 17%; WBC, 1500/mm^3; platelet count, 50,000/mm^3; and reticulocyte count, 0.3%. Bone marrow aspiration is normal. The most likely diagnosis is

(A) leukemia
✓(B) lymphoma
(C) Blackfan-Diamond syndrome *(red cell aplasia)*
(D) Gaucher's disease
(E) Fanconi's anemia — *pancytopenia Aplac. Late No splenomegaly*

176. Characteristics of congenital aplastic anemia (Fanconi's anemia) include all of the following EXCEPT

(A) autosomal dominant transmission
✓(B) presentation of the anemia in infancy
(C) an increased likelihood of leukemia
(D) skeletal malformation *(radial)*
(E) hypogenitalism

177. All of the following tests can be expected to be useful in diagnosing a hemolytic anemia EXCEPT

✓(A) determination of serum folic acid levels
(B) determination of serum haptoglobin levels
(C) determination of serum LDH levels
(D) a peripheral blood smear
(E) a urinalysis

178. Sickle cell anemia screening programs are LEAST effective when applied to

(A) infants of mothers who are known carriers
(B) siblings of affected children
(C) schoolchildren who understand the implications of the carrier state
✓(D) all newborn infants *HbF*
(E) students in health education classes

179. Which of the following values is abnormal for the given age?

(A) Hemoglobin of 8.5 g/100 ml in a 5-week-old premature infant
(B) Hemoglobin of 13.0 g/100 ml in a 1-year-old boy
✓(C) Hemoglobin of 14.5 g/100 ml in a 2-year-old girl
(D) Hemoglobin of 14.5 g/100 ml in an 8-year-old girl
(E) Hemoglobin of 14.5 g/100 ml in a 16-year-old girl

180. In evaluating a patient with a bleeding disorder, all of the following studies are helpful when one is dealing with a platelet defect EXCEPT

(A) bleeding time ↑
✓(B) prothrombin time
(C) clot retraction test
(D) Rumpel-Leede test
(E) peripheral smear examination

181. An 18-month-old girl is brought in to the clinic for a routine visit. A hematocrit and lead screening test are obtained by the capillary method; the results are:

	Patient	Normal Value (for age)
Hct	37%	35%
Lead	40 µg/100 ml	30 µg/100 ml
Free erythrocyte proto-porphyrin (FEP)	150 µg/100 ml	60 µg/100 ml

The tests are repeated on blood obtained by venipuncture, confirming the above results. An abdominal x-ray (shown below) is obtained. The next step in the management of this child is to

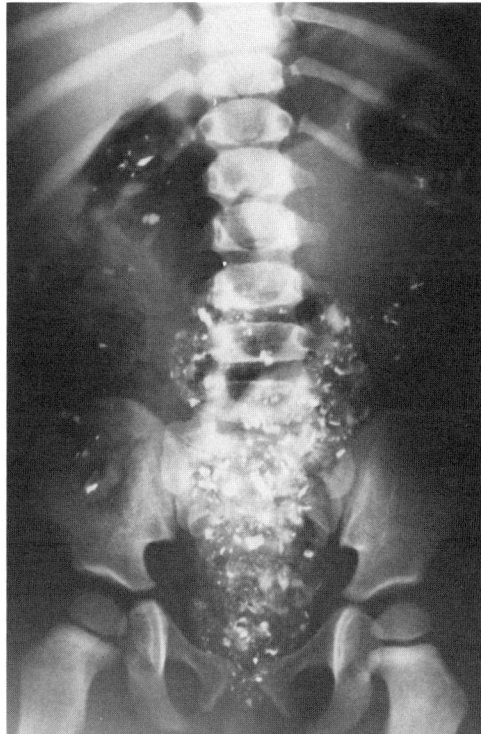

(A) repeat the blood tests immediately
(B) repeat the blood tests in three months
(C) start penicillamine therapy to increase renal excretion of lead
(D) administer psychologic testing for evidence of central nervous system effects
(E) none of the above

dimercaprol.

---

182. The most sensitive and accurate laboratory determination in the diagnosis of iron-deficiency anemia and in monitoring the treatment of the disease is

(A) the serum iron level
(B) the serum ferritin level
(C) the hemoglobin level
(D) the total iron-binding capacity
(E) hemoglobin electrophoresis

183. Children with unilateral Wilms' tumor differ from children who have bilateral Wilms' tumor in all of the following respects EXCEPT that

T (A) they are older at the time of discovery
T (B) their mothers, on average, are younger
F (C) they have a higher incidence of associated anomalies
T (D) their pattern of inheritance is less constant
T (E) they are far more numerous

Aniridia *horse shoe kidneys*
Hemihypertrophy

184. The risk of infection increases dramatically in the presence of which of the following white blood cell (WBC) or differential counts?

(A) The absolute polymorphonuclear (PMN) count is 700/mm^3

√(B) The band forms and PMNs make up 15 percent of 3000 WBC/mm^3 (PMN < 500 + infectia)

(C) The total WBC is 2500 WBC/mm^3

(D) The total WBC is 50,000 WBC/mm^3

(E) Lymphocytes make up 12 percent of 2500 WBC/mm^3

185. A 14-month-old child is being treated for iron-deficiency anemia without success. Upon repetition of the laboratory tests, it is discovered that the patient continues to have a hypochromic, microcytic anemia. The test results are: RBC = 8.8 x 10^6/mm^3; MCV = 77 cu μm; FEP = 70 mg/100 ml; blood lead level = 31 mg/100 ml; and MCV/RBC = 8.7. The patient probably has

(A) iron deficiency anemia

√(B) thalassemia

(C) lead poisoning

(D) folate deficiency

(E) none of the above

186. All of the following statements about Burkitt's lymphoma are true EXCEPT that it is

(A) an extranodal tumor

(B) a multicentric tumor

√(C) a slow growing tumor

(D) a radiosensitive tumor

(E) associated with Epstein-Barr virus antibodies

187. A lymph node biopsy will disclose the maximum amount of information as a consequence of all the following procedures EXCEPT

(A) biopsing the largest node

(B) removing the node intact

(C) making an imprint of the node

(D) biopsing an upper cervical node

(E) fixing the node in 10% formaldehyde

188. Childhood carcinoma of the thyroid usually presents

(A) as a solitary nodule

√(B) with euthyroidism

(C) in association with thyroiditis

(D) with pulmonary metastases

(E) following head or neck irradiation in infancy

Papillary - Good prognosis.

189. A six-year-old child being treated for acute lymphocytic leukemia is admitted to the hospital with a fever. Temperature is 39.2°C (102.5°F). Physical examination reveals no abnormalities beyond malnutrition and drug induced alopecia. There has been no travel or exposure to febrile disease. Test results are as follows: WBC = 900: 56% segmented forms, 10% band forms, 20% monocytes, 10% lymphocytes, 4% eosinophils; chest x-ray, normal. After doing blood cultures, which of the following antibiotics should be initiated for suspected bacterial infection?

(A) Ampicillin plus kanamycin

(B) Cephaloridine plus kanamycin

(C) Trimethoprim-sulfamethoxazole

√(D) Penicillinase-resistant penicillin plus gentamicin

(E) Erythromycin plus gentamicin

190. Treatment of an eosinophilic granuloma of a facial bone would include which of the following?

(A) Local excision

(B) Radiation therapy

(C) Chemotherapy

(D) Local excision and radiation therapy

(E) Local excision and chemotherapy

191. A patient with Hodgkin's disease has just completed his initial staging workup. His presenting complaints included fatigue, fever, and night sweats, but no weight loss. Hodgkin's disease was found in biopsies of the supraclavicular nodes, para-aortic nodes, and spleen. His stage (by the Ann Arbor Method), therefore, is

(A) II

(B) II$_E$B

(C) IIIA

√(D) III$_E$B

(E) IVB

192. A six-year-old, 22 kg (48 lb, 8 oz) boy with acute lymphocytic leukemia presents to the emergency room immediately following an acute bleeding episode. Laboratory values include hemoglobin, 4.0 g/100 ml; hematocrit, 17%; and platelet count, 12,000/mm^3. The decision is made to transfuse the patient with packed red blood cells and platelets to increase his hemoglobin to 10 g/100 ml and his platelets by 60,000-90,000/mm^3. In order to achieve these levels, the child should receive

(A) 360 ml packed red blood cells and 4.4 units platelets

(B) 450 ml packed red blood cells and 4.4 units platelets

(C) 450 ml packed red blood cells and 2.2 units platelets

(D) 600 ml packed red blood cells and 2.2 units platelets

(E) 750 ml packed red blood cells and 6.6 units platelets

DIRECTIONS: Each question below contains four suggested answers of which **one** or **more** is correct. Choose the answer

A	if	**1, 2, and 3**	are correct
B	if	**1 and 3**	are correct
C	if	**2 and 4**	are correct
D	if	**4**	is correct
E	if	**1, 2, 3, and 4**	are correct

193. Which of the following substances can cause hemolysis in a person with glucose-6-phosphate dehydrogenase deficiency?

(1) Acetylsalicylic acid
(2) Tetracycline
(3) Nitrofurantoin
(4) Acetaminophen

194. Sideroblastic anemias are distinguished by the presence of

(1) hypochromia
(2) hyperferremia
(3) microcytosis
(4) normal iron stores

195. An eight-year-old child presents with findings of anemia and thrombocytopenia. The most likely diagnosis is

(1) idiopathic thrombocytopenic purpura
(2) disseminated intravascular coagulation
(3) lead poisoning
(4) bone marrow depression secondary to chloramphenicol toxicity

196. Lack of response in anemic individuals to oral iron therapy may occur in which of the following situations?

(1) Iron given with milk
(2) Presence of thalassemia
(3) Presence of plumbism
(4) Presence of sickle cell trait

197. Eosinophilia is found in association with which of the following disorders?

(1) Hodgkin's disease
(2) Periarteritis nodosa
(3) Eczema
(4) *Trichuris trichiura* infestation

198. A low erythrocyte sedimentation rate is associated with

(1) sickle cell disease
(2) anorexia nervosa
(3) congestive heart failure
(4) hereditary spherocytosis

199. A hemoglobin electrophoresis report showing approximately 70% hemoglobin S in a two-year-old black male with clinically moderate sickle cell disease implies that he may have which of the following sickle syndromes?

(1) SS
(2) S-high F
(3) SC
(4) S-thalassemia

200. Possible etiologies for the infectious mononucleosis syndrome include

(1) Epstein-Barr virus
(2) herpes simplex virus
(3) cytomegalovirus
(4) sulfones

201. Chemotherapeutic agents useful in the treatment of neuroblastoma in children include

(1) vincristine sulfate
(2) doxorubicin
(3) cyclophosphamide
(4) cytosine arabinoside

202. Correct statements about ovarian masses in young girls include which of the following?

(1) They are usually malignant teratomas
(2) They are easily felt on rectal exam
(3) They are usually located on the left side
(4) They are commonly associated with abdominal pain

203. The patient whose picture is shown below has the accompanying lateral skull x-ray. The findings are consistent with

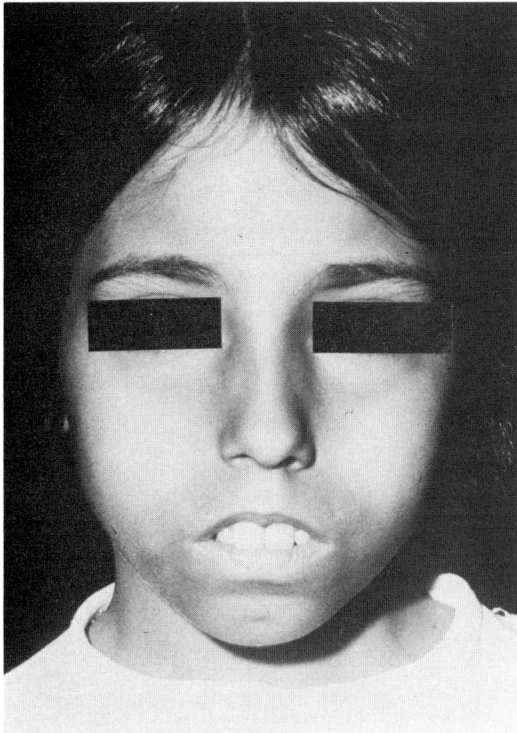

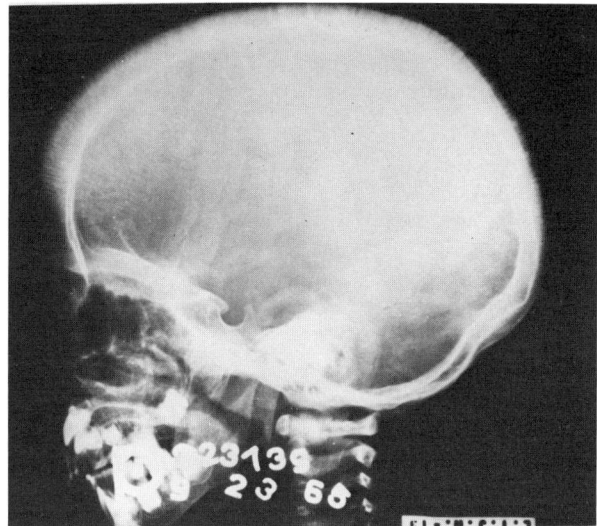

Used with permission of McGraw-Hill Book Company, from *Principles of Pediatrics: Health Care of the Young* (p 1002), by Hoekelman RA et al, ©1978 McGraw-Hill Inc.

(1) hereditary spherocytosis
(2) hereditary stomatocytosis
(3) thalassemia major
(4) thalassemia minor

204. In acute lymphocytic leukemia, an unfavorable prognosis is associated with

(1) an age of less than two or more than ten years
(2) an initial white blood cell count less than 20,000/mm³
(3) the presence of an anterior mediastinal mass
(4) the Caucasian race

DIRECTIONS: The groups of questions below consist of lettered choices followed by several numbered items. For each numbered item select the **one** lettered choice with which it is **most** closely associated. Each lettered choice may be used once, more than once, or not at all.

Questions 205-208

For each statement below, select the peripheral blood smear with which it is most likely to be associated.

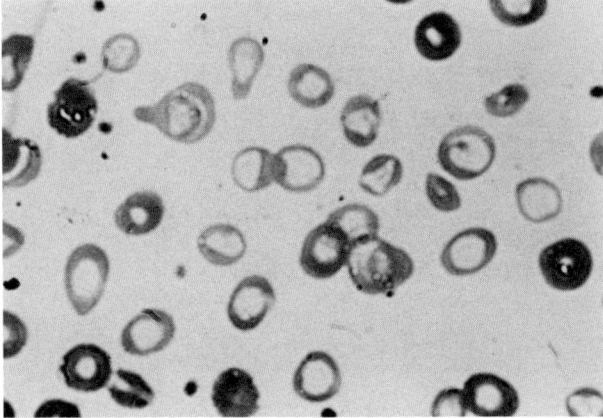

A

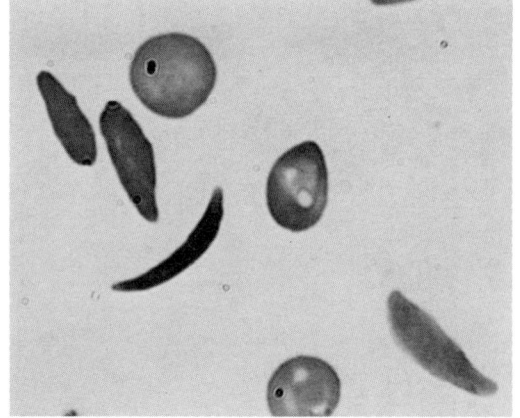

B

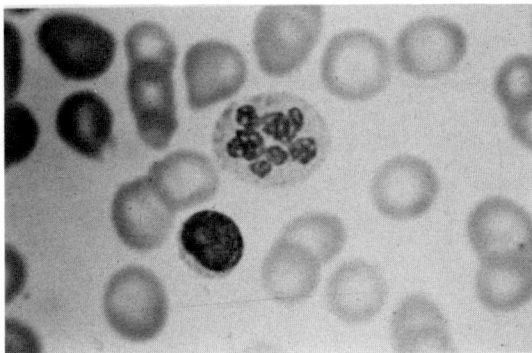

C

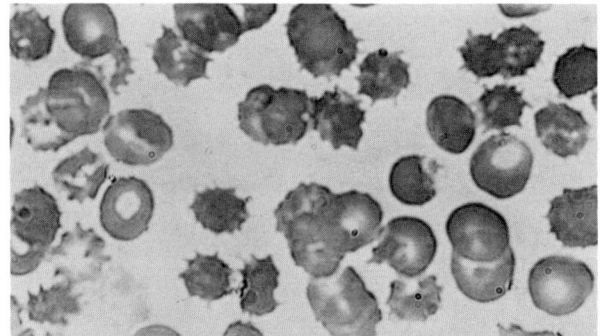

D

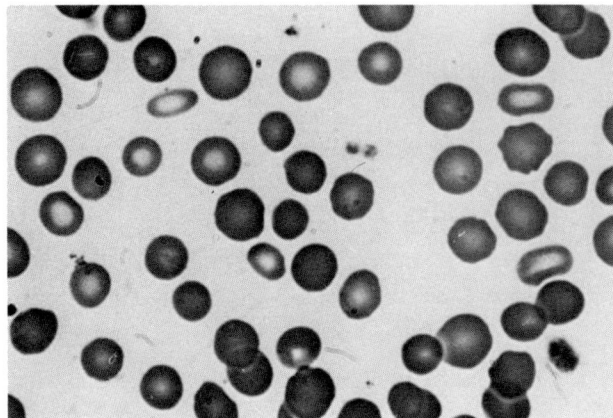

E

Used with permission of McGraw-Hill Book Company, from *Principles of Pediatrics: Health Care of the Young* (pp 989, 1004, 1006, 1016), by Hoekelman RA et al, © 1978 McGraw-Hill Inc.

205. The patient with this smear may derive great benefit from a splenectomy

206. The patient with this smear may have associated neurologic, ophthalmic, and/or gastrointestinal diseases

207. The patient with this smear has been receiving methotrexate therapy

208. The patient with this smear suffered a resection of his terminal ileum as a result of a volvulus

Questions 209-212

In counseling families and patients with certain diseases or conditions, information regarding an increased risk of malignancy associated with the disease should be presented. For each disease below, select the malignancy with which it is most likely to be associated.

(A) Glioma
(B) Leukemia
(C) Retinoblastoma
(D) Rhabdomyosarcoma
(E) Gonadoblastoma

A 209. von Recklinghausen's disease

B 210. Down's syndrome

211. 13q syndrome

E 212. Turner's syndrome

Hematology and Oncology

Answers

173. The answer is C. *(Hoekelman, pp 990-991.)* Children throughout the world suffer from iron-deficiency anemia. In most cases, the response to oral iron therapy is quick and dramatic. The peak reticulocyte response usually will occur between seven and ten days, although the rise in reticulocyte count occasionally begins as early as five days after the onset of therapy. The associated hemoglobin rise depends upon the initial hemoglobin level, but averages around 0.25 to 0.40 g/100 ml per day. This rise in hemoglobin represents a one percent per day rise in hematocrit.

174. The answer is A. *(Hoekelman, pp 1023-1027.)* The goal of therapy for treating bleeding occurrences in hemophiliac patients is to control the bleeding by providing the missing coagulation factor. All therapy must be individualized, depending on the site and severity of the bleeding as well as the particular patient's usual response to treatment. In general, however, a spontaneous bleed into a joint or muscle can be treated by giving 10-15 units of factor VIII per kilogram of body weight for two days. This therapy should produce a desired factor VIII level of 5-20 percent immediately following the infusion. For more severe hematomas or multiple dental extractions, a level of 20-40 percent is desired. In the case of major surgery or serious accidents, one should try to achieve a factor VIII level of 100-150 percent.

175. The answer is B. *(Hoekelman, pp 981-982.)* The child presented in the question exhibits pancytopenia, splenomegaly, and a normal bone marrow aspiration. The differential diagnosis of this combination of findings includes other lymphomas or hypersplenism (due to such etiologies as a connective tissue disorder, portal hypertension, or primary splenic disease). Had the bone marrow aspiration been abnormal, a diagnosis of leukemia or one of the storage diseases, such as Gaucher's or Niemann-Pick, would be plausible. Aplastic anemia (congenital or acquired) or leukemia are considerations if there is pancytopenia without splenomegaly.

176. The answer is B. *(Hoekelman, p 995.)* Fanconi's anemia is a congenital aplastic anemia that presents in association with multiple congenital anomalies. It is transmitted as an autosomal dominant trait, though multiple chromosomal abnormalities have been found in these patients. The anemia usually presents between the ages of 4 and 12 years, and bone marrow biopsy will show generalized hypocellularity with fatty replacement. Associated anomalies include short stature, skeletal defects, hyperreflexia, hypogenitalism, microcephaly, microphthalmia, renal abnormalities, and abnormal skin pigmentation. Frequently, the diagnosis can be made, before the anemia presents, on the basis of the congenital anomalies or the family history.

177. The answer is A. *(Hoekelman, pp 996-1003.)* Many inherent red blood cell structural defects (e.g., hemoglobin, red blood cell enzymes, red blood cell membrane defects) may shorten the life span of such cells (the normal life span of a red blood cell is 120 days.) In addition, extra-corpuscular processes may cause premature or accelerated red blood cell destruction. When diagnosing a hemolytic anemia, the approach should include evaluating the clinical features, detecting the hemolytic process, and determining the exact etiology. The serum haptoglobin will decrease in hemolytic anemias as it becomes saturated with hemoglobin dimers and the complex is cleared by the reticuloendothelial system. The serum lactic dehydrogenase level will rise with hemolysis. A peripheral blood smear will demonstrate changes in red blood cell morphology, such as spherocytes or red blood cell fragments, polychromasia, and nucleated red blood cells, all of which are indicative of a hemolytic process. The urinalysis often will show hemoglobinuria, hemosiderinuria, and urobilinogenuria. Although the serum folic acid level may decrease in hemolytic anemias, it is not helpful in the differential diagnosis.

178. The answer is D. *(Hoekelman, p 187.)* In order to determine the best strategy for a sickle cell screening test, it is necessary to decide what information is needed and the population to which it is most likely to apply. Inasmuch as the major implication of the sickle cell carrier state is transmission to an offspring, it seems that individuals who are not at known risk for the disease state should be screened for carrier status in late childhood or early adolescence, at an age when the results of the screening test can be understood by those being screened. Sickle cell screening is not a procedure that should be applied indiscriminately to large populations.

179. The answer is C. *(Dallman, J Pediatr 94:26-31, 1979.)* As a child grows and develops, the normal blood values change. Hemoglobin levels normally begin to decrease in the first few weeks of life, reaching a nadir at approximately two to five months of age; they then slowly rise. Premature infants will reach their nadirs sooner than full term infants. Most children will reach adult normal values by adolescence, with girls having slightly higher hemoglobins than boys until approximately ages 10 to 12. All of the values given in the question are age-appropriate except for the hemoglobin level of 14.5 g/100 ml in a two-year-old girl; normally it should be between 11 and 14.0 g/100 ml.

180. The answer is B. *(Hoekelman, p 1033.)* The hemostatic process depends on the interaction of the vascular wall and its response to injury, platelet activity, and the blood coagulation factors. Platelet disorders may be a result of either a qualitative or a quantitative defect, or both. The bleeding time will be prolonged when the platelet count is less than 50,000/mm³ or when there is abnormal platelet adhesion or aggregation. Examination of the peripheral smear will provide evidence of platelet numbers and morphology. Both quantitative and qualitative platelet disorders will produce a positive capillary fragility (Rumpel-Leede) test, whereas defective clot retraction is more often an indication of thrombocytopenia. The prothrombin time test measures the activity of the extrinsic secondary hemostatic mechanism and is unaffected by platelet numbers or activity.

181. The answer is E. *(Hoekelman, pp 192-193, 1832-1834.)* An 18-month-old child with an elevated lead level (40 µg/100 ml) and a markedly elevated free erythrocyte protoporphyrin (FEP) level (150 µg/100 ml) should receive chelation therapy. Regardless of symptoms (inasmuch as overt signs of plumbism may be absent), treatment should be initiated to avert permanent damage of subtle central nervous system functions (for example, impairment of learning). Chelating agents used to treat plumbism include dimercaprol (BAL), calcium disodium edetate (CaNa₂EDTA), and D-penicillamine. Because chelation therapy is inherently dangerous, the choice of chelating agent should be made only after the patient has been fully evaluated and all factors are taken into account. Penicillamine therapy is contraindicated in this child because of the presence of radiopaque material (lead paint) on the abdominal x-rays. In addition to increasing the renal excretion of lead, penicillamine will enhance its intestinal absorption.

182. The answer is B. *(Nathan, p 117.)* The serum ferritin test has gained wide acceptance as an excellent reflection of the body's iron status. The measurement is reliable, accurate, and requires only a small volume of blood. Because serum ferritin levels parallel iron stores directly, the serum ferritin test will show change before the other tests included in the question. Serum iron and iron-binding capacity will not become abnormal until after the iron stores are depleted. Of the standard measures of iron deficiency, the hemoglobin level is the last to change as the disease develops or in response to therapy. Hemoglobin electrophoresis is of no use in monitoring treatment in iron-deficiency anemia.

183. The answer is C. *(Hoekelman, p 1048.)* Approximately five to ten percent of children with Wilms' tumor have simultaneously occurring bilateral tumors. Inasmuch as children with unilateral tumors rarely develop a metastasis in the opposite kidney, the best explanation for bilateral tumors is that they are a result of multiple primary tumors. Several features differentiate patients with unilateral Wilms' from patients with bilateral disease; unilateral Wilms' tumor patients generally present at an older age, have a lower mean maternal age, and exhibit a sporadic inheritance pattern. Bilateral aniridia, hemihypertrophy, horseshoe kidney, urinary tract duplications, and renal aplasia or hyperplasia occur more frequently (45 percent) in patients with bilateral Wilms' tumors.

184. The answer is B. *(Hoekelman, pp 1035-1038.)* Leukopenia is diagnosed when the total white blood cell count is below $4000/mm^3$, whereas neutropenia exists when the granulocyte count is less than $1500/mm^3$. The risk of infection increases when a patient has a severe neutropenia—an absolute granulocyte count of less than $500/mm^3$. Neutropenia sometimes occurs when the total white blood cell count is in the normal range (5000 to $10,000/mm^3$). Severe neutropenic patients may complain of fever, chills, irritability, and then may develop necrotic or ulcerative lesions. They are most susceptible to staphylococcal or gram-negative septicemia, usually from their own flora. Lymphocytosis or lymphopenia, unlike the neutropenias, are not associated with increased risk of infection.

185. The answer is B. *(Hoekelman, pp 979-992. McMillan, vol 1. pp 222-223.)* Anemia is one of the most common problems that bring children to the pediatrician. Hypochromic, microcytic anemias are the most common type, and iron deficiency the most frequent etiology. However, if a child does not respond to appropriate iron therapy, one must look for other causes. The next most common etiologies are thalassemia and plumbism. The free erythrocyte protoporphyrin (FEP) level may help, as it is increased in both iron deficiency and plumbism. The mean corpuscular volume (MCV) also can be quite useful in a simple situation. The Mentzer formula (MCV/red blood cell count) has been proposed as an aid in the diagnosis of thalassemia. Values greater than 13.5 strongly suggest that the patient has iron deficiency; values less than 11.5 indicate the presence of thalassemia. Used together, the FEP and MCV also may be of use. A MCV $>$ 77 and normal FEP levels are found in normal individuals; a MCV $<$ 77 and normal FEP levels usually are seen with thalassemia or iron deficiency, and an increased FEP level regardless of the MCV value occurs with iron deficiency anemia and plumbism. Folate deficiency is associated with a megaloblastic anemia.

186. The answer is C. *(Hoekelman, pp 1050-1051.)* Burkitt's lymphoma is an undifferentiated malignant lymphoma. First described in Africa, where an association was discovered with the Epstein-Barr virus, it is in fact found throughout the world. Burkitt's lymphoma occurs in the pelvic or abdominal viscera, retroperitoneal soft tissues, and the facial and long bones. A rapidly growing, multicentric, extranodal tumor, it often presents with concomitant bone marrow involvement. Though it is radiosensitive, its multiple sites preclude radiotherapy alone. It is usually treated with a combination of chemotherapy and radiotherapy.

187. The answer is D. *(Hoekelman, pp 976-977.)* Although enlarged lymph nodes are very common in children, it is sometimes necessary to biopsy a node for diagnosis. A decision to biopsy should be based on an affected child's history (e.g., duration of lymphadenopathy), on the location, size, and character of the lymphadenopathy (e.g., localized or generalized, consistency), on results of any prior investigations (e.g., cultures, blood tests, skin tests), and on the response to a therapeutic trial, if appropriate. If a decision for biopsy is made, in general more information can be obtained if one avoids the upper cervical or inguinal areas and removes the largest, though not necessarily the most accessible, node intact. Once removed, the node is imprinted, cultured for bacteria and fungi, and fixed in 10% formaldehyde for microscopic sectioning and examination.

188. The answer is B. *(Hoekelman, p 1275. Scott, Pediatrics 58:521-523, 1976.)* Thyroid carcinoma in children is equally likely to present as a solitary nodule or as a diffusely enlarged gland or hard lobe. Although thyroid nodules are rare in children, the incidence of carcinoma in a solitary nodule ranges from 17 to 57 percent; consequently, such nodules demand careful examination. Most children with thyroid carcinoma are euthyroid, and many have no history of local irradiation. Most present with cervical node metastases, although pulmonary metastases are present in a few. Association with thyroiditis is rare.

189. The answer is D. *(Hoekelman, p 1158.)* Because staphylococci and enteric gram-negative organisms are the most frequent bacterial causes of febrile episodes in neutrogenic patients, empiric therapy must be directed toward those microorganisms. Most authorities recommend a penicillinase-resistant penicillin and gentamicin in this situation. If *Pseudomonas* species are involved, carbenicillin should be added. Given in combined doses, carbenicillin and gentamicin have a synergistic activity against *P. aeruginosa.* However, inasmuch as this organism has a tendency to develop resistance to gentamicin, this agent should not be used alone for treatment of *P. aeruginosa* infections.

190. The answer is B. *(Hoekelman, p 1862. Geiser, Pediatr Ann 8:54-64, 1979.)* Eosinophilic granuloma, the most benign form of the histiocytosis X disease group, usually presents as a localized, irregular lytic, "punched-out" lesion. It occurs most frequently in older children, producing local pain and swelling. However, it is often asymptomatic. The lesions do not respond to chemotherapy. Low dose radiotherapy (less than 1,000 rads) is usually sufficient for cure. Because the lesions involve several layers of bone, curettage does not always result in complete excision; also, some lesions are difficult to reach. Lesions of the facial bones may encroach upon the teeth and obviate curettage. Radiotherapy, therefore, is the treatment of choice.

191. The answer is D. *(Nathan, p 740.)* In the Ann Arbor classification of the staging of Hodgkin's disease, stages I (involvement limited to a single lymph node region or extralymphatic organ) and II (two or more lymph node regions or localized involvement by direct extension of the same side of the diaphragm) are considered early stages. Stages III (lymph node involvement on both sides of the diaphragm with or without splenic or extralymphatic organ involvement) and IV (disseminated disease) carry a poorer prognosis. Extranodal involvement due to extension is also a less favorable prognostic sign and is designated by the subscript E. The subclassification "A" or "B" refers to the absence or presence, respectively, of the systemic symptoms of night sweats, unexplained fever greater than 38°C (100.4°F), or weight loss of more than 10 percent of body weight within six months of diagnosis. The patient described in the question has systemic symptoms, involvement of lymph nodes on both sides of the diaphragm, and splenic involvement, which place him in stage III$_E$B.

192. The answer is B. *(Hoekelman, p 284. McMillan, vol 1. pp 234-235.)* Despite the occasional risks of transfusions, it frequently is necessary to provide patients with specific blood components. When other therapy is unlikely to increase the intravascular red blood cell mass and a transfusion is necessary, packed red blood cells are preferred. Patients receiving a packed red blood cell transfusion should receive no more than 10% of their blood volume at a time, given at an even rate over a period of not less than three hours. The formula utilized to calculate the appropriate volume of packed red blood cells to be transfused (in ml) is:

$$\frac{\text{Wt (in kg) x Assumed Blood Volume (75 ml/kg) x Desired Rise in Hemoglobin (g/100 ml)}}{22 \text{ g/100 ml (assumed packed red blood cell hemoglobin content)}}$$

If whole blood is necessary, or if the packed red blood cell hemoglobin content is not 22 g/100 ml, appropriate corrections can be made. Platelet concentrates should be given if a patient is thrombocytopenic and bleeding actively, as in the child presented in the question. The goal is to raise the platelet count at least above 20,000/mm^3 in an attempt to control the bleeding. The amount of platelets to be transfused in order to provide a post-infusion rise in the platelet count of approximately 60,000 to 90,000/mm^3 is equal to 0.2 units/kg. Therefore, this patient should receive

$$\frac{\text{Weight (22 kg) x Assumed Blood Volume (75 ml/kg) x Desired Rise in Hemoglobin (6 g)}}{22 \text{ g/100 ml}}$$

= 450 ml of packed red blood cells; and 22 kg x 0.2 units of platelets/kg = 4.4 units.

193. The answer is B (1, 3). *(Hoekelman, pp 1008-1009.)* Glucose-6-phosphate dehydrogenase (G6PD) deficiency is an X-linked disorder that affects approximately 15 percent of black American males and approximately 100 million individuals worldwide. There are over 70 varients, not all of which produce a hemolytic anemia. The most common form (A+), found in black Americans, results in a hemolytic anemia when affected individuals are stressed by a variety of oxidant drugs or metabolites. The various drugs include analgesics and antipyretics (including acetylsalicylic acid), antimalarials, sulfonamides, nitrofurans, sulfones, naphthalene, and others. In contrast, the type of G6PD deficiency (B+) found in Caucasians (primarily of Mediterranean descent) and Orientals may produce a chronic congenital hemolytic anemia, as well as episodes of acute hemolysis precipitated by various oxidant agents.

194. The answer is A (1, 2, 3). *(Hoekelman, p 994.)* Sideroblastic anemias, both congenital and acquired, have many varied etiologies. The anemia is quite similar, clinically and hematologically, to thalassemia. Indeed, diagnostic differentiation between sideroblastic and other anemias, such as thalassemia, is frequently difficult. The problem appears to be one of decreased utilization of available iron due to inefficiency or inactivity of various enzymes. Consequently, these patients will have a hypochromic, microcytic anemia with increased serum iron and iron stores.

195. The answer is D (4). *(Hoekelman, pp 1029-1031, 1833.)* The diagnosis of idiopathic thrombocytopenic purpura requires the presence in the bone marrow of normal granulopoiesis and erythropoiesis as well as a normal number of megakaryocytes. Anemia is not a feature. Disseminated intravascular coagulation is associated with abnormalities of prothrombin and partial thromboplastin times, low fibrinogen levels, thrombocytopenia, and the presence of fibrin split products. Anemia occurs only if bleeding is profound. Lead poisoning may result in anemia secondary to its effect on heme biosynthesis; however, there is no thrombocytopenia. Bone marrow depression secondary to chloramphenicol toxicity results in pancytopenia with anemia and thrombocytopenia as prominent manifestations.

196. The answer is A (1, 2, 3). *(McMillan, vol 2. p 201.)* Among the many reasons for anemic patients not responding to oral iron therapy, failure to receive the iron prescribed is the most common. Other common reasons include: (1) improper administration of the iron (it will not be absorbed if given with milk or other substances with high phosphorus or phytate content); (2) improper dosage (a child should receive 2-3 mg of elemental iron per kilogram of body weight 2-3 times/day); (3) malabsorption of iron (up to 20 percent of children will not absorb iron adequately); (4) inability to utilize iron (if there is associated chronic disease such as a chronic infection, or if there is associated plumbism, the patient may not be able to utilize the iron absorbed); (5) continuing blood loss (for example, from continued gastrointestinal bleeding); and (6) improper diagnosis (plumbism and thalassemia minor frequently are difficult to differentiate from iron deficiency anemia). A patient with sickle cell trait will not be as anemic as an iron-deficient child and will respond to iron therapy, properly given, if associated iron deficiency anemia is present.

197. The answer is A (1, 2, 3). *(Foung, Pediatr Ann 8:47, 1979.)* The major causes of eosinophilia (> 700 eosinophils/mm^3) in children include atopic and allergic diseases, adrenal insufficiency, collagen vascular diseases, parasitic infections, neoplasms, and miscellaneous etiologies. Significantly high levels of eosinophilia are seen in Hodgkin's disease, eosinophilic leukemia, drug hypersensitivity, periarteritis nodosa, invasive helminthic infestations—including *Toxocara* and *Trichinella*—and the idiopathic hypereosinophilic syndrome. Eosinophilia is not usually seen with common helminthic infestations, such as whipworms (*Trichuris trichiura*) or pinworms (*Enterobius vermicularis*).

198. The answer is E (all). *(McMillan, vol 1. pp 226-227.)* The erythrocyte sedimentation rate (ESR) is influenced by many factors, such as serum levels of fibrinogen, α_1 globulin, IgM, cholesterol, as well as the surface characteristics of the erythrocyte and factors still unknown. Many diseases will cause an increased ESR, generally on the basis of inflammation. However, in other situations the ESR is lowered, including anorexia nervosa, sickle cell disease, congestive heart failure, nephrotic syndrome, corticosteroid or aspirin therapy, serum sickness, hypofibrinogenemia, and hematologic disorders such as pyruvate kinase deficiency and hereditary spherocytosis. In these instances, it may be difficult to screen for an associated inflammatory disease, and other indices of inflammation (for example, reactive protein) may have to be utilized.

199. The answer is C (2, 4). *(Nathan, p 421.)* Deoxygenation causes red blood cells with sickle hemoglobin to change shape and form "tractoids." Blood viscosity is altered and anemia and vaso-occlusive phenomena occur. The combination of hemoglobin S with other hematologic conditions (e.g., other hemoglobins, thalassemia) alters the ability of the red blood cells to sickle, thereby modifying the clinical severity of the manifestations of the sickle syndrome. Hemoglobin SS, with 85-95% hemoglobin S (and 5-15% hemoglobin F) on electrophoresis is the most severe syndrome. Hemoglobin S-thalassemia has 60-90% hemoglobin S and is moderately severe, whereas hemoglobin S-high F, with 70% hemoglobin S, is less so. Hemoglobin SC, with 50% hemoglobin S, also has a mild clinical course.

200. The answer is E (all). *(Hoekelman, pp 1038-1040.)* Children with infectious mononucleosis may have lymphadenopathy, fever, pharyngitis, and, occasionally, hepatosplenomegaly. An increase in the total number of atypical lymphocytes is the characteristic laboratory finding. There is evidence that all the agents listed in the question are possible etiologies for the infectious mononucleosis syndrome. Although no agent has been positively identified as the actual cause of the disease, the Epstein-Barr virus frequently is cited as the most likely. Affected individuals who previously lacked antibodies against the Epstein-Barr virus are particularly susceptible to infectious mononucleosis. The presence of these antibodies has been repeatedly demonstrated in persons who have the disease. Indeed, a demonstration of high antibody titers against the Epstein-Barr virus—when available—is one of the more conclusive findings in favor of a diagnosis of infectious mononucleosis.

201. The answer is A (1, 2, 3). *(Hoekelman, pp 1046-1047.)* Neuroblastoma is one of the more common childhood tumors. It arises from the sympathetic nervous system and may occur anywhere in the body. The most common sites are the adrenal glands and cervical, thoracic, and abdominal sympathetic ganglia. Age appears to be the most significant factor in prognosis: the younger the child, the better the prognosis. Cyclophosphamide, vincristine sulfate, and doxorubicin have been used successfully in the treatment of neuroblastoma. Doxorubicin has been shown to be particularly effective against disseminated disease. Cytosine arabinoside is used in the treatment of acute myelocytic leukemia. Children with cervical, thoracic, or pelvic primary tumors do better than do those with tumors located in the abdominal retroperitoneal area, primarily because of earlier detection; some unsubstantiated data show that tumors above the diaphragm are associated with increased survival.

202. The answer is C (2, 4). *(Hoekelman, pp 1330-1331.)* Abdominal pain is a common complaint of girls with ovarian tumors. The pain may result either from torsion of the ovary or from pressure exerted by the pelvic mass on the abdominal viscera. Ovarian tumors and cysts in children may be felt by abdominal examination because of the small size of the premenarchal pelvis and the high position of the ovaries. Smaller tumors are best felt by abdominorectal examination. Because ovarian tumors and cysts arise on the right side more often than the left, acute appendicitis and appendiceal abscess may have to be considered in the differential diagnosis. Teratomas are common ovarian tumors, but they are usually benign; malignant tumors are very rare.

203. The answer is A (1, 2, 3). *(Hoekelman, pp 996-1001.)* The skull x-ray shown in the question exhibits the broad cheekbones and "hair on end" appearance typical of a patient with a chronic hemolytic anemia. These changes, in association with the biconcave vertebrae, are a result of the increase in bone marrow space associated with an intensified erythropoiesis. Hereditary spherocytosis, hereditary stomatocytosis, and thalassemia major (Cooley's anemia) are all chronic, severe hemolytic anemias that may lead to these changes. Thalassemia minor usually produces only a mild anemia.

204. The answer is B (1, 3). *(Hoekelman, pp 1040-1046. Pinkel, Pediatr Clin North Am 23: 117-130, 1976.)* Approximately 75 percent of childhood leukemias are of the acute lymphyocytic type. As more and more children with acute lymphocytic leukemia undergo both initial and complete remissions, certain prognostic factors are being developed. The major unfavorable factors include (1) an initial white blood cell count greater than 25,000/mm^3, (2) an age incidence of less than two years or greater than ten years, (3) central nervous system involvement at the time of diagnosis, (4) presence of an anterior mediastinal mass, (5) presence of significant organomegaly at the time of diagnosis, and (6) being a member of the black race. When lymphocytes from patients with these factors are typed, in about 20 percent of cases the cells are found to be T cells (thymic cells). In addition, these T cell-containing patients more often than not are older males. Although they may undergo an initial remission, frequent relapses within a year are common. The remaining 80 percent of patients with acute lymphocytic leukemia have no detectable immunologic markers on their lymphocytes ("null cells"), have an equal sex ratio, are generally younger, and have a better prognosis than is the case with the T cell group.

205-208. The answers are: 205-E, 206-D, 207-C, 208-C. *(Hoekelman, pp 992-993, 1001-1003, 1005.)* Hereditary spherocytosis (figure E accompanying the question) is an autosomal dominant disorder of the red blood cell membrane. However, there is no familial incidence in 10 to 20 percent of cases. Although it may present in infancy, the disorder often is not detected until the patient is one to two years old; it frequently presents with splenomegaly. These children may suffer hypoplastic, reticulocytopenic crises (usually in association with infections), repeated episodes of hyperbilirubinemia, and sometimes gall-stones. Splenectomy is the treatment of choice for the prevention of these complications. Patients with β-lipoprotein deficiency (figure D) have an inherited deficiency of plasma β-lipoproteins, the major carriers of phospholipids. This plasma deficiency is reflected in the production of acanthocytes, the "thorny," "spiky" cells seen in figure D. The membranes of these cells contain increased sphingomyelin, decreased lecithin, and mildly increased or normal cholesterol and total phospholipids. Affected children may suffer from a mild hemolytic anemia, with mild reticulocytosis, and slightly increased autohemolysis. In addition, these children may have retinitis pigmentosa, mental retardation, and celiac syndrome.

Megaloblastic anemia (figure C) may develop from a number of causes; the most frequent is a deficiency of either vitamin B_{12}, folic acid, or both. The common pathway is the impairment of DNA synthesis, producing delayed nuclear maturation and cell division but not affecting cytoplasmic maturation. The result is large cells with immature nuclei. Vitamin B_{12} deficiency may result from inadequate intake, as with infantile nutritional B_{12} deficiency, or from decreased absorption, as with juvenile addisonian pernicious anemia and other forms of intestinal malabsorption. Inasmuch as vitamin B_{12} is absorbed almost exclusively in the terminal ileum, inflammatory bowel disease or surgical resection in this area will result in malabsorption. Similarly, folic acid deficiency may result from inadequate intake or malabsorption. In addition, deficiency may result from increased demand for folic acid, as seen with hemolytic anemias or leukemia, and when folic acid antagonists such as methotrexate or anticonvulsant drugs are given.

Figure A, from a child with iron deficiency, shows the typical hypochromic and microcytic red blood cells. Figure B shows the irreversibly sickled cells of a patient with sickle cell anemia.

209-212. The answers are: 209-A, 210-B, 211-C, 212-E. *(Hoekelman, pp 347-348, 352, 354. Vaughan, ed 11. pp 1949-1951.)* Patients with von Recklinghausen's disease (neurofibromatosis) have an increased incidence of neuroblastomas, gliomas, and other tumors. Leukemia is seen more frequently in ataxia telangiectasia, Fanconi's anemia, and Down's syndrome. The 13q syndrome patient is at increased risk for retinoblastoma, as are Turner's syndrome patients for gonadoblastoma. Although the rhabdomyosarcoma is the most common malignancy of soft tissues in children, it has not been associated with any genetic disease.

Endocrinology and Metabolism

DIRECTIONS: Each question below contains five suggested answers. Choose the **one best** response to each question.

213. A 12-year-old white boy is admitted to a hospital with a diagnosis of diabetic ketoacidosis. His serum electrolytes are as follows: Na, 130; K, 5; CO_2, 3; and Cl, 106. A serum glucose is 920 and the BUN, 25. What would you expect his serum osmolality to be?

(A) 260
(B) 285
(C) 300
√(D) 325
(E) 340

214. All of the following children would be expected to have tetany secondary to decreased ionized calcium concentration EXCEPT

(A) an 11-year-old child with hypoparathyroidism
(B) a 2-week-old child who has been on whole cow's milk since one day of age
√(C) a 4-year-old child with hypoalbuminemia secondary to cirrhosis
(D) a 13-year-old child who is hyperventilating
(E) a 6-year-old child with chronic renal failure

215. All of the following signs and symptoms of Addison's disease are due to deficient excretion of aldosterone EXCEPT for

√(A) fasting hypoglycemia
(B) a low voltage electrocardiogram
(C) a craving for salt
(D) hyperkalemic acidosis
(E) muscle weakness

216. A 16-year-old girl has normal breast development and mature distribution of pubic and axillary hair; however, she has not menstruated. Which of the following procedures would provide the most useful information in determining the cause of this patient's primary amenorrhea?

(A) Determination of serum gonadotropin levels
√(B) A pelvic examination
(C) Radiologic studies of the pituitary gland
(D) Chromosome analysis of the peripheral blood
(E) None of the above

217. Secondary amenorrhea is associated with all of the following EXCEPT

(A) anorexia nervosa
(B) a brain tumor
√(C) Turner's syndrome
(D) emotional stress
(E) obesity

218. The earliest clinical evidence of disease in the infant shown below is most likely to be

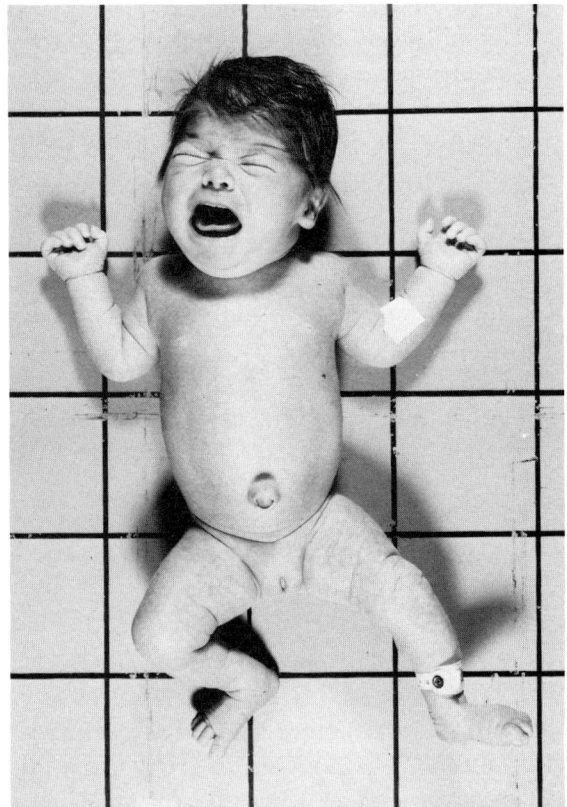

Used with permission of McGraw-Hill Book Company, from *Principles of Pediatrics: Health Care of the Young* (p 1274), by Hoekelman RA et al, © 1978 McGraw-Hill Inc.

(A) a hoarse cry
(B) a cardiac murmur
(C) jaundice
√(D) a large posterior fontanel
(E) low birth weight for gestational age

76

219. All of the following statements concerning cystinuria are correct EXCEPT that

(A) the serum concentrations of cystine, lysine, arginine, and ornithine are elevated
(B) the urine concentrations of cystine, lysine, arginine, and ornithine are elevated
(C) infections of the urinary tract are common complications
(D) the treatment of choice for prevention of complications includes the use of penicillamine
(E) most patients develop renal calculi before the age of 30 years

220. A 15-year-old boy comes to a physician because he is concerned about being only 152 cm (5 feet) tall. According to the boy, his perinatal and childhood history were normal except that he has always been a "little" shorter than his friends; two years ago his friends grew rapidly, but he did not. There is no history of chronic illness, and his parents are of average height. To identify the etiology as soon as possible, it would be necessary to determine

(A) his bone age
(B) his alkaline phosphatase level
(C) the Tanner stage he is in
(D) the heights of his grandparents and siblings
(E) the results of a urinalysis

221. A diagnosis of primary hyperparathyroidism is confirmed by which of the following laboratory findings?

(A) An elevated serum phosphorus level
(B) A decreased alkaline phosphatase level
(C) A decreased serum vitamin D level
(D) An elevated total serum calcium level
(E) An increased urine calcium level

222. One complication of insulin therapy in juvenile diabetes mellitus is termed the Somogyi effect. This form of insulin resistance is characterized by all of the following EXCEPT

(A) hypoglycemia
(B) glucosuria
(C) ketonuria
(D) improved control by large doses of insulin
(E) fluctuating blood sugar levels

223. Neonatal screening for phenylketonuria is used widely to prevent the mental retardation seen in untreated individuals. Of 100 infants whose (blood) screening tests are positive and require further evaluation, what percentage are likely to have the disease?

(A) 5-10 percent
(B) 25-30 percent
(C) 45-50 percent
(D) 65-70 percent
(E) 85-90 percent

224. A four-week-old girl weighing 3.6 kg (7 lb, 15 oz) has a three week history of nonprojectile vomiting. She has not had diarrhea, fever, or any other problems and does not appear dehydrated. No other family members have been ill. The child has been fed a cow's milk-based formula since birth, except for a five-day, clear liquid diet at age two weeks. While receiving clear liquids, the vomiting subsided. Her birth weight was 3.3 kg (7 lb, 4 oz). The next step in the management of this child is to

(A) add cereal to the cow's milk-based formula
(B) change the child to an evaporated milk formula
(C) change the child to a soy-based formula
(D) obtain a urinalysis and a urine ferric chloride test
(E) obtain a urine culture

225. A 14-month-old white female is evaluated because of failure to thrive. Bone age, determined by the Sonntag method, is found to be greater than 2 standard deviations below the mean for chronologic age. The most likely etiology of this patient's failure to thrive is

(A) gonadal dysgenesis
(B) congenital toxoplasmosis
(C) fetal alcohol syndrome
(D) hypothyroidism
(E) Cockayne's syndrome

226. Metabolic acidosis occurs in association with all of the following conditions EXCEPT

(A) diabetic ketoacidosis
(B) diarrhea
(C) dehydration
(D) pyloric stenosis
(E) renal failure

227. A ten-year-old boy is admitted to the hospital
with sudden onset of right-sided hemiparesis. He
has a history of frequent grand mal seizures, mental
retardation, and ectopia lentis. The most likely
diagnosis is

(A) cystinuria
√(B) homocystinuria
(C) phenylketonuria
(D) argininosuccinicaciduria
(E) methylmalonic acidemia

DIRECTIONS: Each question below contains four suggested answers of which **one** or **more** is correct. Choose the answer

A	if	1, 2, and 3	are correct
B	if	1 and 3	are correct
C	if	2 and 4	are correct
D	if	4	is correct
E	if	1, 2, 3, and 4	are correct

228. An 11-year-old girl is brought in for a physical examination. At 162 cm (5 feet, 4 inches), she is considerably taller than her classmates. The girl and her parents are concerned that she will grow to be excessively tall. Information that can be used to arrive at a prediction of growth potential includes

(1) bone age
(2) length at birth
(3) age at menarche
(4) height of siblings

229. Hypothyroidism occurring after two years of age results in

(1) reduced velocity of linear growth
(2) delayed dental development
(3) delayed sexual maturation
(4) irreversible central nervous system damage

230. A newborn infant presents with ambiguous genitalia. It appears that the baby is a female with masculinization of the external genitalia. Which of the following laboratory tests would provide the most useful information for arriving at a diagnosis?

(1) Nuclear chromatin determination
(2) Determination of serum gonadotropin level
(3) Measurement of 24-hour urinary 17-keto-steroid excretion
(4) Determination of serum estrogen level

231. Clinical presentations seen in association with chronic lymphocytic thyroiditis (Hashimoto's thyroiditis) include which of the following?

(1) A firm goiter
(2) Signs and symptoms of hyperthyroidism
(3) Serum antibodies against thyroglobulin
(4) An elevated T_4 level

232. A 14-year-old boy presents with no evidence of testicular enlargement. If constitutional delay is suspected, which of the following tests should be requested?

(1) Bone age x-rays
(2) Chromosome analysis
(3) Determination of serum gonadotropin level
(4) Skull x-rays

233. Clinical presentations characteristic of Cushing's syndrome in children include which of the following?

(1) Arrested growth and retarded bone age
(2) Decreased 24-hour urinary 17-ketosteroid excretion
(3) Elevated urinary cortisol levels
(4) A normal serum adrenocorticotropic hormone (ACTH) level

234. Thyrotoxicosis (Graves' disease) is characterized by which of the following statements?

(1) It is more common in females than in males
(2) It is more common in patients under five years of age
(3) The thyroid-stimulating hormone (TSH) level is decreased
(4) The goiter is nodular

235. A ten-year-old boy presents with findings that suggest a feminizing adrenal tumor. Clinical manifestations compatible with that diagnosis include

(1) advanced bone age
(2) advanced height age
(3) bilateral gynecomastia
(4) enlarged penis and testes

SUMMARY OF DIRECTIONS

A	B	C	D	E
1, 2, 3 only	1, 3 only	2, 4 only	4 only	All are correct

236. An eight-year-old girl presents with bilateral breast development and pubic hair. The suspected diagnosis is idiopathic (constitutional) isosexual precocity. An increase in which of the following measurements would be compatible with the suspected diagnosis?

(1) Bone age
(2) Serum gonadotropins
(3) Growth rate
(4) Gonadal steroids

237. Hypoparathyroidism with onset in later infancy and childhood may be associated with

(1) adrenal insufficiency
(2) cataracts
(3) moniliasis
(4) pernicious anemia

238. A four-day-old infant weighing 3,162 g (6 lb, 15 oz) at birth is found to have ambiguous genitalia. The phallus is a normal size, but the urethral orifice is at its base. The labioscrotal fold is fused, and testes are not palpable. The infant is taking 90-120 ml of a 20 cal/ounce formula per day. An intravenous pyelogram is performed to define renal and urinary anatomy; it shows normal excretory capacity for a newborn and normal anatomy. During the voiding cystourethrogram, however, the infant becomes hypotensive, tachycardiac, mottled, and gray-ashen in appearance. With aggressive intravascular fluid volume administration and intravenous dopamine 10 μ/kg/min, the infant's condition improves. Which of the following laboratory tests should be performed?

(1) Determination of serum Na, K, Cl, CO_2, and pH
(2) Measurement of 24-hour urinary 17-ketosteroid excretion
(3) Chromosome analysis
(4) Administration of desoxycorticosterone

239. On examination a 36-hour-old infant, the product of a normal pregnancy and delivery, is found to be lethargic and hypotonic. He has mild jaundice and a liver edge palpable at 4 cm below the right costal margin. Bilateral cataracts are noted. Besides vomiting the last two feedings of breast milk, the infant has had four liquid brown stools within the last two hours. Although the urine dipstick was negative, the clinitest was five percent. Correct statements concerning this infant include which of the following?

(1) If a positive blood culture was obtained, the most likely organism would be a gram-negative rod
(2) Each sibling of the same parents would have approximately one chance out of four of having the same disease
(3) A change to a soy-based formula in the future would be appropriate
(4) Even with appropriate therapy, the outlook for the intellectual development of this infant is very poor

DIRECTIONS: The groups of questions below consist of lettered choices followed by several numbered items. For each numbered item select the **one** lettered choice with which it is **most** closely associated. Each lettered choice may be used once, more than once, or not at all.

Questions 240-243

For each of the neonatal metabolic disorders listed below, select the appropriate laboratory determination that would confirm or support the diagnosis.

(A) Elevated plasma isoleucine, valine, and leucine
(B) Methyl citrate in the urine
(C) Positive urine cyanide nitroprusside reaction
(D) Hypercholesterolemia
(E) None of the above

E 240. Citrullinemia

B 241. Propionic acidemia

A 242. Maple syrup urine disease

C 243. Homocystinuria

Questions 244-247

Children with inherited metabolic disorders often present with nonspecific symptoms and findings, including vomiting, lethargy, jaundice, seizures, and poor growth. Simple urine screening tests can aid in establishing the likelihood of a metabolic disease. For each of the abnormal urinary substances listed below, select the test with which it is most likely to be detected.

(A) Dipstix
(B) Clinitest tablets
(C) Ketostix
(D) Ferric chloride test
(E) None of the above

D 244. Amino acids

B 245. Any reducing substance

A 246. Glucose only

D 247. Organic acids

Questions 248-252

The growth percentile curves shown in the graph below define the parameters of linear growth for 90 percent of children. Four other growth patterns are included on the graph and are labeled A, B, C, and D. For each of the conditions listed below, select the growth pattern that depicts the type of linear growth expected.

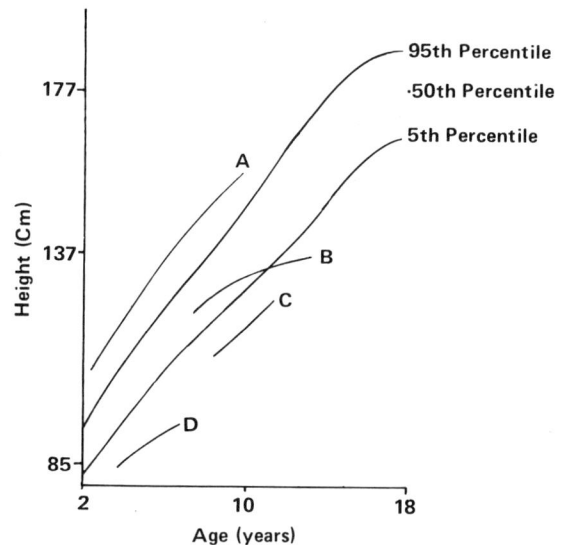

Used with permission of W.B. Saunders Company, from *Symposium on Pediatric Endocrinology* (vol 26, no 1, p 2, February 1979) by Douglas FS.

(A) Curve **A**
(B) Curve **B**
(C) Curve **C**
(D) Curve **D**
(E) None of the above curves

D 248. Growth hormone deficiency, congenital

B 249. Acquired hypothyroidism

C 250. Constitutionally delayed growth

B 251. Chronic renal disease

C 252. Familial short stature

Endocrinology and Metabolism

Answers

213. The answer is D. *(Hoekelman, pp 250-251.)* A simple method of estimating serum osmolality is to double the serum sodium concentration. However, any additional substances that contribute to the hypertonicity of serum must also be considered. For instance, glucose and urea both increase serum osmolality. The following formula can be used for quick estimates:

$$\text{Serum osmolality (mosm/kg of body water)} \cong$$

$$(2\ [Na^+]\ mEq/L) + \frac{\text{glucose mg}/100\ ml}{18} + \frac{\text{BUN mg}/100\ ml}{2.8}$$

The serum osmolality of 325 in this case is very high and has probably led to significant extracellular fluid shifts at the expense of intracellular fluid content. Considerable care must be taken to decrease the glucose concentration slowly so that rapid fluid shifts from extra- to intracellular space do not occur. The latter may result in cerebral edema and convulsions.

214. The answer is C. *(Hoekelman, p 252.)* The primary clinical manifestation of decreased **ionized** calcium concentration is tetany. The ionized fraction is decreased in hypoparathyroidism either primary or secondary to renal failure. The ionized fraction is also decreased in alkalosis when it accompanies hyperventilation and in phosphate overload when it occurs in very young children given whole cow's milk, which has a high absolute amount of phosphate and a high phosphate/calcium ratio. Although the total serum calcium, as measured in the laboratory, is decreased in hypoalbuminemia, the ionized concentration remains at a normal level, and the patient remains asymptomatic.

215. The answer is A. *(Hoekleman, pp 1292-1294.)* Aldosterone acts on the renal tubules to increase reabsorption of sodium. When aldosterone production is decreased, there is loss of sodium and chloride, retention of potassium, and development of hyperkalemic acidosis. The metabolic disturbance causes a craving for salt, muscle weakness, and low voltage changes on electrocardiogram. Blood sugar levels are not affected. Other cardiovascular disorders associated with aldosterone deficiencies include decreased heart size, hypotension, and decreased blood volume. Additional gastrointestinal involvement includes anorexia, nausea, vomiting, and diarrhea.

216. The answer is B. *(Hoekelman, p 1325. Dewhurst, Pediatr Clin North Am 19:605, 1972.)* Primary amenorrhea in a 16-year-old girl with good secondary sexual development is usually due to an anatomic defect. A pelvic examination would reveal the two most likely anatomic causes of amenorrhea—vaginal obstruction due to an imperforate membrane or absence of the vagina. If secondary sexual development is poor (or absent), amenorrhea is usually due to failure of the pituitary to produce gonadotropin or failure of the ovary to respond to gonadotropin. Knowledge of gonadotropin levels and pituitary anatomy is important in the diagnosis of conditions characterized by poor or absent secondary sexual development. Ovarian failure is one of the symptoms of Turner's syndrome, which is diagnosed by a karyotype.

217. The answer is C. *(Hoekelman, pp 354-355, 1325-1326. Grodin, Pediatr Clin North Am 19:619, 1972.)* Turner's syndrome is characterized by congenital gonadal dysgenesis. Most patients will not enter adolescence and menstruate without cyclic estrogen treatment. Thus, the amenorrhea associated with this condition is termed primary. The menstrual cycle is induced by replacement hormone therapy. With each of the other conditions listed in the question, amenorrhea may be present as a secondary event. The mechanisms involved with each are not well understood.

218. The answer is D. *(Hoekelman, pp 483-484, 1274. Smith, J Pediatr 87:959-961, 1975.)* The infant in the figure accompanying the question has congenital hypothyroidism or cretinism. Neonatal screening is an effective means of early detection of this condition; clinical findings are frequently present in the newborn period. A large posterior fontanel can be felt on the initial physical examination; this fontanel measures less than 0.5 cm in 97 percent of normal infants born at term. A variety of other signs may be present in the newborn with hypothyroidism, including hypothermia, hypoactivity, peripheral cyanosis, and delay in stooling. Jaundice is not present at birth but appears, if at all, during the first week of life, sometimes lasting for several weeks or months. A hoarse cry is usually evident at a later age. Cardiac murmurs are not characteristic of neonatal hypothyroidism. These infants tend to be large for gestational age.

219. The answer is A. *(Hoekelman, pp 1590-1591, 1621-1623. Rudolph, ed 16. p 689.) Vaughan, ed 11. p 1522.)* Cystinuria, usually an autosomal recessive disease, is a disorder of renal tubular transport of the dibasic amino acids (cystine, lysine, arginine, and ornithine), which results in an increased urinary excretion of these molecules. However, there is not always an increased serum level of these amino acids. Complications associated with cystinuria are urinary tract infections and renal calculi (usually before the age of 30 years). The treatment of choice for prevention of these problems includes the use of penicillamine, which yields soluble compounds when combined with cystine.

220. The answer is C. *(Hoekelman, pp 1251-1252. Rimoin, J Pediatr 92:523-528, 697-704, 1978. Shenker, Pediatr Ann 7:608-610, 1978.)* Constitutional delayed puberty is one of the most common causes of short stature in adolescence. These youths begin their pubertal changes, including acceleration of growth, later than their peers. There is usually no evidence of chronic illness, and their full adult height is eventually average or above. The height growth spurt in adolescent boys usually occurs between Tanner stages III and IV; thus, a youth with this history, who has a normal physical examination and a Tanner II to III appearance, often has short stature because of constitutional delayed puberty. The bone age will be delayed, and the alkaline phosphatase level will not peak until the maximum growth spurt occurs. Therefore, the Tanner stage is an easier method to help determine growth potential in the adolescent than are the other methods listed in the question. The heights of family members provide only indirect evidence of growth potential, and a urinalysis will not reveal a cause for growth failure unless very severe, chronic renal disease is present.

221. The answer is D. *(Hoekelman, pp 1279-1280. Gardner, pp 400-407.)* Parathyroid hormone has an effect on both bone and kidney that results in the elevation of serum calcium levels. With hyperparathyroidism, there is an elevation of serum calcium, a reduction in serum phosphorus, and either a normal or somewhat elevated alkaline phosphatase. Normal urinary calcium levels are usual. While vitamin D deficiency may be seen with secondary hyperparathyroidism, it is not characteristic of primary hyperparathyroidism.

222. The answer is D. *(Hoekelman, p 1265. Gardner, p 958.)* The Somogyi effect is one form of insulin resistance. It is brought about by insulin dosages in excess of two units per kilogram of body weight per day, a dosage that produces hypoglycemia. The hypoglycemia often is not apparent clinically and is followed by hyperglycemia, glucosuria, and ketonuria. An insensitivity to insulin develops. If the hyperglycemia is interpreted as representing poor control and is treated with more insulin, the condition will worsen. Treatment consists of gradual reduction of the insulin dosage until good control is achieved. Other manifestations of the Somogyi effect are rapid fluctuations in the levels of urine glucose when hypoglycemia (or hypoglycemic symptoms) occurs, despite the presence of glucosuria occurring when continued increase of the insulin dose does not lead to improvement and when the total insulin dose is greater than 2 units/kg/day.

223. The answer is A. *(Hoekelman, p 185.)* Only one of every 15 to 20 infants with a positive screening test for phenylketonuria (PKU) will have the disease. The test measures the blood level of phenylalanine, which may be transiently elevated in the neonate. Those infants with a false-positive PKU test require a thorough evaluation to establish that they are normal. Screening carried out after the first five days of life is much more likely to detect PKU than screening carried out earlier. Between five and ten percent of infants with PKU could be missed if they are screened before they are five days old. When newborns are tested and discharged before the fifth day, a follow-up test should be carried out before the age of two weeks. For every dollar spent on PKU screening, four dollars are saved on the long-term care of individuals with the disease.

224. The answer is D. *(Hoekelman, pp 888-892.)* This child's persistent vomiting while receiving formula **may** be a manifestation of a metabolic disease. The urinary ferric chloride test is abnormal in most aminoacidopathies, and ketones frequently are found on urinalysis. Urine tests and blood tests should be performed before any dietary changes are made. A urinary tract infection at three weeks of age would be unlikely, particularly as a cause for isolated persistent vomiting; therefore, a urine culture would not be indicated in the initial investigation of this patient.

225. The answer is D. *(Hoekelman, p 1844.)* X-rays of the skull, chest, and long bones are valuable in the evaluation of failure to thrive, both to determine bone age and to detect any radiologically-apparent lesions such as intracranial calcifications and the bony changes seen with metabolic or hereditary diseases. Bone age should be compared to both height age and chronologic age. Bone age is less than height age and less than chronologic age in only a few conditions, most notably, hypothyroidism, hypopituitarism, and malnutrition. In failure to thrive secondary to intrauterine infections, such as congenital toxoplasmosis, or maternal drug ingestion, such as in the fetal alcohol syndrome, the bone age is usually equal to chronologic age and the height is retarded. This is also true for Cockayne's syndrome and gonadal dysgenesis.

226. The answer is D. *(Hoekelman, pp 254, 754-755. Pitts, ed 3. p 219.)* A metabolic acidosis can be caused by one of several combinations of situations involving the production and excretion of hydrogen ions (H) and bicarbonate ions (HCO_3). These situations are: (1) a production of hydrogen ions at a rate faster than can be excreted; (2) a disease-induced decrease of hydrogen ions and renewed bicarbonate production by the kidney; and (3) excessive bicarbonate losses from the kidney or intestinal tract. When there is either overproduction or underexcretion of hydrogen ions, the consumption of body fluid bicarbonate ions is increased to buffer the hydrogen ions. The loss of bicarbonate involves the disassociation of carbonic acid, an event that leaves hydrogen ions behind in body fluids. The results of these imbalances include: (1) a fall in serum bicarbonate ion concentration; (2)

a fall of the bicarbonate/carbonic acid ratio to below 20:1; and (3) an increase in hydrogen ion concentration. The respiratory center responds rapidly to the fall in pH and there is hyperventilation. In diabetic ketoacidosis, there is an increased production of hydrogen ions; in diarrhea, there is an excessive loss of bicarbonate ions in the stools; in dehydration, there is decreased renal perfusion and therefore decreased excretion of hydrogen ions; and in renal failure there is decreased excretion of titratable acid. Pyloric stenosis usually results in a hypochloremic alkalosis, since there is a significant loss of chloride and potassium from the gastrointestinal tract. The kidneys will compensate by reabsorbing bicarbonate ions and excreting hydrogen ions (paradoxical aciduria).

227. The answer is B. *(Hoekelman, pp 939-940. Rudolph, ed 16. pp 673-687.)* Homocystinuria is the second most common disorder of amino acid metabolism; phenylketonuria is the most common. Homocystinuria is an autosomal recessive disorder characterized by the absence of cystathionine synthetase, which is necessary for the interaction of homocystine with serine to produce cystathionine. The most common clinical findings include mental retardation, ectopia lentis, thromboembolic phenomena, a Marfan-like appearance, and orthopedic malformations. Mental retardation is a common finding in phenylketonuria, argininosuccinicaciduria, and methylmalonic acidemia. However, these children do **not** exhibit ectopia lentis or thromboembolic phenomena. Patients who have cystinuria are **not** usually mentally retarded, but they do have significant renal disease secondary to cystine stones. This condition can lead to renal failure. These stones are caused by a renal tubular defect which prevents normal resorption of cystine.

228. The answer is B (1, 3). *(Hoekelman, pp 646-647. Wettenhall, J Pediatr 86:603-604, 1975.)* Excessive height in the female adolescent is often noted with displeasure by both the child and her parents. The physician may be asked by the early adolescent female about her growth potential. When menarche occurs, as it usually does in the late Tanner III or the early Tanner IV stage, it is generally an indication that the individual will not grow more than a few inches thereafter. A bone age of 12 years or less, despite the chronologic age, indicates that there is still growth potential in the individual patient. Length at birth provides no indication of adult height, and the height of siblings gives only indirect evidence of a person's eventual height. Treatment with estrogen over several years has been used in some patients to reduce growth.

229. The answer is A (1, 2, 3). *(Hoekelman, pp 1274-1275.)* Hypothyroidism with onset after two years of age causes reduction in growth rate and delay in tooth eruption and sexual maturation. These abnormalities are always severe, but the degree of severity depends on the extent and duration of the disease. Contrary to the effect of thyroid deficiency in infancy (cretinism), hypothyroidism occurring after age two does not have a lasting effect on mental development.

230. The answer is B (1, 3). *(Hoekelman, pp 1285-1287. Gardner, pp 476-495.)* The major cause of virilization of the external genitalia of the female fetus is congenital adrenal hyperplasia, a condition associated with decreased cortisol production and an increased production of adrenocorticotropic hormone (ACTH). The resulting hyperplasia of the adrenals leads to excess androgen production and masculinization of the external genitalia. In this situation, study of the nuclear sex chromatin pattern in a buccal smear and measurement of the 24-hour urinary 17-ketosteroid excretion are the most helpful laboratory tests in establishing the gender and the existence of an excess production of adrenal steroids. Knowing the serum levels of estrogen and gonadotropin does not help in establishing this diagnosis.

231. The answer is B (1, 3). *(Hoekelman, pp 1272-1273. Gardner, pp 317-323.)* The goiter with lymphocytic thyroiditis is firm and variable in texture; the most helpful laboratory finding is the presence of antibodies against thyroglobulin in the blood serum; however, antibody production can also be stimulated by other proteins found in the microsomal fractions of thyroid cells. The clinical presentation is usually one of either hypothyroidism or euthyroidism, rarely hyperthyroidism. Often the T_4 level is decreased and the thyroid-stimulating hormone level increased.

232. The answer is B (1, 3). *(Hoekelman, pp 1259-1260. Gardner, pp 66-82.)* A diagnosis of constitutional delay is justified in this patient if the bone age is delayed and the serum gonadotropins are appropriate for the extent of sexual development but lower than expected for the patient's age. If the serum gonadotropin level and bone age do not support a diagnosis of constitutional delay, other causes of delayed sexual development must be considered. These include either primary gonadal dysgenesis or failure in pituitary gonadotropin production. Failure of gonadotropic production may be related to a neoplasm in the region of the pituitary gland, in which case skull x-rays would be useful. Primary gonadal dysfunction may be a result of a chromosomal abnormality (e.g., Klinefelter's syndrome), which can be documented by a karyotype.

233. The answer is B (1, 3). *(Hoekelman, pp 1294-1295. Gardner, pp 500-506.)* The clinical manifestations of Cushing's syndrome are due to excess cortisol production, which may arise either from increased ACTH production, causing adrenal hyperplasia, or from a primary adrenal tumor (benign adenoma or carcinoma). The most notable clinical manifestations of excess cortisol production in childhood are retarded bone age and arrested growth. The increase in cortisol production is reflected by increased urinary excretion of cortisol, and there is usually an increase in the urinary excretion of 17-ketosteroids as well. Serum ACTH levels are either high or low, rather than normal. In the case of adrenal hyperplasia, the serum ACTH level is high; with an autonomous adrenal tumor, the serum ACTH level is low. Cushing's syndrome is rare in children. When it occurs in infancy and early childhood, the cause is most likely to be malignant adrenal tumors. After the age of eight, the etiologic factors are similar to those in adults.

234. The answer is B (1, 3). *(Hoekelman, pp 1273-1274. Gardner, pp 295-313.)* About one-third of children with goiters will be hyperthyroid. With thyrotoxicosis, the gland acts autonomously to produce excessive thyroid hormone; this serves to suppress the production of thyroid stimulating hormone (TSH) by the pituitary gland. The goiter in thyrotoxicosis is diffuse and not nodular. This disorder is rarely seen in those below the age of five years and is encountered with increasing frequency toward the second decade. Goiters, as well as all forms of thyroid disease, are more common in females. Exacerbations and remissions are characteristic. Children with this disease do not present with the characteristic triad of Graves' disease of adulthood—that is, goiter, ophthalmopathy, and pretibial myxedema. The goiter occurs in childhood thyrotoxicosis, but myxedema does not; the ophthalmopathy may or may not occur.

235. The answer is A (1, 2, 3). *(Hoekelman, p 1297.)* Adrenal tumors that have a feminizing effect are rare. They are possibly a variant of virilizing adrenal tumors. They produce amounts of estrogen that are appropriate for an adult woman but excessive for prepubertal children. In both males and females increased estrogen secretion results in breast enlargement, advanced height age, and advanced bone age. In most patients of either sex, there is also increased androgen production, but this causes no clinical signs. The male genitalia remain normal for the child's age.

236. The answer is E (all). *(Hoekelman, pp 1260-1261.)* Isosexual precocity, the premature development of secondary sexual characteristics appropriate for the child's phenotype, occurs twice as often in females as males. Sexual development is considered to be premature if it occurs before the age of eight in females and nine and a half in males. Isosexual precocity occurs when there is a stimulation or early maturation of hypothalamic pituitary function. The resultant secretion of gonadotropins will stimulate the secretion of gonadal steroids. The premature production of gonadal steroids may be due to several causes, such as tumors, neurologic lesions, and hypothyroidism. It can occur with or without the secretion of gonadotropins. The latter occurs when the tumor or lesion is gonadal, adrenal, or exogenous. When the cause of precocious secretion of gonadotropins is unknown, the isosexual precocity is termed constitutional, idiopathic, or cryptogenic. Increased growth rate and advanced bone age are diagnostic of sexual precocity.

237. The answer is E (all). *(Hoekelman, p 1276.)* Hypoparathyroidism that presents later than the newborn period is presumed to be due to autoimmunity and may be associated with similar damage to other secretory systems, including the adrenal cortex and gastric mucosa. This type of hypoparathyroidism is also called idiopathic hypoparathyroidism. Adrenal insufficiency and pernicious anemia may result. Chronic hypocalcemia is damaging to ectodermal tissues. Hair loss, nail abnormalities, and cataracts may also be present. Chronic infections with *Candida albicans* occur in the abnormal skin and nails, and systemic moniliasis has also been noted.

238. The answer is E (all). *(Hoekelman, pp 1296-1297. Avery, pp 960-962.)* The adrenogenital syndrome is a genetic disorder involving impaired synthesis of adrenal steroid hormones. Defects in mineralocorticoid synthesis result in aldosterone deficiency, and defects in glucocorticoid synthesis result in cortical deficiency; a reduction in androgenic hormone synthesis causes a variety of clinical manifestations based upon end-product deficiencies. Approximately 90 percent of all virilizing forms are due to a lack or depletion of the 21-hydroxylase enzyme. Female infants with virilization of the developing genitalia may become acutely ill because of sodium depletion secondary to aldosterone insufficiency with a concomitant rise in potassium. Impaired synthesis of cortisol makes these infants susceptible to acute shock, peripheral collapse, and death, especially during any induced physiologic stress. Management includes restoration of intravascular fluid volume and blood pressure, determination of serum electrolytes with appropriate correction of acid-base disequilibrium, and prompt administration of a glucocorticoid with some mineralocorticoid effect such as deoxycorticosterone acetate. Measurement of pregnanetriol, cortisol, and 24-hour urinary excretion of 17-ketosteroids will assist in establishing the site of the enzymatic defect. Chromosome analysis (karyotype) will permit a determination of genetic sex for purposes of further psychosocial and surgical management.

239. The answer is A (1, 2, 3). *(Hoekelman, pp 185, 349, 771. Aleck, Pediatr Clin North Am 25:431-451, 1978. Burton, Pediatrics 61:398-405, 1978.)* The acute onset of illness in a healthy newborn after the initiation of feeding has a broad differential diagnosis. However, jaundice, hepatomegaly, anorexia, vomiting, diarrhea, lethargy, and hypotonia suggest a metabolic disorder, sepsis, or both. The presence of congenital cataracts and the detection of nonglucose reducing sugar in the urine are almost certainly diagnostic of galactosemia. This autosomal recessive disorder is correctable with galactose and lactose-free formulas such as those made with a soybean base. If appropriate therapy is instituted early, the outlook for future development is good. It should be kept in mind, however, that a frequent cause of death in these infants is gram-negative sepsis.

240-243. The answers are: 240-E, 241-B, 242-A, 243-C. *(Hoekelman, pp 887-905. Burton, Pediatrics 61:398-405, 1978. Nyhan, Curr Probl Pediatr 7:6-12, 1977.)* Citrullinemia is an inborn error of metabolism of the urea cycle with reduced or absent argininosuccinate synthetase. Elevations of citrulline are found in the urine and plasma. In addition, plasma ammonia levels rise and cause a clinical syndrome characterized by somnolence, lethargy, vomiting, alternating hypertonia and hypotonia, respiratory distress, seizures, coma, and death. Onset of symptoms relates to temporal protein intake.

Propionic acidemia is an autosomal recessive organic acidemia in which there is a defect in the activity of propionyl-CoA carboxylase. Clinically, the disorder presents with vomiting, ketosis, metabolic acidosis, and coma. It is characterized by the propionic acidemia, hyperglycinemia, and hyperammonemia. A number of abnormal metabolites of propionic acid, including methyl citrate and 3-hydroxypropionate, are excreted in the urine of patients with propionic acidemia.

Maple syrup urine disease and its variants are due to deficiencies in the branched-chain ketoacid olecarboxylase complex resulting in elevations in serum and urine leucine, isoleucine, and valine. The burnt sugar odor of the urine in these patients is due to high concentrations of branched-chain α-ketoacids. In addition to ketosis and acidemia, these infants frequently exhibit hypoglycemic attacks and elevated plasma lactates. Patients require parenteral fluid and electrolyte therapy prior to feedings of synthetic amino acids low in the branched-chain forms. Milder variants of the disease have been reported to respond to large doses of thiamine.

Homocystinuria results from deficiencies of cystathionine synthetase, the enzyme required for conversion of homocysteine to cystathionine, both sulfur-containing amino acids. Urine from these patients has a positive cyanide nitroprusside reaction. Ectopia lentis, presumably a result of pathologic weakness of the lental suspensory ligament, is also seen.

244-247. The answers are: 244-D, 245-B, 246-A, 247-D. *(Hoekelman, p 890. Burton, Pediatrics 61:398, 1978.)* The **Dipstix** will detect glucose in the urine, but not any other reducing substances. The **Clinitest** tablets, however, will identify any reducing substance. Urinary-reducing substances are present in many inborn errors of metabolism. These conditions include galactosemia, hereditary fructose intolerance, renal glycosuria, and Fanconi's syndrome. In the latter two conditions, glucose is present in the urine and will yield a positive Dipstix test as well. The **Ketostix** detects the presence of ketones. A large number of the metabolic disorders result in urinary ketones. The **ferric chloride test** is useful, since many substances react with Fe^{+++}, producing color compounds. The substances found in the urine in many metabolic disorders result in an abnormal ferric chloride test. This circumstance makes the test an extremely useful screening tool for infants suspected of having a metabolic disorder. A negative ferric chloride test, however, does not rule out the presence of a metabolic disorder, since a sufficient quantity of the abnormal substance must be present in the urine to produce a color change. The test is easy to perform, and the reagents are readily available in most general hospitals.

248-252. The answers are: 248-D, 249-B, 250-C, 251-B, 252-C. *(Hoekelman, pp 1252, 1254, 1257. Frasier, Pediatr Clin North Am 26:1-2, 1979.)* Growth pattern A depicts a child with constitutional tall stature, a variant of the normal pattern of child growth. These children grow at a rate that is parallel to, but above, the normal growth curve. The growth curve in patients with excessive secretion of growth hormone caused by a functioning pituitary tumor is not only more rapid than expected, but progressively deviates above normal compared to the parallel increased rate of growth seen in constitutional tall stature.

The growth curve represented by curve B shows acquired growth failure as seen with acquired hypothyroidism or chronic renal disease. After a period of normal growth, the acquired disorder causes the child's growth to fall below normal. In acquired hypothyroidism, the amount of reduction in growth rate varies; however, the height age is not usually delayed to the extent that the bone age is. Gastrointestinal as well as renal disorders commonly present with short stature.

Growth pattern C describes a short individual with a normal rate of growth. This pattern is seen both with familial short stature, where the adult height will be below normal, and constitutional delays, where the adult height will eventually be in the normal range. Children with constitutional delay in growth lag behind their peers until they have transcended adolesence, which for them occurs later and lasts longer than normal.

Growth pattern D is seen with congenital conditions that interfere with growth. It shows a deviation from normal at an early age, as occurs with congenital deficiency of growth hormone. Congenital forms of growth hormone deficiency (e.g., pituitary dysgenesis), however, are less common than acquired forms, such as craniopharyngioma and basilar skull fracture.

Cardiology and Pulmonology

DIRECTIONS: Each question below contains five suggested answers. Choose the **one best** response to each question.

253. The generally accepted estimate of the incidence of congenital heart disease in infants alive at birth is

(A) 0.5 percent
✓(B) 1.0 percent
(C) 2.0 percent
(D) 5.0 percent
(E) 10.0 percent

254. All of the following cyanotic congenital cardiac lesions are usually associated with increased pulmonary blood flow EXCEPT

(A) total anomalous pulmonary venous return
(B) transposition of the great vessels
(C) truncus arteriosus
✓(D) tetralogy of Fallot
(E) aortic atresia

255. Acceptable management of a large patent ductus arteriosus with congestive failure in a premature infant includes all of the following EXCEPT

(A) diuretic therapy
(B) fluid restriction
(C) indomethacin
(D) digitalis
✓(E) prostaglandin E_1

256. A 48-hour-old male infant with a previously benign perinatal history is found to be mildly cyanotic and tachypneic with grunting respirations. Further examination reveals a pale, mottled, somewhat irritable infant with diffuse rales, a prominent gallop rhythm, an enlarged firm liver, and barely palpable pulses with a marked delay in capillary filling. Blood pressure could not be obtained. An electrocardiogram shows normal right ventricular forces for age, but a septal Q wave was not detected. Mild cardiomegaly with pulmonary venous congestion is noted on a chest x-ray. The most likely diagnosis is

(A) a ventricular septal defect
(B) a truncus arteriosus
(C) septic shock
(D) coarctation of the aorta
✓(E) an underdeveloped left ventricle

257. A three-month-old acyanotic girl presents with tachypnea, a hyperdynamic precordium, a grade III pansystolic murmur of even amplitude at the lower left sternal border, a mildly accentuated pulmonary closure sound, a soft grade I apical mid-diastolic murmur, a firm liver palpable 3 cm below the right costal margin in the midclavicular line, and adequate but not full pulses. An electrocardiogram reveals an axis of +90° and combined ventricular hypertrophy. This infant's chest x-ray is shown below. The most likely diagnosis is

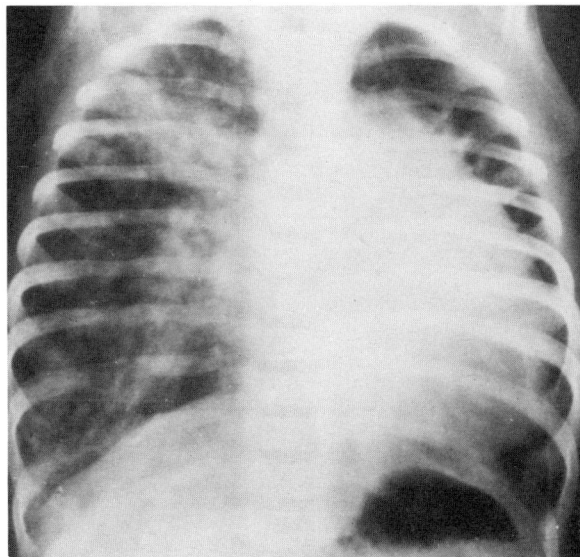

Used with permission of McGraw-Hill Book Company, from *Principles of Pediatrics: Health Care of the Young* (p 1514), by Hoekelman RA et al, © 1978 McGraw-Hill Inc.

(A) an atrial septal defect
✓(B) a ventricular septal defect
(C) a total anomaly of pulmonary venous return
(D) a complete atrioventricular canal defect
(E) a patent ductus arteriosus

258. Ventricular premature contractions may be considered to be benign if

✓(A) the ectopic beats disappear with exercise
(B) the ectopic beats occur in association with organic heart disease
(C) the ectopic beats are multifocal in origin
(D) four or more premature beats occur in a row
(E) the premature beats fall on the peak of the T wave

259. A four-year-old acyanotic girl presents with a recent history of mild fatigue upon vigorous exertion. Examination reveals a small child with clear lungs, a hyperdynamic precordium, a grade II systolic flow murmur at the upper left sternal border, a persistently split second sound of normal intensity, and a soft grade I mid-diastolic murmur at the lower left sternal border. Her liver is not enlarged, and the peripheral pulses are normal. Her electrocardiogram and chest x-ray are shown below. The most likely diagnosis is

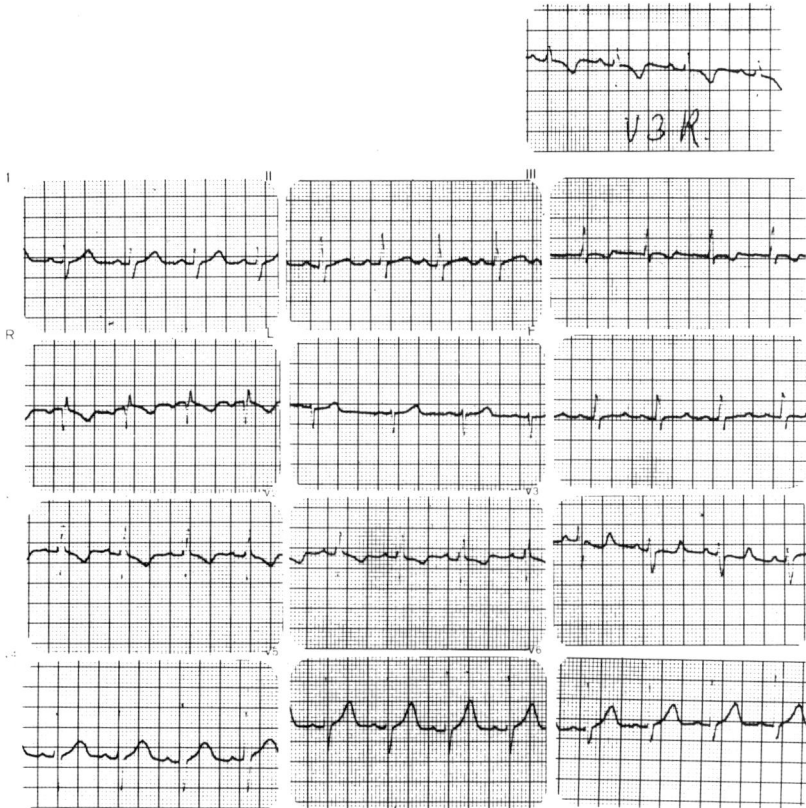

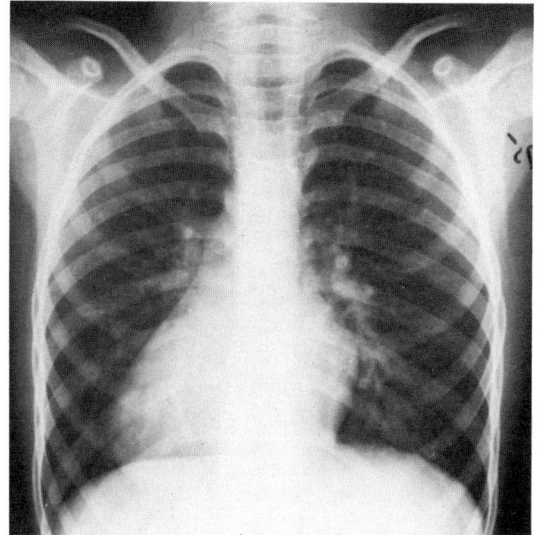

- ✓(A) an atrial septal defect
- (B) a tetralogy of Fallot
- (C) valvular pulmonary stenosis
- (D) tricuspid atresia
- (E) a functional murmur

---

260. Bacterial endocarditis would be LEAST likely to occur in a patient with

- ✓(A) an atrial septal defect
- (B) a ventricular septal defect
- (C) aortic valve stenosis
- (D) a tetralogy of Fallot
- (E) a patent ductus arteriosus

261. Eight days after surgical closure of a typical secundum atrial defect, a six-year-old girl develops fever to 38.9°C (102°F), lethargy, decreased breath sounds over the right posterior lung base, and somewhat muffled heart tones. A blood count reveals a leukocytosis with a left shift. The erythrocyte sedimentation rate is 80 mm/hour. An increase in heart size with loss of the usual cardiac silhouette and a small right pleural effusion are noted on a chest x-ray. The most likely diagnosis is

- (A) acute bacterial endocarditis
- (B) acute rheumatic fever
- (C) postperfusion syndrome
- ✓(D) postpericardiotomy syndrome
- (E) none of the above

262. The cardiac anomaly most likely to be present in a child with the electrocardiogram shown below is

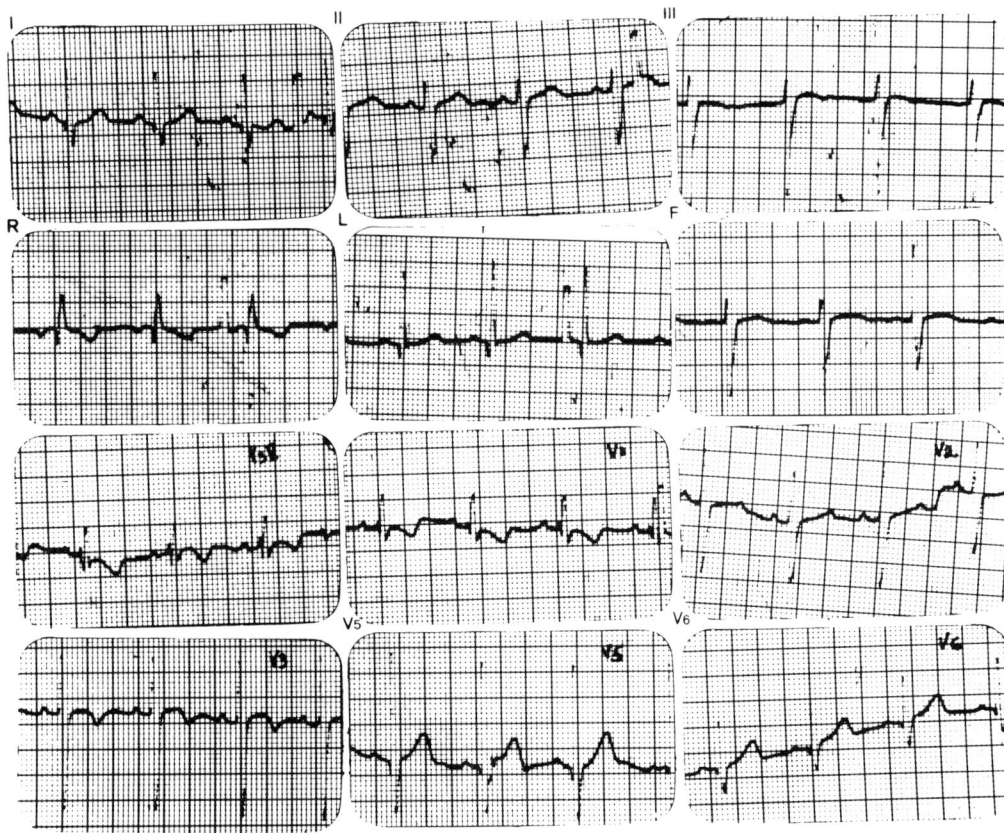

(A) an atrial septal defect
(B) a tetralogy of Fallot
(C) aortic valve stenosis
√(D) a partial atrioventricular canal defect
(E) a partial anomaly of pulmonary venous return

---

263. All of the following are characteristic features of tetralogy of Fallot EXCEPT

(A) a large ventricular septal defect
(B) an overriding aorta
√(C) an enlarged left atrium
(D) pulmonic stenosis
(E) right ventricular hypertrophy

264. A three-year-old healthy acyanotic boy is found to have a continuous whistling murmur in the right and left infraclavicular areas. The murmur varies somewhat with respiration and disappears in the supine position and with a Valsalva maneuver. The aortic and pulmonary closure sounds are of normal intensity, and the remainder of his cardiovascular examination is within normal limits. The most likely diagnosis is

(A) a patent ductus arteriosus
(B) a pulmonary arteriovenous fistula
(C) a cerebral arteriovenous fistula
(D) mild aortic stenosis and insufficiency
√(E) a venous hum

265. Purulent pericarditis in childhood most likely is caused by

(A) *Hemophilus influenzae* or beta-hemolytic streptococcus
(B) *Staphylococcus aureus* or beta-hemolytic streptococcus
(C) *Hemophilus influenzae* or *Streptococcus (Diplococcus) pneumoniae*
(D) *Neisseria meningitidis* or viridans streptococci
(E) *Hemophilus influenzae* or *Staphylococcus aureus* ✓

266. The chest x-ray shown below reveals all of the following EXCEPT

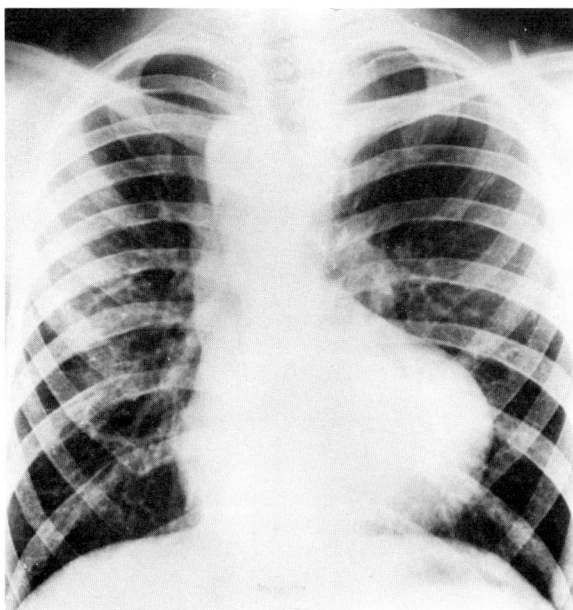

Used with permission of McGraw-Hill Book Company, from *Principles of Pediatrics: Health Care of the Young* (p 1515), by Hoekelman RA et al, © 1978 McGraw-Hill Inc.

(A) a normal heart size
(B) a prominent main pulmonary artery ✓
(C) a right aortic arch
(D) an uptilted apex
(E) decreased pulmonary blood flow

267. All of the following factors increase the susceptibility of infants to lower respiratory tract infection EXCEPT

(A) relative immunologic incompetence
(B) narrow peripheral airways
(C) fewer conducting airways than an adult ✓
(D) inefficient collateral ventilation
(E) ineffective cough mechanism

268. Cystic fibrosis is classified primarily as a

(A) chronic progressive pulmonary disease
(B) disorder of mucociliary clearance
(C) gastrointestinal malabsorption syndrome
(D) disorder of exocrine gland function ✓
(E) disorder of endocrine and exocrine pancreatic function

269. A four-year-old boy is admitted to the hospital because of wheezing, which was unresponsive to subcutaneous epinephrine administered previously by his physician. The child is alert and oriented but frightened. The mother indicates that the child has had no other medication and has had little to eat or drink in the preceding 24 hours because of respiratory distress and vomiting. Physical examination reveals mild acrocyanosis in addition to moderate respiratory distress. Initial patient management could include all of the following EXCEPT

(A) intravenous theophylline to reduce bronchospasm
(B) intravenous fluids to maintain hydration
(C) parenteral sedatives to reduce anxiety ✓
(D) supplemental oxygen to correct hypoxia
(E) aerosolized β-adrenergics to reduce bronchospasm

270. At the present time, the diagnosis of the cystic fibrosis carrier state is best determined by

(A) quantitative analysis of sweat sodium and chloride
(B) measurement of sweat conductivity
(C) duodenal intubation and pancreatic enzyme quantitation
(D) pulmonary function testing
(E) obtaining a family history ✓

Now isoelectric focussing · CF Protein band (Trypsin-)

271. The most common infectious etiology for bronchiolitis is

(A) adenovirus
(B) *Hemophilus influenzae* type B
(C) influenza virus
(D) respiratory syncytial virus ✓
(E) parainfluenza virus

272. The clinical feature most commonly associated
with the lower respiratory tract infection revealed
in the chest x-ray shown below is

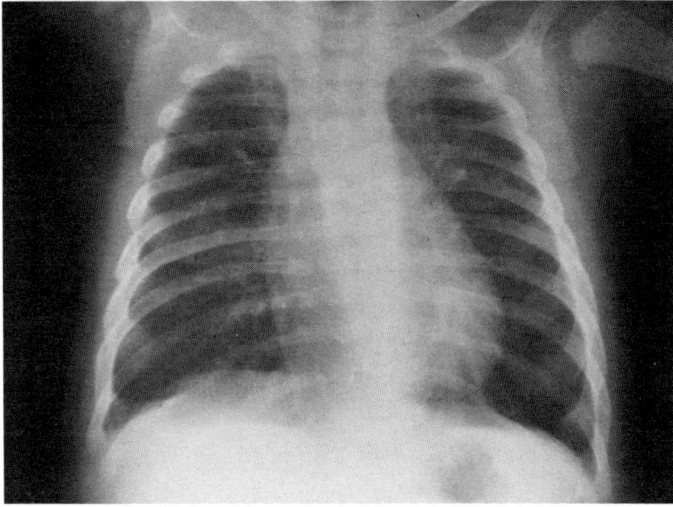

√(A) tachypnea
 (B) cyanosis
 (C) leukocytosis
 (D) hepatomegaly
 (E) fever

DIRECTIONS: Each question below contains four suggested answers of which **one** or **more** is correct. Choose the answer

A	if	**1, 2, and 3**	are correct
B	if	**1 and 3**	are correct
C	if	**2 and 4**	are correct
D	if	**4**	is correct
E	if	**1, 2, 3, and 4**	are correct

273. The electrocardiogram shown below could have been obtained from a patient with

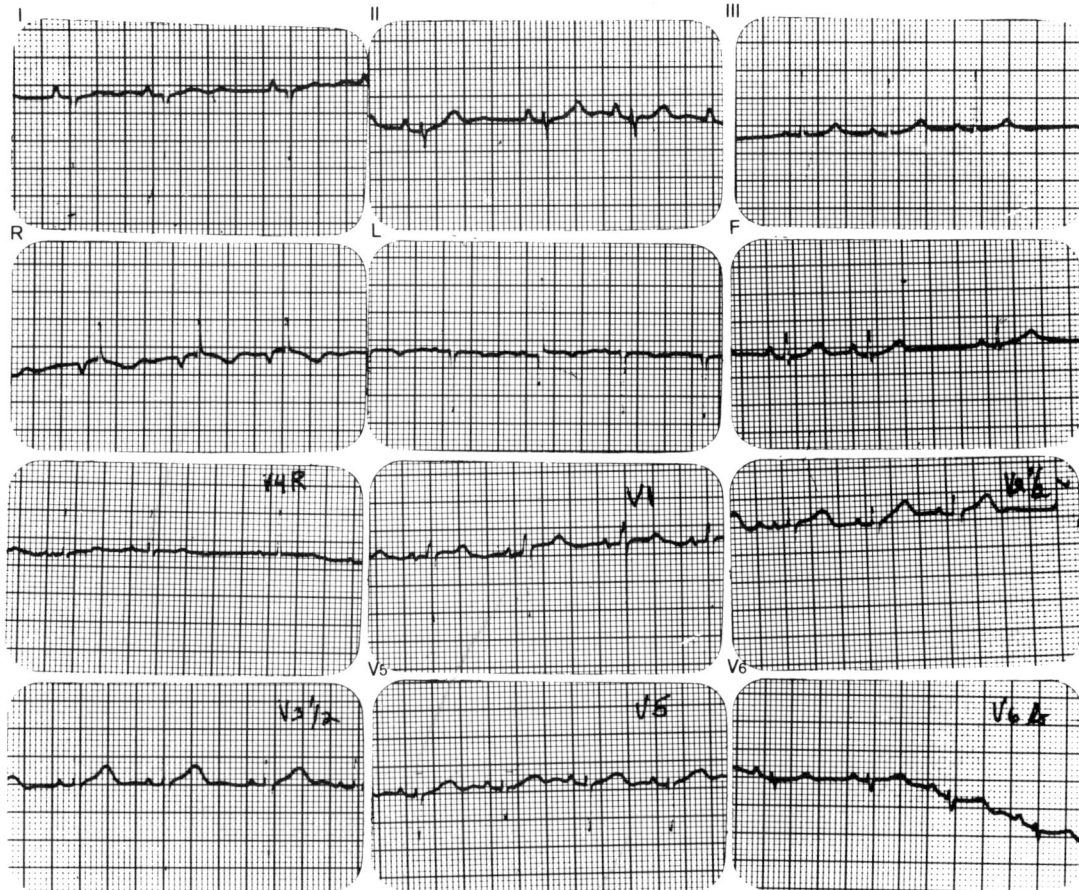

(1) tetralogy of Fallot
(2) transposition of the great arteries
(3) severe pulmonary valve stenosis
(4) tricuspid atresia

---

274. Which of the following entities can be associated with intermittent or persistent cyanosis of the newborn infant?

(1) Central nervous system disease
(2) Severe polycythemia
(3) Atrial septal defects
(4) Tricuspid atresia

275. Management of hypercyanotic spells in a patient with a severe tetralogy of Fallot includes

(1) morphine sulfate
(2) propranolol
(3) oxygen
(4) knee-chest position

276. A ten-year-old boy with suspected myocarditis is admitted to the hospital. On his second hospital day he suddenly begins to exhibit brief, generalized seizures with loss of consciousness. Up to this point, he has been managed with bed rest and diuretic agents. Serum electrolytes, calcium, and magnesium, blood sugar, and blood urea nitrogen are within normal limits. Continuous electrocardiographic monitoring reveals intermittent episodes (see rhythm strip below). Management at this point should include

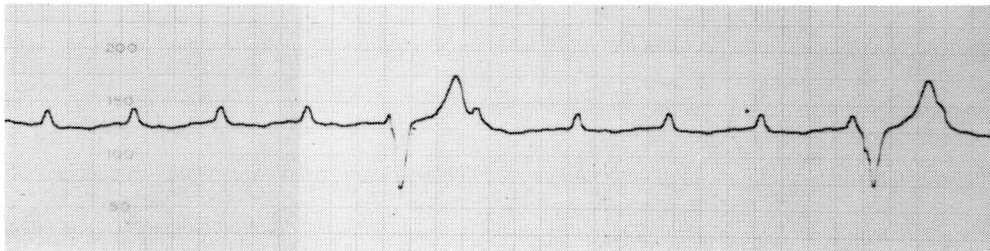

 (1) digitalis
 ✓(2) an isoproterenol infusion
 (3) atropine
 ✓(4) temporary transvenous pacing

277. A small patent ductus arteriosus should be closed (electively) in early childhood because of the risk of the subsequent development of

 (1) congestive heart failure
 (2) cardiac arrhythmias
 (3) pulmonary vascular disease
 ✓(4) bacterial endocarditis (arteritis)

278. The natural history of a significant ventricular septal defect may include

 ✓(1) congestive heart failure
 ✓(2) infundibular hypertrophy
 ✓(3) spontaneous closure
 ✓(4) aortic insufficiency

279. A five-month-old boy is admitted to the hospital with bronchiolitis. Over the course of several hours he develops peripheral cyanosis despite the use of 40 percent oxygen. Which of the following clinical signs may also be associated with impending respiratory failure?

 ✓(1) Decreased muscle tone
 ✓(2) Decreased expiratory wheezing
 ✓(3) Changes in mental status
 ✓(4) Decreased inspiratory breath sounds

280. A ten-year-old boy presents with a history of chronic cough and recurrent pneumonias. Serial chest x-rays reveal persistent left lower lobe atelectasis, increased pulmonary markings, and dextrocardia. Other features associated with this syndrome include

 ✓(1) nasal polyposis
 (2) dysgammaglobulinemia
 ✓(3) chronic sinusitis
 (4) recurrent aspiration

Questions 281-282

A three-week-old girl is brought to the emergency room with a two-day history of fever, nonproductive cough, and tachypnea. Physical examination reveals marked intercostal retractions and nasal flaring. Rhonchi are audible over both lung fields. The patient is inactive and has poor muscle tone. The total white blood cell count is 20,000/mm^3 with a marked shift to the left. This infant's chest x-ray is shown below.

281. Laboratory investigations that may be beneficial in determining the etiologic agent for this patient's lower respiratory tract infection include

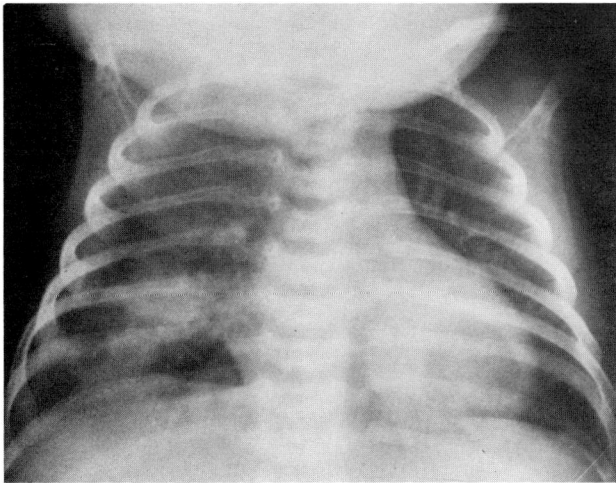

  ✓(1) blood culture
  (2) rapid cold agglutinins test
  ✓(3) counter immunoelectrophoresis
  (4) nitroblue tetrazolium dye test

282. This infant's chest x-ray is consistent with a diagnosis of

  (1) chlamydial pneumonia
  (2) pneumococcal pneumonia
  (3) *Pneumocystis carinii* pneumonia
  ✓(4) staphylococcal pneumonia

283. In a nonatopic child, asthma may be associated with

  ✓(1) aspirin
  ✓(2) food dyes
  ✓(3) a history of influenza
  ✓(4) exercise

284. A 12-year-old boy with seasonal allergic rhinitis and asthma is evaluated for a two-week history of mild wheezing. He is noted to have some wheezing bilaterally before isoproterenol inhalation; however, after isoproterenol inhalation, the wheezing is partially cleared. Wheezing in this patient is most likely due to

  ✓(1) peripheral airway smooth muscle contraction
  ✓(2) peripheral airway mucosal edema
  ✓(3) mucus in the peripheral airways
  (4) absence of β-adrenergic receptors in peripheral airway smooth muscle

285. An 18-year-old patient presents with a sudden onset of shortness of breath and left-sided chest pain. The patient's symptoms and his chest x-ray shown below demonstrate a condition that

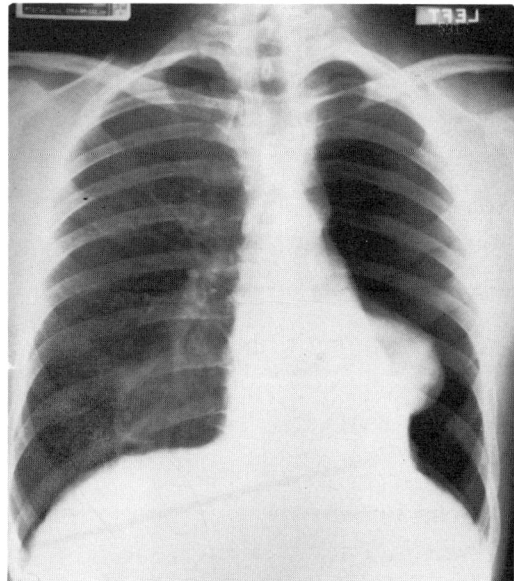

  (1) is unusual except in late adolescence
  ✓(2) can be a complication of status asthmaticus
  (3) is more frequent in adolescent girls than in adolescent boys
  ✓(4) is similar pathologically to pulmonary interstitial emphysema

286. Valuable maneuvers in pediatric cardiopulmonary resuscitation include

  ✓(1) the application of direct pressure over the cricoid cartilage during endotracheal intubation
  (2) intratracheal administration of sodium bicarbonate
  ✓(3) intratracheal administration of epinephrine
  (4) precordial thump in a witnessed cardiac arrest

DIRECTIONS: The groups of questions below consist of lettered choices followed by several numbered items. For each numbered item select the **one** lettered choice with which it is **most** closely associated. Each lettered choice may be used once, more than once, or not at all.

Questions 287-290

For each clinical description below, select the expiratory spirogram in the figure below with which it is most likely associated.

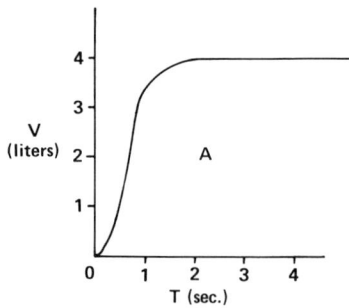

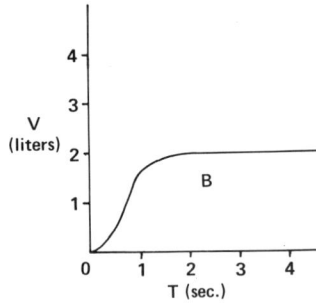

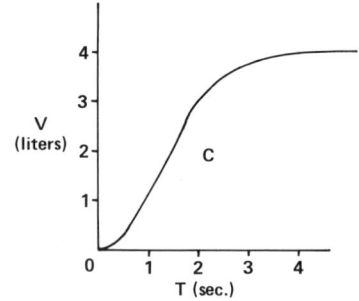

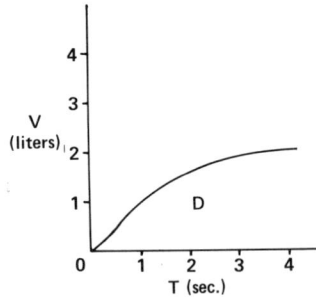

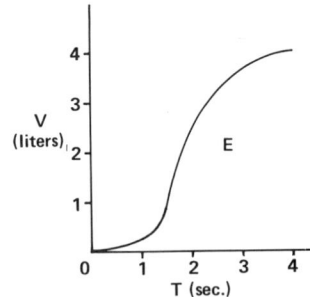

287. A 15-year-old boy with marked kyphoscoliosis

288. A 15-year-old boy who has a history of asthma and is having an acute attack of bronchospasm

289. A 15-year-old boy with pectus excavatum

290. A 15-year-old boy who has a history of asthma and who had an acute attack of bronchospasm five days ago

Questions 291-294

For each syndrome below, select the cardiac defect with which it most often is associated.

(A) Supravalvular aortic stenosis
(B) Aortic aneurysm
(C) Cardiomyopathy
(D) Pulmonary stenosis
(E) Atrioventricular canal defect

291. Trisomy 21

292. Hypercalcemia syndrome

293. Noonan's syndrome

294. Marfan's syndrome

Questions 295-298

For each syndrome below, select the cardiac defect with which it is most often associated.

(A) Ventricular septal defects
(B) Arterial thromboses
(C) Coronary artery aneurysms
(D) Coarctation of aorta
(E) Patent ductus arteriosus

295. Turner's syndrome

296. Fetal alcohol syndrome

297. Rubella syndrome

298. Mucocutaneous lymph node syndrome

Questions 299-301

The oxygen-carrying capability of blood varies with age and disease states. For each clinical situation listed below, select the oxyhemoglobin dissociation curve shown in the graph below with which it is most likely to be associated. (Assume that curve B reflects normal hemoglobin, pH, and body temperature.)

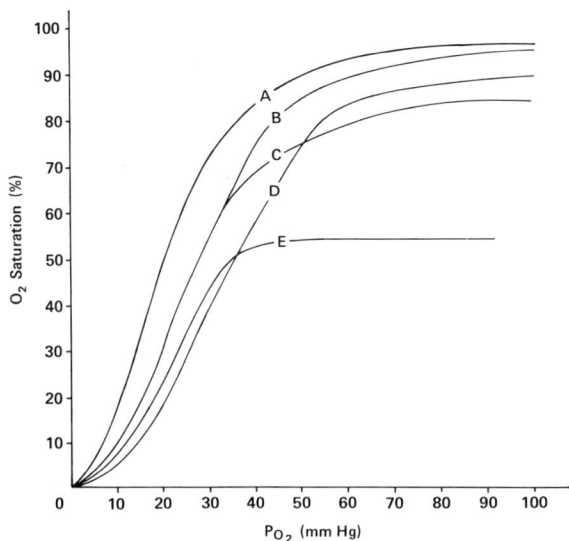

299. A normal fetus at eight months gestation

300. A three-year-old child with fever and acidosis

301. A five-year-old child with an increased concentration of D-2-3-diphosphoglycerate

Questions 302-304

For each clinical situation below, select the arterial blood gas description with which it is most likely to be associated.

(A) Normal pH, normal P_{CO_2}, elevated HCO_3
(B) Elevated pH, decreased P_{CO_2}, normal HCO_3
(C) Normal pH, elevated P_{CO_2}, elevated HCO_3
(D) Decreased pH, elevated P_{CO_2}, normal HCO_3
(E) Decreased pH, decreased P_{CO_2}, elevated HCO_3

302. An 18-year-old girl with slowly-progressive, severe cystic fibrosis

303. A five-year-old boy with acute status asthmaticus and impending respiratory failure

304. A ten-year-old boy with hyperventilation secondary to a central nervous system infection

Cardiology and Pulmonology

Answers

253. The answer is B. *(Hoekelman, p 1530.)* The incidence of congenital heart disease is estimated to be 1 per 100 live births. This figure may well be an underestimate in view of the high frequency of spontaneous closure of small ventricular septal defects in the neonatal period. Furthermore, aortic valve stenosis due to a congenital bicuspid aortic valve may not become clinically apparent until adulthood.

254. The answer is D. *(Hoekelman, p 1516.)* Tetralogy of Fallot usually is characterized by **decreased** pulmonary blood flow because the resistance to right ventricular emptying imposed by the infundibular stenosis is greater than systemic vascular resistance. Therefore, a significant fraction of the right ventricular stroke volume will pass through the ventricular defect into the ascending aorta with resultant arterial hypoxemia. The decrease in systemic vascular resistance seen with exercise results in a larger right-to-left shunt and an accentuation of cyanosis. Increased pulmonary blood flow is seen in total anomalous pulmonary venous return, truncus arteriosus, transposition of the great vessels, and aortic atresia.

255. The answer is E. *(Rudolph, ed 16. pp 1410-1411, 1480-1484.)* Digitalis, diuretics, and fluid restriction are the major components of therapy for congestive heart failure and are usually employed as initial therapy for a premature infant with heart failure due to a large patent ductus arteriosus. Recent experience has demonstrated that indomethacin inhibits the production of prostaglandin synthetase, with a resultant drop in the level of circulating prostaglandins and consequent closure of the patent ductus in preterm infants. The exact mechanism by which ductal closure occurs is as yet unknown, but pharmacologic closure of the ductus is successful in a significant percentage of premature infants with a symptomatic ductus. Prostaglandin E_1 has been shown to dilate the ductus arteriosus, particularly in infants who are dependent upon the ductus as a source of pulmonary blood flow. Therefore, prostaglandin E_1 would be contraindicated in the management of congestive failure due to a large patent ductus in a preterm infant.

256. The answer is E. *(Kawabori, Pediatr Clin North Am 25:790-792, 1978. Rudolph, ed 16. pp 1466-1467.)* The underdeveloped or hypoplastic left heart syndrome is the most common cause of severe, low output congestive heart failure in the first week of life. Infants may appear normal for a brief time after birth. The entity becomes clinically manifest when the ductus arteriosus, which supplies systemic blood flow, begins to constrict. Inability to locate a septal Q wave and therefore true left ventricular forces is a characteristic feature of this syndrome; it serves to differentiate an underdeveloped left heart from other entities such as septic shock and coarctation of the aorta, both of which can be associated with a low systemic blood flow. Congenital heart lesions such as a ventricular septal defect or truncus arteriosus usually do not present with heart failure until later in infancy when pulmonary vascular resistance is lower than in early infancy.

257. The answer is B. *(Hoekelman, pp 1512-1514. Rudolph, ed 16. pp 1413-1416.)* A pansystolic murmur of even amplitude at the lower left sternal border is quite characteristic of a ventricular septal defect. A similar murmur can result from atrioventricular valve insufficiency, but left ventricular hypertrophy would not be expected in a patient with tricuspid regurgitation, and the murmur of mitral insufficiency usually is audible at the cardiac apex. A pansystolic regurgitant murmur and left ventricular hypertrophy are not features of an atrial defect or a total anomaly of pulmonary venous return. Most patients with a complete atrioventricular canal defect do not have a normal axis on an electrocardiogram, but instead exhibit an extreme left axis deviation. The absence of a continuous murmur at the upper left sternal border and full or bounding pulses would dictate against a patent ductus arteriosus.

258. The answer is A. *(Hoekelman, pp 1538-1539. Rudolph, ed 16. pp 1400-1401.)* Unifocal atrial or ventricular premature beats, occurring in healthy children or adolescents, that are not related closely to the preceding T wave and that disappear with exercise, usually are considered to be benign entities. On the other hand, ventricular ectopic beats occurring in the setting of organic heart disease, multifocal premature beats, ectopic beats occurring in sequence, and ventricular premature contractions that fall on or near a preceding T wave should be considered as serious and potentially life-threatening dysrhythmias. A patient with one or more of the latter abnormalities should be referred quickly to a cardiologist for further investigation. Ventricular dysrhythmias occur most often in the first few months of life. These dysrhythmias are also observed in preadolescent children, most often males with apparently normal hearts.

259. The answer is A. *(Hoekelman, pp 1512-1513. Rudolph, ed 16. pp 1418-1419.)* Children with significant secundum-type atrial defects frequently are not referred to a cardiologist until a heart murmur is noted on a routine examination or an enlarged heart is detected on a chest x-ray obtained for other reasons. Most children with atrial defects are asymptomatic, but occasionally there is a history of fatigue with exertion or recurrent lower respiratory infections. Physical examination usually reveals a small child with precordial hyperactivity, a systolic flow murmur at the upper left sternal border due to relative pulmonary stenosis, and a wide, fixed splitting of the second sound, which is probably related to a prolongation of right ventricular ejection. If a large left-to-right shunt is present, a soft mid-diastolic murmur at the lower left sternal border due to relative tricuspid stenosis may be audible. Electrocardiograms reveal a normal or mild right axis and right ventricular hypertrophy with a typical RS-R pattern. On chest x-ray, cardiomegaly with prominence of the right heart and increased pulmonary blood flow are seen.

260. The answer is A. *(Hoekelman, p 1509. Rudolph, ed 16. pp 1469-1471.)* Bacterial endocarditis is a very rare complication in patients with a typical secundum atrial defect. Generally, a high velocity, turbulent blood flow, which occurs with the other four choices, is thought to be important in the pathogenesis of infective endocarditis. Growth of microorganisms may be encouraged by an abnormal jet of blood striking the opposite endocardium, causing a thickening called a jet lesion. Since the velocity of blood flow across an atrial defect is low and associated with very little turbulence, the integrity of the endocardium remains intact and the incidence of endocarditis is extremely low.

261. The answer is D. *(Hoekelman, p 1528.)* The postpericardiotomy syndrome is a relatively common, but usually quite benign, complication of cardiac surgery in which the pericardium is opened. The usual findings include the presence of persistent fever beyond the first postoperative week, pleural and pericardial reactions, fatigue, leukocytosis with a mild left shift, and an elevated sedimentation rate. Pleural and pericardial effusions are often present, and in the presence of pericardial fluid, a pericardial friction rub may not be audible. The presence of antiheart antibodies in significant titers in a patient with a suspected postpericardiotomy syndrome has raised the question of an autoimmune reaction. However, a viral illness may play an important role as well. While there is usually only one episode of illness, there may be recurrences months or even years later. Therapy includes bed rest and the administration of anti-inflammatory agents such as aspirin or steroids. The postperfusion syndrome characterized by the fever, splenomegaly, and atypical lymphocytosis does not appear until three to six weeks after cardiac surgery. Bacterial endocarditis is associated with a high velocity, turbulent blood flow. Rheumatic heart disease is not usually associated with surgery.

262. The answer is D. *(Hoekelman, pp 1513-1514.)* Electrocardiographic findings of an extreme left axis deviation, prolongation of atrioventricular conduction, and a right ventricular conduction delay as shown in the electrocardiogram that accompanies the question are characteristic of an atrioventricular canal defect. Right ventricular hypertrophy is seen on the electrocardiograms of patients with an atrial defect or a partial anomaly of the pulmonary venous return. Occasionally, a prolonged P-R interval can be seen, but the electrical axis in the frontal plane is normal or more commonly is placed to the right in these anomalies. Patients with aortic valve stenosis will have either normal forces or evidence of left ventricular hypertrophy. Right axis deviation, right ventricular hypertrophy, and a normal atrioventricular conduction time are found in tetralogy of Fallot patients.

263. The answer is C. *(Hoekelman, p 1516.)* Characteristic features of tetralogy of Fallot include a large high ventricular septal defect, pulmonary stenosis at the infundibular and occasionally the valvular level, overriding of the ventricular septum by the aorta, and hypertrophy of the right ventricular musculature. A patent foramen ovale, right aortic arch, and a prominent conus coronary artery are other less common anatomic findings in this entity. Since pulmonary blood flow usually is reduced in patients with tetralogy, enlargement of the left atrium would not be expected. Although the heart is not enlarged, a boot-shaped contour is often seen on x-ray.

264. The answer is E. *(Hoekelman, p 1496. Rudolph, ed 16. pp 1363-1364.)* Venous hums are a frequent benign finding in childhood and are thought to arise from turbulent flow among the cervical veins entering the superior thoracic cavity. A venous hum is a continuous low-pitched murmur that can be grade III-IV/VI in intensity. Maneuvers that reduce or abolish the velocity of flow in these venous channels, thus causing the venous hum to disappear, are compression of the veins, a Valsalva maneuver, and assumption of a supine position. The murmur of a patent ductus usually does not vary with changes in position and typically is louder in systole, whereas a venous hum usually is more prominent in diastole. Pulmonary arteriovenous fistulae are associated with cyanosis and frequently are silent. Murmurs arising from cerebral arteriovenous fistulae and from a ventricular defect with aortic insufficiency typically are louder in systole, do not vary significantly with positional changes, and usually are associated with a hyperdynamic precordium.

265. The answer is E. *(Feldman, Am J Dis Child 133:641-644, 1979.)* *Staphylococcus aureus* and *Hemophilus influenzae* are the most common etiologic agents in acute bacterial pericarditis during childhood. This is a rare but potentially life-threatening disease. It occurs with greatest frequency among children under the age of four. Usually an organ system other than the heart is infected, and the pericarditis probably occurs as a result of a bacteremia. Surgical drainage of the pericardial space and appropriate systemic antibiotic therapy constitute management.

266. The answer is B. *(Hoekelman, p 1515.)* Chest x-rays of patients with tetralogy of Fallot characteristically reveal a normal heart size, an uptilted apex, decreased pulmonary blood flow, and a small or concave conus of the main pulmonary artery. Hypoplasia of the right ventricular outflow tract, which may include the proximal main pulmonary artery, is an essential feature of tetralogy. A right aortic arch is seen in approximately 25 percent of patients with this anomaly. A boot-shaped heart contour is frequently seen in x-rays of tetralogy of Fallot patients.

267. The answer is C. *(Hoekelman, p 1467. Kendig, ed 3. pp 177-183.)* There are numerous factors that predispose the young infant to lower respiratory tract infection. The cough reflex of infants is less effective than that of adults because of underdeveloped accessory muscles of respiration. There is a relative immunologic incompetence and inexperience with exposure to infectious agents, as well as numerous contacts with other infants of similar age with respiratory infections. Airway resistance is 15 times greater than in adults, primarily because the infant has relatively narrow peripheral airways. Collateral ventilation is also suboptimal, as collateral pathways, such as the pores of Kohn, are not fully developed in early childhood. The total number of conducting airways in an infant, however, is the same as in an adult after about the third month of gestation.

268. The answer is D. *(Hoekelman, pp 1845-1846.)* Cystic fibrosis involves multiple organ systems. In addition to the pathophysiologic hallmarks of (1) pancreatic enzyme deficiency, (2) progressive, chronic, obstructive, infective, and destructive pulmonary disease, and (3) elevated sweat sodium and chloride concentrations, numerous other manifestations have been described, generally secondary to thick mucus secretions or abnormal secretory electrolyte concentrations. When taken together, these manifestations generally point to cystic fibrosis being a generalized disease of exocrine gland function. Despite vigorous investigation, however, the basic defect has not yet been determined. While the other problems listed do occur, they are secondary manifestations of the underlying defect.

269. The answer is C. *(Hoekleman, pp 1479-1480.)* Sedatives and tranquilizers are contraindicated in patients with status asthmaticus because they depress respirations, increase pulmonary-vascular resistance, and may enhance the release of histamine. All the other therapeutic measures listed are indicated to treat the specific problems associated with status asthmaticus. Bronchospasm may be treated with intravenous theophylline and aerosolized β-adrenergic agents. Corticosteroids will also aid bronchodilatation. Hypoxia can be a problem because of the development of ventilation-to-profusion mismatch. Humidified oxygen should be used in sufficient concentrations to keep the arterial P_{O_2} above 60 mm Hg. Hydration must be monitored, as these patients tend to become dehydrated due to decreased intake as well as increased losses from vomiting, diaphoresis, and hyperventilation.

270. The answer is E. *(Hoekleman, pp 1848-1849.)* Neither sweat testing nor any other laboratory test presently available accurately determines the cystic fibrosis carrier state. The only definitive means of identifying the carrier is by family history. Cystic fibrosis is an autosomal recessive disease. Both parents must be carriers in order for a child to have cystic fibrosis. Healthy siblings of cystic fibrosis patients have a 66 percent chance of being a carrier. Assuming that each of the parents is a carrier and not a victim of the disease, the chance of the same parents producing a carrier with a subsequent pregnancy is 50 percent.

271. The answer is D. *(Hoekelman, pp 1472-1474.)* Bronchiolitis is predominantly a viral disease, although on rare occasions bacteria may produce a similar syndrome. The most common etiology is respiratory syncytial virus (RSV). Attempts have been made to produce a vaccine against RSV; however, it has been found that killed RSV vaccines predispose to more serious illness following subsequent natural infection with this virus. Live attenuated RSV virus vaccines have also been studied. These will produce intranasal immunity when given by that route but will not produce immunity in the lower respiratory tract. Other viruses, including parainfluenza 1 and 3 and influenza, have been associated with bronchiolitis, although less commonly than has RSV.

272. The answer is A. *(Hoekelman, pp 1472-1473.)* The x-ray that accompanies the question shows the typical roentgenographic appearance of bronchiolitis—that is, hyperinflated lungs without significant infiltrates in a young infant. Infants with bronchiolitis uniformly are tachypneic. The disease is most common in infants under six months of age. It is rarely diagnosed after the age of two years. Cyanosis is a common but not a universal feature. Fever is not present consistently and is usually low grade when it is present. The white count is usually within normal limits. Hepatomegaly is generally not present unless heart failure develops as a complication. Sometimes lobar consolidation or atelectasis is found. The possibility exists that small areas of infiltrate or atelectasis are canceled out by radiopaque areas, an effect that gives a general appearance of a normal lung.

273. The answer is A (1, 2, 3). *(Rudolph, ed 16. p 1386.)* Right axis deviation and significant right ventricular hypertrophy, manifested by a pure tall R wave in the right precordial leads, are commonly seen in cardiac anomalies that have, as part of their pathophysiology, systemic pressure in the right ventricle. Examples include tetralogy of Fallot, transposition of the great arteries, and severe pulmonary valve stenosis. In the latter instance, suprasystemic right ventricular pressures may be present with a strain pattern, sharply inverted T waves, and ST segment depression present in the right precordial leads. Electrocardiograms (like the one presented in the question) obtained from patients with an underdeveloped right ventricle, as found in tricuspid atresia, will have a paucity of right ventricular forces.

274. The answer is E (all). *(Rudolph, ed 16. pp 1446-1447.)* Diseases of the central nervous system in neonates can cause respiratory depression and, consequently, alveolar hypoventilation and arterial hypoxemia. Peripheral cyanosis can be seen in polycythemic infants, but central cyanosis also can occur with red blood cell sludging in small vessels of the central nervous system and pulmonary vascular bed. Intermittent bi-directional atrial level shunting can occur through a patent foramen ovale as a result of similar atrial afterloads in the early neonatal period. Since all systemic venous return bypasses the tricuspid valve and flows into the left atrium in patients with tricuspid atresia, cyanosis is present; however, the degree of desaturation is dependent upon the magnitude of pulmonary blood flow. Reports of cyanosis (blueness or duskiness) in newborns require immediate attention. Many of the causes of cyanosis can result in rapid deterioration of the infant.

275. The answer is E (all). *(Hoekelman, p 1524.)* The knee-chest position, oxygen, and morphine sulfate constitute the standard acute management of a hypercyanotic spell in a tetralogy of Fallot patient. If these measures are unsuccessful and a severe spell with loss of consciousness, seizures or bradycardia persists, intravenous bicarbonate and propranolol may be necessary to relieve the spell. Oral propranolol has been shown to decrease the frequency and severity of such episodes, but palliative or reparative surgery should be performed to ensure adequate pulmonary blood flow.

276. The answer is C (2, 4). *(Hoekelman, pp 1540-1546. Rudolph, ed 16. p 1403.)* Conduction disturbances such as complete atrioventricular dissociation with a slow idioventricular rate can occur in the setting of diffuse or focal myocarditis and can result in Stokes-Adams attacks with loss of consciousness and seizure activity due to an inadequate cerebral blood flow. Management includes the insertion of a temporary transvenous pacemaker to ensure a satisfactory ventricular rate and cardiac output. Until a pacing wire is inserted, an infusion of isoproterenol can be given to increase the idioventricular rate. Digitalis prolongs atrioventricular conduction and therefore would be relatively contraindicated in the presence of intermittent complete heart block. Atropine has less of an effect on the distal or ventricular conduction system than it has on atrial or junctional tissue and is usually of little benefit in third degree heart block.

277. The answer is D (4). *(Rudolph, ed 16. p 1411.)* Elective closure of a small patent ductus arteriosus during early childhood generally is advised because of the risk of developing bacterial arteritis (endocarditis) in later life. The infection usually occurs on the wall of the pulmonary artery at the site of a jet lesion opposite the orifice of the ductus. Since pulmonary blood flow is only mildly increased and, consequently, the cardiac hemodynamic burden is slight, congestive heart failure, atrial arrhythmias, and pulmonary vascular disease would not be expected.

278. The answer is E (all). *(Rudolph, ed 16. pp 1414-1416.)* Congestive heart failure is a relatively frequent feature in the natural history of significant ventricular defects, usually occurring between one and three months of age, when pulmonary vascular resistance reaches its nadir. Spontaneous closure as a consequence of growth of tissue at the margins of the defect, or apposition of the septal leaflet of the tricuspid valve to the defect is another event quite frequently associated with significant ventricular events. The development of infundibular hypertrophy is unusual. However, when it does occur the development is rapid, and left-to-right shunting may be present for a short period. Cyanosis, occurring initially on exercise, soon follows but gradually becomes more persistent. Features similar to those of tetralogy of Fallot can develop. Aortic insufficiency, due to prolapse of either the right or noncoronary cusp, also is uncommon, but occurs more frequently with supracristal ventricular septal defects.

279. The answer is E (all). *(Hoekelman, pp 1468, 1472-1473, 1480.)* Several sets of criteria for assessing the possibility of respiratory failure have been developed for infants and children. These are usually broken down into clinical and laboratory or physiologic criteria. The clinical criteria usually considered are: (1) a decrease or loss of audible inspiratory breath sounds, (2) increased severity of retractions and use of accessory musculature, (3) changes in mental status ranging from depression or agitation to coma, (4) reduced skeletal muscle tone, and (5) observable cyanosis despite the administration of supplemental oxygen. In obstructive lung disease, such as bronchiolitis or asthma, an increase in wheezing is usually associated with increased respiratory distress and potential respiratory failure. However, with severe obstruction, wheezing may actually diminish with impending respiratory failure because of the decreased air exchange.

280. The answer is B (1, 3). *(Kendig, ed 3. pp 447-448.)* The triad of sinusitis, situs inversus, and bronchiectasis was first described by Kartagener in 1933; however, not all patients who exhibit this triad of symptoms have Kartagener's syndrome. Later, investigators noted an increased frequency of nasal polyposis in these patients. The frequency of bronchiectasis in patients with congenital dextrocardia may be as high as 20 percent. Although patients with gamma globulin deficiencies or recurrent aspiration still may present with recurrent pneumonia and bronchiectasis, these two findings are not associated with Kartagener's syndrome.

281. The answer is B (1, 3). *(Hoekelman, pp 1469-1470.)* It is generally recommended that children being evaluated for pneumonia have at least one blood culture prior to starting antibiotic therapy, as this culture may yield a definitive pathogen. This information would be much more valuable than the results of a culture of the upper respiratory tract. Likewise, counter immunoelectrophoresis performed on the blood and urine may detect bacterial antigens in these patients. Staining white blood cells with nitroblue tetrazolium is not as useful as previously thought because it does not distinguish between viral and bacterial etiologies. In addition, the cold agglutinin determination is nonspecifically positive in patients with numerous types of viral illnesses, as well as those with *Mycoplasma pneumoniae* infections.

282. The answer is D (4). *(Kendig, ed 3. p 391.)* The presence of patchy consolidation and pneumatocele formation is most consistent with the diagnosis of staphylococcal pneumonia. The fluid-filled and air-filled cysts which develop may persist for months following acute infection. Complications can include pneumothorax and bronchopleural fistula. In one series of staphylococcal pneumonia patients, 21 percent developed pneumothorax and 13 percent developed an abscess or pneumatoceles. Pneumococcal pneumonia, while it does produce patchy consolidation or lobar consolidation, usually does not result in pneumatocele formation. Chlamydial pneumonia and *Pneumocystis* pneumonia also tend to produce more diffuse bilateral infiltrates in this age group.

283. The answer is E (all). *(Kendig, ed 3. pp 633-638.)* Asthma may be divided into allergic and nonallergic types, although both may coexist in a single child. Included in the nonallergic etiologies are postinfectious asthma, aspirin-induced asthma, and exercise-induced asthma. Postinfectious asthma is most common after measles, bronchiolitis, or influenza. After the initial insult to the lung, these children seem more prone to develop subsequent asthma attacks. Although some may have respiratory difficulties for the remainder of their lives, many tend to outgrow their problem. Aspirin-induced asthma is a well-known syndrome in adults, but may also be found in the pediatric age group. In addition to aspirin, other nonsteroidal anti-inflammatory agents and certain food dyes, such as tartrazine, may produce a similar syndrome. Exercise-induced bronchospasm is one of the most frequently described causes for wheezing in children. This syndrome is believed to be a manifestation of increased bronchial lability, which may be a genetic trait.

284. The answer is A (1, 2, 3). *(Hoekelman, pp 1083-1084, 1475.)* The pathophysiologic changes seen with asthma include mucosal edema, bronchospasm, and increased intraluminal secretions. These changes can all be secondary to a type I hypersensitivity reaction to specific allergens. Mediators released with the degranulation of mast cells can (1) increase vascular permeability with resultant tissue edema, (2) change smooth muscle tone with resultant bronchoconstriction, and (3) increase production of viscous mucus by bronchial goblet cells. The failure of a bronchodilating agent such as isoproterenol to reverse this patient's wheezing completely and the prolonged two-week history of wheezing suggest that mucosal edema and mucus in peripheral airways are probably present in addition to pure smooth muscle bronchoconstriction. However, the presence of a positive, although partial, response to isoproterenol inhalation indicates that there must be some β-adrenergic receptor function in this patient's peripheral airway smooth muscle.

285. The answer is C (2, 4). *(Hoekelman, pp 1482-1483.)* Pneumothorax in the pediatric age group occurs most frequently in the newborn period, although there is a second peak of increased incidence in late adolescence and early adulthood. The pathophysiologic mechanism of pneumothorax is thought to be an air leak from the alveolus into the interstitial tissues, secondary to the positive pressure gradient between these two spaces. The air, once having entered the interstitial tissue, can migrate along the vascular ray, producing pulmonary interstitial emphysema. The air can also dissect into the mediastinum, producing pneumomediastinum, or can rupture into the pleural space, producing pneumothorax. Conditions that predispose to the development of these conditions, therefore, include disorders such as status asthmaticus in which there is an increase in pressure gradient between the alveolus and the interstitial tissue. The reason for the increased incidence of spontaneous pneumothorax in adolescents is unclear. It has been found statistically to be more common in adolescent males than in females. It is not associated with any known underlying respiratory disease, although it is postulated that some structural weakness of the pulmonary tissues or pleura exists.

286. The answer is B (1, 3). *(Hoekleman, pp 1813-1819. Safar, pp 132-137. JAMA Suppl 227:847, 1974.)* After infancy, the trachea usually has sufficient rigidity to be able to occlude the potential space of the esophagus when direct pressure is applied on the cricoid cartilage. With this maneuver, even stomach contents under pressure may be prevented from entering the hypopharynx. The American Heart Association has never endorsed the precordial thump in the pediatric age group because the hazards involved outweigh the possible benefits. Several authors also question its usefulness in adults because of the likelihood of inducing ventricular fibrillation. The intrapulmonary route of drug administration is still experimental, but it has been shown to be extremely effective for certain medications. Slightly less effective, but still well absorbed from pulmonary circulation, are drugs delivered by the intratracheal route (via endotracheal tube). Epinephrine as well as lidocaine are thus absorbed, but sodium bicarbonate is too damaging to the pulmonary surfactant to be administered by this route. Sodium bicarbonate, administered intravenously, is often useful in the treatment of acidosis associated with cardiopulmonary arrest. However, sodium bicarbonate should not be used in situations where the removal of CO_2 is inadequate in the absence of adequate ventilation, or when cardiac arrest has been of such brief duration as to make acidosis unlikely.

287-290. The answers are: 287-B, 288-D, 289-A, 290-C. *(Polgar, 213-239.)* The expiratory spirogram is a graphic representation of the cumulative volume of air expelled during a forced expiratory maneuver. Three important measurements which can be obtained from the expiratory spirogram are: (1) forced vital capacity (FVC), (2) forced expiratory volume in the first second (FEV_1), and (3) forced expiratory volume in the first second as a percentage of total forced vital capacity ($FEV_1\%$). A normal 15-year-old boy of average height (170 cm or 5 feet 6 inches) should have a vital capacity of between 3 and 5 liters. The FEV_1 should be at least 75 percent of vital capacity.

Patients with marked chest deformities secondary to kyphoscoliosis have a restrictive type of lung disease characterized by a decrease in the total forced vital capacity and FEV_1, but a relatively normal $FEV_1\%$. On the other hand, patients with pectus excavatum, a relatively mild thoracic deformity, generally have normal pulmonary function, although gradual stiffening of the thorax can occur, a circumstance that may result in abnormalities in later life.

Patients with asthma have an obstructive type of pulmonary function abnormality, which is characterized by a decrease in the FEV_1 and the $FEV_1\%$. This decrease may persist even during clinically asymptomatic periods. During an acute attack of bronchospasm, a total forced vital capacity is also usually reduced.

291-294. The answers are: 291-E, 292-A, 293-D, 294-B. *(Noonan, Pediatr Clin North Am 25:797-816, 1978.)* Cardiac defects occur in approximately 40 percent of patients with Down's syndrome (trisomy 21) and account for a significant degree of morbidity during the infancy of these patients. Atrioventricular canal defects and ventricular defects are the anomalies most commonly associated with this syndrome, but atrial defects and tetralogies also occur.

The hypercalcemia syndrome is characterized by "elfin" facies, mental retardation, hypercalcemia during infancy, and supravalvular aortic stenosis. Other cardiovascular anomalies associated with this entity include peripheral pulmonary stenosis and stenosis of other major arterial vessels.

Valvular pulmonary stenosis is the most common cardiac lesion seen in patients with Noonan's syndrome, although atrial defects and aortic stenosis may also occur. Chromosomal studies are usually done when this syndrome is suspected. However, the diagnosis rests upon clinical recognition of the typical features, especially the facies, which resemble those found in Turner's syndrome.

Cystic medial necrosis with resultant aortic dilatation and the possibility of a dissecting aneurysm are features of Marfan's syndrome. Mitral valve prolapse is also a common finding in this connective tissue disorder. Cardiomyopathy is not associated with any of the syndromes in the question.

295-298. The answers are: 295-D, 296-A, 297-E, 298-C. *(Hoekelman, pp 355, 1525, Fujiwara, Pediatrics 61:100-107, 1978. Noonan, Pediatr Clin North Am 25:797-815, 1978.)* Twenty to thirty percent of patients with Turner's syndrome have congenital heart disease, usually coarctation of the aorta. Aortic stenosis may also occur and should receive early surgical treatment. Coarctation of the aorta in these patients should also be surgically corrected early in infancy if medical management is unsuccessful.

The incidence of cardiac defects in those with fetal alcohol syndrome ranges from 30 to 40 percent. The most frequent types of cardiac defects seen in this syndrome are ventricular and atrial septal defects. Tetralogy of Fallot also has been detected in a significant number of these patients. The effect of alcohol on the developing fetal heart probably is related to a genetic predisposition to heart disease.

Approximately 50 percent of patients with rubella syndrome have congenital heart defects, most commonly patent ductus arteriosus. Peripheral pulmonary artery stenosis and myocarditis are also found. Early surgical treatment is usually called for in patent ductus arteriosus.

One to two percent of patients with mucocutaneous lymph node syndrome (Kawasaki disease) die from the disease, usually because of cardiac lesions. Coronary artery aneurysms, which may be transient in nature, are a feature of Kawasaki disease. Rupture of an aneurysm, occlusion of a major coronary vessel, inflammation of the conduction system, and myocarditis can result in sudden death in these patients.

299-301. The answers are: 299-A, 300-D, 301-D. *(Kendig, ed 3. pp 32-35.)* The oxygen carrying capability of blood depends on the strong affinity of hemoglobin for oxygen, not on the solubility of oxygen in plasma. The steepness of the curve reflects the large changes in saturation that are possible with small changes in oxygen tension. This characteristic allows uptake of large quantities of oxygen in the lung, and release of similarly large quantities in the peripheral tissues, with only small changes in the P_{O_2}.

Fetal hemoglobin has an even higher affinity for oxygen, and this affinity is reflected by a shift of the curve to the left. This assures that, despite fetal P_{O_2} levels in the 30's, sufficient oxygen will be delivered to fetal tissues.

On the other hand, several factors that are present in respiratory disease states tend to shift the curve to the right, thereby decreasing the oxygen-carrying capability of the blood. Among these factors that shift the curve to the right are fever, acidosis, and increased P_{CO_2}. This property is of some benefit to the body, however, in that the (1) higher temperature, (2) lower pH, (3) and higher P_{CO_2} present in the peripheral tissues do help to increase oxygen extraction. However, when there is a generalized increase in these three factors throughout the body, total oxygen-carrying capacity is definitely reduced.

In a similar fashion, increased levels of D-2-3-diphosphoglycerate, which are found in red cells in certain conditions such as anemia, also tend to shift the oxyhemoglobin dissociation curve to the right. This shift aids in extraction of oxygen in the tissues in anemic states.

302-304. The answers are: 302-C, 303-D, 304-B. *(Hoekelman, p 1947.)* Measurement of arterial pH and P_{CO_2} and determination of bicarbonate (HCO_3), which can be done directly or calculated from the Henderson-Hasselbach equation, yield useful information regarding both respiratory and metabolic acid-base disturbances. In acute respiratory acidosis, as might be seen with acute respiratory insufficiency or failure from any etiology, the pH is usually decreased and the P_{CO_2} elevated. There usually has not been sufficient time for renal compensation for the acidosis; hence, bicarbonate is usually in the normal range.

In contrast, in the patient with long-standing respiratory insufficiency as might be seen with cystic fibrosis, although the P_{CO_2} can be elevated, the pH is usually maintained in the normal range by a compensatory increase in bicarbonate.

In patients with acute hyperventilation, either voluntary or induced by central nervous system disease such as infection or tumor, the P_{CO_2} is decreased with a concurrent rise in pH. However, if the hyperventilation is prolonged, pH may return to normal or near-normal levels, as total bicarbonate is reduced secondary to renal excretion.

Immunology and Infectious Diseases

DIRECTIONS: Each question below contains five suggested answers. Choose the **one best** response to each question.

305. In a private pediatric practice, what percentage of children with culture-proven GABHS tonsillitis can be expected to complete a ten-day course of penicillin as prescribed?

(A) 25 percent
(B) 45 percent
(C) 66 percent
(D) 80 percent
(E) 95 percent

306. A six-year-old boy presents with fever and isolated axillary lymphadenopathy. There is a 2 cm x 3 cm moderately tender, nonfluctuant node that is palpable. There is also a 2 mm papule on the upper arm. The boy has two kittens which he plays with frequently. The pediatrician should recommend which of the following treatment regimens?

(A) A ten-day course of dicloxacillin
(B) A ten-day course of tetracycline
(C) Needle aspiration for culture
(D) Observation for one month
(E) Surgical excision

307. A 16-year-old girl has low abdominal pain, fever, leukocytosis, and a vaginal discharge containing gram-negative intracellular diplococci. The initial treatment of this patient should include

(A) symptomatic treatment while awaiting culture results
(B) high dose intravenous penicillin therapy in the hospital
(C) 4.8 million units procaine penicillin intramuscularly with 1 g probenecid
(D) 3.5 g ampicillin with 1 g probenecid
(E) a surgical consultation

308. The most frequently encountered complication of mumps is

(A) pancreatitis
(B) thyroiditis
(C) meningoencephalitis
(D) deafness
(E) myocarditis

309. A ten-year-old child receives an appropriate dose of intramuscular benzylpenicillin for culture-proven streptococcal pharyngitis, which has been symptomatic for 24 hours. Ten days later, the child develops fever, generalized urticaria, migratory polyarthralgias, and lymphadenopathy. He is somewhat uncomfortable, but not acutely ill. The pediatrician should tell the parents that the child

(A) is not at risk for future similar symptoms
(B) may develop permanent joint damage
(C) will require corticosteroid therapy
(D) will recover without sequelae
(E) none of the above

310. All of the following statements concerning pertussis are true EXCEPT that

(A) pneumonia is the most frequent complication
(B) transplacental immunity does not exist
(C) antibiotic therapy does not shorten the duration of the paroxysmal cough
(D) the syndrome is associated with *Bordetella bronchiseptica* infections
(E) fever is characteristically present in the paroxysmal cough stage

311. Gram-positive rods are seen in the cerebrospinal fluid of an ill three-day-old infant. The most likely pathogen is

(A) *Clostridium tetani*
(B) *Listeria monocytogenes*
(C) *Corynebacterium diphtheriae*
(D) *Lactobacillus* species
(E) none of the above

312. A patient with documented immediate-type penicillin hypersensitivity requires parenteral therapy for a serious infection caused by penicillinase-producing *Staphylococcus aureus*. Which of the following drugs should be prescribed?

(A) Clindamycin
(B) Erythromycin
(C) Vancomycin
(D) Cephalosporin
(E) Trimethoprim-sulfamethoxazole

313. A three-year-old boy experiences the onset of a maculopapular rash following an upper respiratory infection. The rash, located on the buttocks and lower legs, starts out as an urticarial maculopapular eruption that becomes purpuric over a period of 24 hours. He complains of intermittent abdominal pain. Physical examination reveals periorbital, knee, and ankle periarticular swelling. All of the following laboratory results are consistent with the most likely diagnosis EXCEPT

(A) a normal platelet count
(B) proteinuria
(C) a decreased C3 level
(D) a negative antinuclear antibody
(E) a positive stool hematest

314. All of the following statements about X-linked hypogammaglobulinemia are true EXCEPT that

(A) the IgG level is less than 100 mg/100 ml
(B) B cells are absent
(C) there is a poor primary antibody response
(D) there is a poor secondary antibody response
(E) symptoms begin during the first three months of life

315. A 13-year-old boy sustains a severe wound of his right foot on a harrow (farm machine). He has received all of his childhood immunizations but has had none since starting school at age 6 years. In addition to debridement, tetanus prophylaxis should include

(A) penicillin, tetanus-diphtheria toxoid (TD), and tetanus immune globulin
(B) tetanus-diphtheria toxoid (TD) and tetanus immune globulin
(C) tetanus-diphtheria toxoid (TD)
(D) tetanus immune globulin
(E) none of the above

316. A child presents with an acute respiratory illness. The clinical feature that suggests ornithosis as the most likely diagnosis is

(A) a history of exposure to poultry
(B) a history of exposure to parrots or parakeets
(C) the presence of headache, fever, and muscle aches
(D) an x-ray finding of a lobar pneumonia
(E) an x-ray finding of an interstitial pneumonia

317. All of the following statements about T cells are true EXCEPT that

(A) they have a surface receptor for sheep red blood cells
(B) they have a surface immunoglobulin as their antigen-binding receptor
(C) they produce lymphokines, such as migration inhibition factor
(D) they respond in a mixed lymphocyte culture
(E) they respond to phytohemagglutinin

318. Which of the following statements about *Pneumocystis carinii* pneumonia is true?

(A) It is treated most appropriately with 25 mg/kg/day of trimethoprim and 100 mg/kg/day of sulfamethoxazole
(B) It should be considered in the differential diagnosis of any child with pneumonia
(C) It is diagnosed best by an endobronchial brush biopsy
(D) It is characterized clinically by fever, tachypnea, and rales
(E) It is characterized by prolonged resistance to reinfection following recovery

319. All of the following statements about immune serum globulin are true EXCEPT that

(A) it provides protection against hepatitis A virus
(B) it has a half-life of 20-30 days
(C) it is given intramuscularly
(D) it may precipitate an anaphylactic reaction
(E) it corrects mucosal antibody deficiency

320. *Mycoplasma pneumoniae* infection has been associated clinically with all of the following manifestations EXCEPT for

(A) Stevens-Johnson syndrome
(B) glomerulonephritis
(C) pneumonia
(D) hemolytic anemia
(E) Guillain-Barré syndrome

321. The antibiotic therapy most likely to be effective against pneumonia due to *Chlamydia trachomatis* would be

(A) amoxicillin
(B) erythromycin
(C) penicillin
(D) trimethoprim-sulfamethoxazole
(E) none of the above antibiotics

322. All of the following statements about IgA deficiency are true EXCEPT that

(A) it occurs in 1 in 500 individuals
(B) it is treated with immune serum globulin
(C) patients form large amounts of IgG antibodies to foreign protein
(D) there is an association with chromosome 18 abnormalities
(E) the greatest number of associated diseases are of an autoimmune nature

323. A nine-month-old infant presents two days after exposure to measles. The immediate management should include

(A) immunization with killed measles virus
(B) immunization with live measles virus
(C) immunization with live measles virus and the administration of killed measles virus
(D) administration of immune serum globulin
(E) observation only, until signs of illness appear

324. A seven-week-old infant presents with coughing for one week and failure to gain weight. Gestation and delivery were uneventful; however, conjunctivitis was noted in the second week of life. There have been no respiratory infections in the family, and there is no family history of allergies. Physical examination reveals a dyspneic and coughing child who does not appear toxic. The tympanic membranes are opaque and bulging, and their landmarks are obscured. The lungs are clear to auscultation. The white blood cell count is 15,000, including 50% segmented forms, 6% band forms, 26% lymphocytes, 7% monocytes, and 11% eosinophils. The chest x-ray is shown below. The most likely diagnosis is pneumonitis caused by

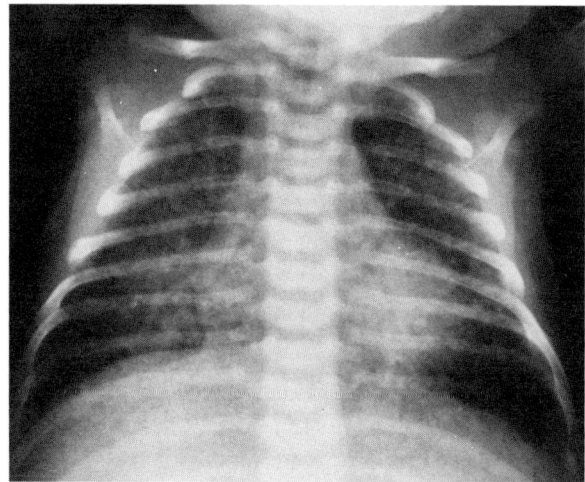

(A) respiratory syncytial virus
(B) a parainfluenza virus
(C) *Streptococcus (Diplococcus) pneumoniae*
(D) *Chlamydia trachomatis*
(E) *Bordetella pertussis*

325. All of the following statements about asplenia or splenic dysfunction are true EXCEPT that

(A) immune serum globulin is indicated in the treatment of this condition
(B) associated sepsis is most commonly caused by *Streptococcus (Diplococcus) pneumoniae* and *Hemophilus influenzae*
(C) it is diagnosed by the finding of Howell-Jolly bodies in peripheral blood smears
(D) the risk of sepsis is less if splenectomy is performed for trauma rather than for thalassemia
(E) immunization with pneumococcal polysaccharide vaccine is indicated if the affected child is older than age two years

326. A family history of a similar disease in a male uncle of a patient is compatible with all of the following EXCEPT for

(A) chronic granulomatous disease
(B) Wiskott-Aldrich syndrome
(C) congenital agammaglobulinemia
(D) severe combined immunodeficiency
(E) DiGeorge's syndrome

DIRECTIONS: Each question below contains four suggested answers of which **one** or **more** is correct. Choose the answer

A	if	**1, 2, and 3**	are correct
B	if	**1 and 3**	are correct
C	if	**2 and 4**	are correct
D	if	**4**	is correct
E	if	**1, 2, 3, and 4**	are correct

327. A three-year-old child who has had age-appropriate immunizations and whose last diphtheria booster was at 18 months of age is bitten on the hand by the family's pet cat. The area around the bite rapidly develops signs of cellulitis. The treatment regimen for this child should include

(1) human rabies immune globulin and duck embryo rabies vaccine
(2) human tetanus immune globulin
(3) chloramphenicol
(4) penicillin

328. A two-year-old previously well child presents in the emergency room with an acute onset of petechiae and fever. Initial workup of this child should include

(1) a blood culture
(2) a buffy coat examination
(3) a bone marrow aspiration
(4) an antinuclear antibody test

329. Mebendazole is effective therapy for infestations caused by

(1) *Trichuris trichuria*
(2) *Enterobius vermicularis*
(3) *Ascaris lumbricoides*
(4) *Ancylostoma duodenale*

330. Viral encephalitis is characterized by which of the following statements?

(1) It is most frequently associated with common childhood infections—measles, mumps, rubella, and varicella—when the cause is known
(2) It is fatal in approximately 25 percent of the cases caused by arboviruses
(3) It is characteristically associated with increased cerebrospinal fluid (CSF) pressure, CSF pleocytosis of 40-400 mononuclear cells, and normal or slightly elevated CSF glucose and protein
(4) It is best treated with corticosteroids

331. True statements about Rocky Mountain spotted fever include which of the following?

(1) Ampicillin plus gentamicin is effective therapy
(2) It is caused by a tick-borne rickettsia
(3) It is most common in the Rocky Mountain states
(4) If untreated, the fatality rate is about five percent

332. Components of the immune system known to respond to *Hemophilus influenzae* infection include which of the following?

(1) IgG antibody
(2) Polymorphonuclear white blood cells
(3) Complement
(4) T killer cells

333. Pneumonia caused by *Klebsiella pneumoniae* is characterized by which of the following statements?

(1) It occurs primarily in debilitated individuals
(2) It commonly is spread by contaminated humidification equipment
(3) It frequently is associated with bacteremia
(4) It may be suspected by the appearance of lobar consolidation with bulging fissures on x-ray

334. Correct statements concerning lymphocytic choriomeningitis virus include which of the following?

(1) It may cause an influenza-like syndrome
(2) It may be isolated from pet hamsters
(3) It may be isolated from cerebrospinal fluid
(4) It is usually transmitted by person-to-person contact

335. Hereditary angioneurotic edema is characterized by

(1) decreased C4 and C2 during attacks
(2) decreased functional C1 esterase inhibitor
(3) nonpruritic subcutaneous edema precipitated by trauma
(4) relief of symptoms with epinephrine

336. Pending firm diagnosis of the disease in the animal, rabies prophylaxis should be instituted following the bite of a

(1) cat
(2) strange dog
(3) coyote
(4) rabbit

337. A deficiency of serum complement may be associated with

(1) recurrent pyogenic infections
(2) gonococcemia
(3) a systemic lupus erythematosus-like syndrome
(4) chronic moniliasis

338. Patients who are candidates for the pneumococcal polysaccharide vaccine (Pneumovax) would include

(1) a one-year-old child with sickle cell disease
(2) a three-year-old child with SS hemoglobin
(3) an 18-month-old child with nephrotic syndrome
(4) a six-year-old child who has had a posttrauma splenectomy

339. The history, physical examination, and laboratory data found in association with infantile botulism may include

(1) constipation
(2) cranial nerve weakness
(3) botulin toxins in the stool
(4) accentuation of deep tendon reflexes

340. Antibiotic prophylaxis therapy should be prescribed for which of the following individuals?

(1) A healthy 18-year-old boy whose college roommate has meningococcal meningitis
(2) A healthy four-year-old girl whose sister has been hospitalized with epiglottitis caused by *Hemophilus influenzae* type B
(3) a 16-year-old female who is asymptomatic and has a normal physical examination but whose sexual partner has gonorrhea
(4) A healthy ten-year-old child whose sister has leukemia and *Pneumocystis carinii* pneumonia

DIRECTIONS: The groups of questions below consist of lettered choices followed by several numbered items. For each numbered item select the **one** lettered choice with which it is **most** closely associated. Each lettered choice may be used once, more than once, or not at all.

Questions 341-343

For each disease listed below, select the graph that includes data most likely to be associated with it.

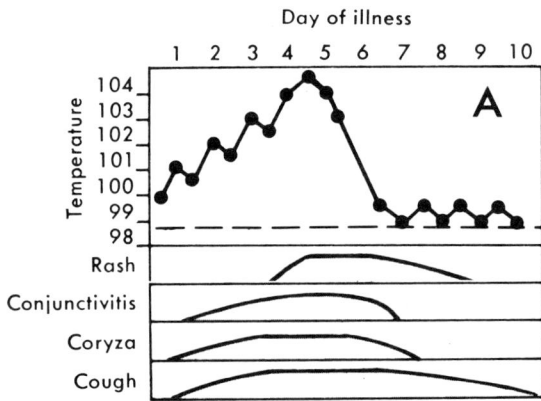

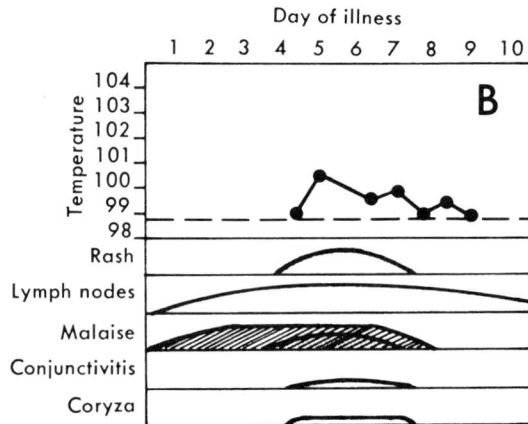

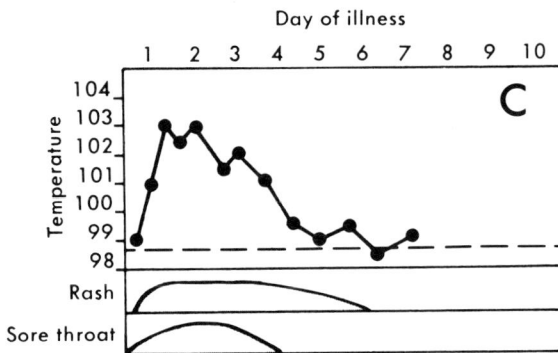

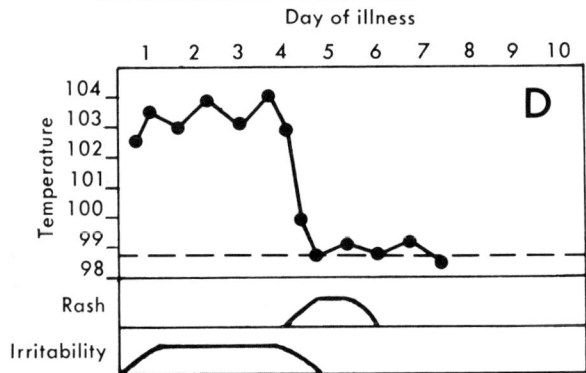

Adapted with permission of C.V. Mosby Company, from *Infectious Diseases of Children* (p 475), by Krugman S et al © 1977.

- (A) Graph **A**
- (B) Graph **B**
- (C) Graph **C**
- (D) Graph **D**
- (E) None of the above graphs

341. Roseola

342. Rubeola (measles)

343. Rubella

Questions 344-346

For each description that follows, select the immunoglobulin class with which it is most likely to be associated.

(A) IgA
(B) IgD
(C) IgE
(D) IgG
(E) IgM

344. Fixes to receptors on mast cells

345. Fixes to receptors on polymorphonuclear neutrophils

346. Covalently binds to a protein, which prevents its degradation by proteolytic enzymes

Questions 347-350

Gram-negative endotoxic shock results in a multisystem insult in which there is a series of pathophysiological events, some of which are listed below. For each pathophysiological event, select the clinical finding that is most likely to result.

(A) Hypotension
(B) Oliguria
(C) Hyperventilation
(D) Bleeding from several sites
(E) Fever

347. Release of endogenous pyrogens

348. Release of kinins, histamine, prostaglandins

349. Release of epinephrine and norepinephrine

350. Metabolic acidosis

Questions 351-353

For each immunoglobulin class listed below, select the curve on the graph with which it is most likely to be associated.

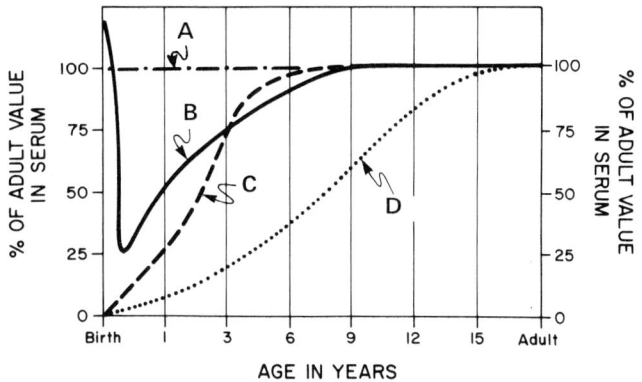

Used with permission of McGraw-Hill Book Company, from *Principles of Pediatrics: Health Care of the Young* (p 1063), by Hoekelman RA et al, ©1978 McGraw-Hill Inc.

(A) Curve A
(B) Curve B
(C) Curve C
(D) Curve D
(E) None of the above curves

351. IgA

352. IgG

353. IgM

Questions 354-356

For each disease listed below, select the combination of signs and symptoms with which it is most likely to be associated.

- (A) It is an influenza-like syndrome with fever, myalgia, headache, and a fine papular erythematous rash that is centrifugal in distribution
- (B) It begins with a low-grade fever and erythematous rash that first appears on the cheeks, spreads to the trunk, and fades to a lacy appearance
- (C) It presents as a high fever with no other sign; a macular rash involving the trunk and extremities appears on the fourth day when the fever fails
- (D) It begins with a posterior cervical, post-occipital lymphadenopathy followed by an enanthem on the soft palate and the development of a downward-spreading maculopapular rash and a low-grade fever
- (E) It presents with a high fever with the appearance of a maculopapular rash on the trunk, arthritis, and dysuria

354. Rubella

355. Early meningococcemia

356. Fifth disease (erythema infectiosum)

Questions 357-360

For each of the conditions listed below, which have an immunologic basis, select the operative immune response.

- (A) Type I reaginic (IgE) hypersensitivity reaction
- (B) Type II cytotoxic reaction
- (C) Type III immune complex reaction
- (D) Type IV T cell hypersensitivity reaction
- (E) None of the above reactions

357. Poststreptococcal glomerulonephritis

358. Reaction to x-ray contrast media

359. Poison ivy rash

360. Anaphylactic reaction to bee venom

Questions 361-364

For each clinical entity below, select the bacterial cause with which it is most likely to be associated.

- (A) *Hemophilus influenzae*
- (B) *Streptococcus (Diplococcus) pneumoniae*
- (C) *Staphylococcus* species
- (D) Group A streptococci
- (E) Group B streptococci

361. Meningitis in a two-year-old child

362. Osteomyelitis in an 18-month-old child

363. Septic arthritis in an eight-year-old child

364. Meningitis in a one-week-old infant

Questions 365-367

For each disease listed below, select the combination of signs and symptoms with which it is most likely to be associated.

- (A) Calcified pulmonary lesions, mediastinal lymph nodes, and a negative tuberculin skin test
- (B) Chills, fever, pneumonitis, macular erythematous rash, and arthralgia
- (C) Pyuria, fever, and flank pain
- (D) Chills, fever, and right upper quadrant pain
- (E) Afebrile episodes of wheezing and expectoration of brown mucus

365. Histoplasmosis

366. Coccidiodomycosis

367. Amebiasis

Immunology and Infectious Diseases

Answers

305. The answer is C. *(Hoekelman, pp 113-114.)* A well-designed study conducted in a private pediatric practice found that only 66 percent of children with tonsillitis due to GABHS completed a ten-day course of penicillin as prescribed. The compliance rate was higher if the child was seen by his or her regular pediatrician rather than a partner who was covering the practice. Compliance was also related to how long the patient had been under the physician's care and to the mother's perception of the seriousness of the illness.

306. The answer is D. *(Hoeprich, ed 2. pp 1194-1198.)* The patient presents with the typical findings of cat scratch fever, a disease that is usually transmitted by the scratch of a young cat. The patient should be observed for one month to ensure that the fever and the lymphadenopathy subside. The primary lesion presents most commonly as a papule, followed by swelling and tenderness of a regional lymph node. Antibiotics are of no value in cat scratch fever. Since the presentation is so typical, aspiration to identify a potentially treatable agent is not warranted, nor is excision of the node to rule out malignancy.

307. The answer is B. *(Hoekelman, p 653.)* This young patient has the features of acute salpingitis due to gonorrhea. The goal of treatment is to preserve patency of the fallopian tubes, and this is best achieved by high dose intravenous penicillin therapy. This therapy often results in the dramatic resolution of symptoms within 24 to 48 hours. However, penicillin therapy for ten days will eradicate all organisms and preserve tubal patency. It would not be prudent to await culture results before beginning penicillin therapy. Surgical intervention is contraindicated in acute pelvic inflammatory disease.

308. The answer is C. *(Hoekelman, p 1188.)* Infection with mumps may involve the pancreas, thyroid, gonads, meninges, cerebral cortex, and myocardium. Meningoencephalitis is the most common clinically evident complication, occurring in about ten percent of cases. The infection is usually mild without sequelae. Deafness is a very rare but serious complication of mumps, and myocarditis is an occasional complication among adults. Pancreatitis, a relatively rare but briefly severe complication, includes the following symptoms: high fever, severe epigastric pain, vomiting, chills, and prostration. These symptoms subside in three to seven days, and the patient usually recovers completely.

309. The answer is D. *(Hoekelman, pp 1346-1347. Middleton, pp 574, 578-581.)* The child described in the question has received adequate therapy parenterally for streptococcal disease. He developed the typical findings of serum sickness at the expected time interval, and he is not unusually ill. This is a self-limited disease from which he can be expected to recover completely. Because he has mild disease, corticosteroids are not indicated unless the patient is not symptomatically improved by salicylates, antihistamines, or both. If a patient has an adverse reaction to a drug, he would be at risk for future episodes of serum sickness or anaphylaxis from drugs or foreign proteins.

310. The answer is E. *(Hoekelman, pp 1211-1212. Vaughan, ed 11. pp 766-768.)* Whooping cough or pertussis has been associated with infection by *Bordetella pertussis* and *B. bronchiseptica* as well as with infection with adenovirus types 1, 2, 3, or 5. There does not appear to be any passive protection transmitted to newborns transplacentally. The disease is usually not accompanied by fever, unless complications (of which pneumonia is most common) occur. Pneumonia is the usual direct cause of deaths associated with pertussis, particularly in infants. Controlled studies have demonstrated that antibiotics do not alter the duration of symptoms, although they do decrease shedding of *B. pertussis.*

311. The answer is B. *(Hoekelman, pp 924, 1218.)* Although *Clostridium tetani, Listeria monocytogenes, Corynebacterium diphtheriae,* and *Lactobacillus* species are all gram-positive organisms, only *L. monocytogenes* is likely to be found in an ill infant's cerebrospinal fluid. This organism is one of the more common causes of meningitis in the neonatal period. *L. monocytogenes* may cause an early postpartum onset disease with pneumonia and shock. It may also present as a late onset illness characterized by meningitis. Therapy is with ampicillin or penicillin. Despite the inclusion of "monocytogenes" in the nomenclature of this organism, lymphocytosis of the cerebrospinal fluid is seen rarely.

312. The answer is A. *(Hoekelman, p 291.)* Although erythromycin, the cephalosporins, vancomycin, and trimethoprim-sulfamethoxazole all have some antistaphylococcal properties, clindamycin is preferred for the situation described in the question. Cephalosporins produce severe reactions in ten percent of penicillin-sensitive patients. Erythromycin and trimethoprim-sulfamethoxazole are not regarded as clinically efficacious against staphylococcal organisms, and resistance may develop during therapy. Most consultants prefer clindamycin to vancomycin, because of the lower incidence of side effects. Unlike vancomycin, clindamycin is not associated with phlebitis or oto- and nephrotoxicity. There have been rare cases, however, of pseudomembranous colitis associated with clindamycin.

313. The answer is C. *(Hoekelman, p 1121. Stiehm, pp 428-429.)* Henoch-Schönlein purpura is manifested by a rash that evolves from erythematous urticarial macules and papules to palpable purpura occurring on the lower extremities and buttocks. Arthritis and abdominal pain occur. Hematuria and proteinuria reflect glomerular involvement. Laboratory tests show a normal C3 level, normal platelet count, and negative antinuclear antibody. The colicky abdominal pain may be accompanied by stools positive for occult blood or by gross rectal bleeding. The etiology of the syndrome is not known.

314. The answer is E. *(Hoekelman, p 1067. Stiehm, pp 178-179, 185-191.)* X-linked hypogammaglobulinemia does not present until the second half of the first year of life. This delay is due to the protection afforded by maternal antibody. These boys suffer from recurrent pyogenic infections, including (1) otitis media, (2) pneumonia, (3) conjunctivitis, (4) sinusitis, (5) sepsis, and (6) meningitis. Arthritis of nonbacterial etiology may occur. Laboratory evaluation reveals that IgG levels are less than 100 mg/100 ml and that IgA and IgM values are low. There is poor antibody response to immunization, and B cells are absent. These findings contrast with those of transient hypogammaglobulinemia of infancy, in which the antibody response to some antigens is intact and B cells are present.

315. The answer is C. *(Yow, ed 18. p 283.)* Recommendations for the prophylaxis of tetanus are based on the characteristics of the wound and on the immunization history of the patient. The child in the question has had the basic series of immunizations—that is, three or four shots of tetanus toxoid completed six or more years before sustaining a severe injury. He has sustained a wound that has probably exposed him to tetanus spores (injury by machine and exposure to animal excreta), and more than five years have elapsed since his primary immunization. This situation requires a "booster" dose of TD only. If his primary immunization were not complete, or if the wound were more than 24 hours old, he would also require tetanus immune globulin. Penicillin is not part of tetanus prophylaxis, although some authorities recommend its use in tetanus therapy.

316. The answer is A. *(Hoeprich, ed 2. pp 289-291.)* In the United States, the most common sources of ornithosis are turkeys and pigeons. The disease may present with symptoms suggesting a mild viral syndrome, such as an influenza-like illness, or the patient may be very ill. However, symptoms of an influenza-like illness may be due to many agents. Pneumonitis is typically interstitial, but this pattern may also be produced by a number of other agents.

317. The answer is B. *(Hoekelman, pp 1054, 1079. Fudenberg, ed 2. pp 89-91, 128-138, 376-383.)* T and B cells are distinguished by surface receptors and in vitro functional assays. T cells have a receptor for (1) sheep red blood cells, (2) the Fc piece of IgG and IgM, and (3) measles virus. There are distinct differentiation antigens on the T and B cell surfaces; these are detectable by antisera. The antigen-binding receptor on T cells is undefined, but it is not the conventional surface immunoglobulin (SIG) which exists on B cells. B cells have receptors for the third component of complement; they also have IgG Fc receptors. T cells proliferate when incubated with antigens, such as phytohemagglutinin and concanavalin A, with a mixed lymphocyte culture, and with specific antigens. Lymphocytes release lymphokines, such as migration inhibition factor, which accounts for the accumulation and activation of macrophages at sites of delayed hypersensitivity.

318. The answer is A. *(Hoekelman, pp 1157-1158. Hughes, N Engl J Med 297:1381-1383, 1977.)* Pneumocystis carinii pneumonia rarely if ever occurs in patients without an immunodeficiency. In fact, among patients receiving immunosuppressive therapy, it is the most commonly diagnosed cause of diffuse alveolar disease. In children with cancer, the incidence of the disease is related directly to the intensity of chemotherapy. Children with acute lymphocytic leukemia are at greatest risk. The disease presents a clinical picture similar to the common causes of pneumonitis, except that rales are not heard. It is best diagnosed by an open-lung biopsy. Trimethoprim-sulfamethoxazole is now the drug of choice for prophylaxis and treatment, rather than the more toxic pentamidine isothionate used previously. The recurrence rate is 15 percent, which is higher than the overall frequency in children with cancer.

319. The answer is E. *(Hoekelman, pp 158-159, 1080-1081. Stiehm, Pediatrics 63:301-319, 1979.)* Immune serum globulin (ISG) is a 16.5 percent solution of gamma globulin overall with IgG constituting 95 percent of the total amount. Prepared by ethanol fractionation of normal human serum, it is injected intramuscularly. The IgG (and, therefore, ISG) has a half-life of 20-30 days. Only trace amounts of IgA and IgM are found in ISG. Deficiency of IgA and IgM without deficiency of IgG should not be treated with ISG. The half-life of these immunoglobulins is three to seven days. If an IgA-deficient patient is treated with ISG, there is a risk of inducing an anaphylactic reaction due to the production of antibody to trace amounts of IgA in the ISG. There is no evidence that the passively-obtained IgG is secreted at mucosal surfaces. ISG can modify hepatitis A and measles infection if given to contacts after exposure to these viruses.

320. The answer is B. *(Vaughan, ed 11. pp 855-856.)* *Mycoplasma pneumoniae* frequently causes an atypical pneumonia syndrome, but it has also been associated with pharyngitis, otitis media, a variety of rashes, Stevens-Johnson syndrome, Guillain-Barré syndrome, meningoencephalitis, and hemolytic anemia. Glomerulonephritis has not been reported to be associated with infection by this organism. Although association with many body sites has been reported, the respiratory tract is the only area of the body where *Mycoplasma* infections have been shown to be constant.

321. The answer is B. *(Beem, Pediatrics 63:198-203, 1979.)* Ampicillin and penicillin are not consistently effective against *Chlamydia trachomatis* in vitro and would not be expected to have clinical efficacy. Data on trimethoprim-sulfamethoxazole are not available. Both erythromycin and sulfasoxazole have been shown to shorten the clinical course of chlamydia pneumonitis and reduce the time of shedding of *C. trachomatis*.

322. The answer is B. *(Stiehm, pp 199-211.)* IgA deficiency is the most common primary immunodeficiency, with an incidence of about 1 in 500 people in the general population. The usual criteria for diagnosis require a serum IgA of less than 5-10 mg/100 ml. A decrease of IgA may cause no symptoms or it may be associated with (1) autoimmune disorders such as rheumatoid arthritis and thyroiditis, (2) recurrent infections usually involving the sinopulmonary system (including bronchiectasis), (3) allergic symptoms such as asthma and allergic rhinitis, and (4) gastrointestinal diseases such as celiac disease, intestinal nodular hyperplasia, ulcerative colitis, and regional enteritis. Large numbers of cases of selective IgA deficiency have been associated with chromosome 18 abnormalities. These include partial deletion of the short arm of the chromosome, and ring chromosome 18. IgA deficiency patients are able to produce large quantities of IgG antibodies to foreign protein. Over 60 percent demonstrate the presence of both precipitating and hemagglutinating antibodies to cows' milk. Therapy is not directed toward replacing IgA. Immune serum globulin will not replace the IgA absent in secretions and may sensitize the patient to develop anti-IgA antibodies, which may cause anaphylaxis.

323. The answer is D. *(Hoekelman, pp 159-160, 164.)* Any child exposed to measles should receive immune serum globulin (ISG), if he or she has not had the disease or the vaccine previously. The ISG should be administered within one week of exposure in order to be effective. If there is no clinical evidence of disease, the ISG should not be followed by immunization with live measles virus until at least three months have elapsed. In the case of a nine-month-old infant, however, the measles immunization should be given at 15 months of age as recommended for all infants. Killed measles vaccine should not be used since the protection is not as effective as live measles vaccine, and children subsequently exposed to the wild virus may develop atypical measles.

324. The answer is D. *(Beem, N Engl J Med 296:306, 1977.)* A young infant with an afebrile, chronic coughing syndrome who also has a middle ear effusion, eosinophilia, and a chest x-ray with diffuse infiltrates is very likely to have *Chlamydia pneumonitis*. The diagnostic features mentioned distinguish this syndrome from diseases caused by respiratory syncytial virus (bronchiolitis), parainfluenza viruses (febrile pneumonia), pneumococci (febrile lobar pneumonia), and whooping cough (afebrile, coughing syndrome with severe paroxysms).

325. The answer is A. *(Hoekelman, p 1070. Stiehm, pp 284-285, 316-319.)* Asplenia or splenic dysfunction may be complicated by fulminant sepsis with *Streptococcus (Diplococcus) pneumoniae, Hemophilus influenzae, Neisseria meningitidis* or *Escherichia coli.* Disseminated intravascular coagulation may complicate the sepsis. The risk of sepsis is increased when the patient is less than five years old, during the first two years after splenectomy, and if splenectomy is associated with a disease that alters the function of the remaining reticuloendothelial system or causes immunosuppression or immunodeficiency. Patients are at risk for years after splenectomy; older children and adults are also at risk. Immunization with pneumococcal polysaccharide vaccine is recommended for patients over two years of age. Immune serum globulin is not a recommended treatment. However, Howell-Jolly bodies are found in the peripheral blood smear in cases of asplenia and splenic dysfunction.

326. The answer is E. *(Hoekelman, p 1066. Stiehm, pp 150-152, 216-218.)* A family history of early deaths, immunodeficiency, unusual or recurrent infections, allergy, autoimmunity, and malignancy should be sought if immunodeficiency is suspected. Immunodeficiencies with an X-linked inheritance include congenital agammaglobulinemia, Wiskott-Aldrich syndrome, chronic granulomatous disease, severe combined immunodeficiency, and immunodeficiency with hyper-IgM. Autosomal inherited disorders include severe combined immunodeficiency with and without adenosine deaminase deficiency, chronic granulomatous disease, ataxia telangiectasia, and Chediak-Higashi syndrome. DiGeorge's syndrome is not inherited, but it is thought to be secondary to a pathologic event in the first trimester of pregnancy affecting the third and fourth pharyngeal pouches.

327. The answer is D (4). *(Hoekelman, pp 297-298, 1795-1796. Smith, Pediatr Alert 4:45-46, 1979. Yow, ed 18. pp 213, 284.)* The rapid development of cellulitis in the area of a bite inflicted by a cat is a sign of infection by *Pasteurella multocida.* This infection is treated effectively by penicillin or ampicillin. The cat should be observed, and if no illness develops within ten days, rabies is not a concern. Tetanus immunization provides protection for at least five years after the 18-month injection. No additional tetanus toxoid or immune globulin is indicated.

328. The answer is E (all). *(Hoekelman, pp 1031, 1042.)* Children with petechiae and fever present a diagnostic problem that requires immediate evaluation. The differential diagnosis includes meningococcemia, enterovirus infection, other infection with shock or disseminated intravascular coagulation, idiopathic thrombocytopenic purpura, other thrombocytopenic states or vasculopathy, leukemia or another neoplasm with metastases, or systemic lupus erythematosus. The initial workup should rule in or out as many of these diseases as possible so that appropriate therapy may be given. This evaluation should include a complete history and physical examination to detect pertinent signs, symptoms, or exposures. Laboratory studies should include (**in order of performance**) the following: (1) examination of the cerebrospinal fluid, (2) multiple cultures, (3) a complete blood count with smear, (4) a reticulocyte count, (5) an erythrocyte sedimentation rate, (6) a buffy coat examination to detect both neoplastic cells and microorganisms, (7) a bone marrow aspiration and biopsy, (8) clotting studies (e.g., prothrombin time, partial thromboplastin time, and bleeding time), (9) an immunogram, and (10) serologic tests for autoimmune disease.

329. The answer is E (all). *(Hoekelman, p 1243.)* Mebendazole (Vermox) is effective therapy for trichuriasis (whipworm), enterobiasis (pinworm), ascariasis (roundworm), and hookworm infestations caused by the *Necator* or *Ancylostoma* species. This oral drug has achieved 90 percent cure rates in single and multiple infestations. It is the drug of choice for multiple infestations.

330. The answer is B (1, 3). *(Krugman, ed 6. pp 25-34.)* The cause of encephalitis is unknown in 60 percent of the reported cases. Of the known causes, the common childhood exanthema—measles, rubella, and chickenpox—and mumps comprise the majority of cases. There are many forms of viral encephalitis, varying from the benign forms resembling aseptic meningitis, such as mumps meningoencephalitis, to the severe forms, such as herpes simplex encephalitis, which has an associated case fatality rate of 35 percent as compared to mumps, which has a 1 percent fatality rate, and arboviruses, which have a 6 percent fatality rate. A diagnosis of viral encephalitis is based on clinical findings in most cases. The lumbar puncture is of great importance because, in addition to an elevation in cerebrospinal fluid pressure, the findings characteristically include a pleocytosis of mononuclear cells with relatively normal glucose and protein concentrations. Viral cultures and serology should be obtained. There is no effective treatment of encephalitis.

331. The answer is C (2, 4). *(Hoekelman, pp 1223-1224.)* Rocky Mountain spotted fever (RMSF) is a rickettsial disease that is transmitted to man by ticks. Although first observed in the Rockies, it is now more commonly seen in the southern Atlantic states. It is characterized by fever, systemic toxicity, and a rash that is centrifugal in distribution. The rash begins as blanching macules and then progresses to papules and petechiae. The diagnosis must be suspected early for antibiotic therapy to be instituted in time to be effective. Diagnosis can be confirmed by the Weil-Felix reaction test three weeks after the illness. Chloramphenicol or tetracycline are effective drugs. Mortality today is approximately 20 percent among untreated individuals.

332. The answer is A (1, 2, 3). *(Hoekelman, p 1059. Fudenberg, ed 2. pp 219-225. Stiehm, pp 557-559.)* Hemophilus influenzae systemic infection is almost always caused by the type B strain, which is encapsulated with a polysaccharide polymer. This capsule prevents surface phagocytosis of the bacteria. However, IgG antibody directed to the capsule will promote phagocytosis by binding to the Fc receptor of white blood cells. This anticapsular antibody fixes complement utilizing the classical complement pathway, and C3b is deposited on the bacteria. The white blood cells also have a receptor for C3b that promotes attachment of the white cells to the bacteria. T killer cells do not play a role in *H. influenzae* infection.

333. The answer is E (all). *(Vaughan, ed 11. pp 1213-1214.)* *Klebsiella pneumoniae* is an uncommon cause of pneumonia and is seen most commonly in the compromised host or as a complication of chronic lung disease. It is a "water bug" that grows well in humidity-producing equipment. Bacteremia is common, as is empyema. X-ray findings are not specific, but a lobar consolidation with bulging fissures should make the clinician consider this organism as an etiologic possibility. Pulmonary abscesses may also be seen. During epidemics, infants, most of whom are asymptomatic, often carry *K. pneumoniae* in their nasopharynges.

334. The answer is A (1, 2, 3). *(Krugman, ed 6. pp 150-151, 233, 256.)* Lymphocytic choriomeningitis virus may cause an aseptic meningitis or an influenza-like illness. It can be established as the etiological agent in aseptic meningitis by isolation of the virus from blood or cerebrospinal fluid or by demonstration of a rise in titer of complement-fixing or neutralizing antibodies. Transmission is from mice, guinea pigs, hamsters, and dogs, but there is no evidence of human-to-human transmission. The house mouse is the most likely source of human infection, although epidemics have been associated with pet hamsters.

335. The answer is A (1, 2, 3). *(Hoekelman, p 1069. Stiehm, pp 289-293.)* Hereditary angioneurotic edema is caused by the absence or dysfunction of the C1 esterase inhibitor. Affected individuals develop sudden attacks of circumscribed subcutaneous edema without discoloration of the overlying skin, pruritus, or pain. Often precipitated by trauma, these attacks evolve quickly and subside in about three to four days. Involvement of the larynx and gastrointestinal tract may cause asphyxiation and colicky abdominal pain, respectively. A rash similar to erythema marginatum may be associated with attacks. Laboratory findings include decreased C2 and C4 levels during attacks and depressed C4 levels at all times. Tracheostomy may be life-saving if there is respiratory compromise. Except in rare circumstances, epinephrine is not useful in controlling the swelling.

336. The answer is A (1, 2, 3). *(Hoekelman, pp 1795-1796. Yow, ed 18. p 212.)* Rabies has been reported following bites from cats, coyotes, wolves, dogs, bats, and skunks. Therefore, until more information is available regarding the involved animal, prophylaxis should be started. There have been no reports of rabies following bites of rabbits, mice, or rats. Since rabies immunization products are not without danger, the choice must be made after careful consideration of the following factors: (1) the extent and site of bites (deep puncture wounds of the face, fingers, neck, and hands are more likely to produce rabies than bites elsewhere), (2) the nature of the attack (unprovoked attacks are more suggestive of rabies than provoked attacks), and (3) the immunization status of the attacking animal.

337. The answer is A (1, 2, 3). *(Hoekelman, pp 1057, 1069. Stiehm, pp 293-299.)* Deficiency of a serum complement component (C) may predispose to recurrent bacterial infections or be associated with autoimmune disease. Absence of C3 or C3b inactivator is associated with recurrent pyogenic infections. The terminal complement components are required for bactericidal activity against *Neisseria;* for example, absence of C6, C7, and C8 is associated with recurrent sepsis with *N. meningitidis* or *N. gonorrhoeae.* Deficiency of C2 or C4 is associated with autoimmune disease—a systemic lupus erythematosus-like syndrome. Absence of C1 esterase inhibitor results in hereditary angioneurotic edema. Chronic moniliasis and other chronic fungal infections have not been associated with serum complement deficiencies.

338. The answer is C (2, 4). *(Klein, Pediatrics 61:321-322, 1978.)* The polyvalent pneumococcal polysaccharide vaccine has been recommended for use in patients with an increased risk of pneumococcal disease such as the sickling syndromes, splenectomized patients, and those with nephrotic syndrome. Since the immunologic response to polysaccharide vaccines is deficient in those under two years of age, the use of this vaccine is recommended for the above indications only in children older than two.

339. The answer is A (1, 2, 3). *(Johnson, Am J Dis Child 133:586-593, 1979.)* Infantile botulism is a recently delineated syndrome associated with the presence of *Clostridium botulinum* and its toxins in the stools of infants. The illness begins with constipation and progresses to generalized weakness with poor cry and decreased sucking and gag reflex. Ptosis, extraocular muscle weakness, facial weakness, and decreased or absent deep tendon reflexes are found on examination. Loss of head control is usually apparent. Treatment is supportive, including respiratory care. Diagnosis is based on the characteristic electromyographic findings and on the isolation of the organism and its toxin from the stool. There is an association with honey intake but with no other foods.

340. The answer is A (1, 2, 3). *(Granoff, Pediatrics 63:397-401, 1979. Ward, N Engl J Med 301:122-126, 1979.)* The use of antibiotic prophylaxis for infectious diseases is a matter of constant controversy. Although not many would question the use of prophylactic medication for someone who has had contact with a person who has venereal disease such as gonorrhea, the necessity for prophylactic medications in those who have had contact with victims of meningococcal and *Hemophilus influenzae* disease is frequently questioned. Among the most recent recommendations is the management of close contacts with sporadic meningococcal disease with the administration of rifampin as a prophylactic measure, especially since there is a rising resistance of this organism to sulfonamides. Rifampin has also been recommended recently for preventing *H. influenzae* type B infections in children less than age four years; the chances in this age group of developing severe disease after close contacts is two to five percent. Exposure of a healthy child to *Pneumocystis carinii* does not usually call for antibiotic prophylaxis, as this organism tends to invade immunosuppressed children with poor host defense mechanisms.

341-343. The answers are: 341-D, 342-A, 343-B. *(Hoekelman, pp 1181-1184, 1188-1190.)* Roseola is an illness that characteristically has a course of three to five days of fever and irritability without rash. A maculopapular rash appears when the fever falls, but soon fades.

Rubeola or measles begins with fever followed by cough, coryza, and conjunctivitis. On the third day, an enanthem (Koplik's spots) may be noted. On the fourth day, a maculopapular rash appears on the face and spreads downward. At that time, the other symptoms usually improve and the rash fades. There may be desquamation of the skin.

Rubella is a mild infection in young children. Malaise and lymphadenopathy (especially cervical, postauricular, and suboccipital) are present three to four days before the rash. The rash presents as discrete pink maculopapules that appear on the face and spread downward. Fever is not very elevated or prolonged.

344-346. The answers are: 344-C, 345-D, 346-A. *(Hoekelman, pp 1054-1059. Fudenberg, ed 2. pp 23-37.)* IgE is secreted by lymphocytes and binds to an Fc receptor on mast cells. Antigen binds to the IgE and activates the release of allergic mediators from the mast cell. Polymorphonuclear neutrophils have a receptor for the Fc piece of IgG. IgG bound to antigen binds to the Fc receptor. Subclasses of IgG are unique in that they are actively transported across the placenta. IgA is secreted at mucosal surfaces covalently bound to a secretory piece, which prevents its degradation by proteolytic enzymes. Polymeric IgM may bind a secretory piece, but the bond is not covalent. IgM, the largest of the immunoglobulins, is the first to appear in fetal life.

347-350. The answers are: 347-E, 348-A, 349-B, 350-C. *(Hoekelman, pp 1201-1203.)* In gram-negative endotoxic shock, endogenous pyrogens are released by the local inflammatory process.This release of pyrogens results in fever. There is also release of vasodilating substances, including kinins, histamine, and prostaglandins, whose actions produce hypotension. As part of the compensatory mechanism for the fall in blood pressure, epinephrine and norepinephrine are released and are responsible for vasoconstriction and subsequent ischemic changes in target organs. The kidney and lung are the organs most severely affected. Oliguria results from poor renal perfusion. Lactic acidosis occurs following poor tissue perfusion and is one cause of hyperventilation. One of the major complications of gram-negative endotoxic shock is disseminated intravascular coagulation, which causes bleeding from several sites, and results from platelet aggregation and depletion of factors in the blood required for clotting.

351-353. The answers are: 351-D, 352-B, 353-C. *(Hoekelman, pp 1062-1064, 1075. Stiehm, pp 60-61.)* At birth, the only immunoglobulin class detectable is IgG. This immunoglobulin class is of maternal origin and will be catabolized with an approximate half-life of 20-30 days. IgG is the only class of immunoglobulins that is actively transported across the placenta. The infant begins to produce its own IgG during the first month of life, due to exposure to antigens in the environment. A nadir is reached at three to five months of age, after which the IgG level slowly increases. At age one, the infant has about 60 percent of the adult IgG level; the adult level is reached by about age ten. IgM synthesis begins during the first weeks of life and approaches 80 percent of adult levels by five to six years of age. Serum IgA increases slowly during the first year of life, reaching 80 percent of adult levels by adolescence. Curve A is not associated with any immunoglobulin class.

354-356. The answers are: 354-D, 355-A, 356-B. *(Hoekelman, pp 1188-1190. Vaughan, ed 11. p 758.)* Rubella is characterized by a relatively mild course. The prominent lymphadenopathy and the downward spreading rash help distinguish this disease from meningococcemia and erythema infectiosum.

Acute meningococcal disease may begin with fever, malaise, myalgia, and a fine papular or morbilliform rash. The rash usually evolves into the more characteristic petechial and purpuric rash associated with this disease within hours or days.

Erythema infectiosum usually manifests as a day or two of mild fever followed by the appearance of a characteristic maculopapular, erythematous rash most marked on the cheeks, giving the patient the "slapped cheek" sign. Discrete morbilliform lesions may be seen on the trunk. The rash fades to a lacy appearance lasting only a few days, but it may reappear during the succeeding few weeks in response to stress, fever, or bathing in warm water.

357-360. The answers are: 357-C, 358-E, 359-D, 360-A. *(Hoekelman, pp 1084-1090. Gell, ed 3. p 761.)* There are several types of distinct mechanisms involved in the production of hypersensitivity reactions. As classified by Gell and Coombs, the type I reaction occurs after an antigen binds antibody (IgE) on the surface of a mast cell, causing the release of mediators from that cell. This is the mechanism that occurs with systemic anaphylaxis.

In type II reactions, antibodies in the serum combine with antigen on the surface of a target cell. This reaction leads to agglutination of the cell, activation of complement, and lysis of the cell, or to attachment to the target cell surface by cells with an Fc receptor and destruction of the target cell. Autoimmune hemolytic anemias are an example of type II reactions.

In type III reactions, antigen-antibody complexes form and are deposited in tissues. Complement is activated and inflammation occurs at the tissue sites; poststreptococcal glomerulonephritis is an example.

In type IV hypersensitivity reactions, T cells recognize antigens and kill them directly or release lymphokines which do so. Poison ivy causes a contact dermatitis, which is a type IV reaction. A history of poison ivy rash suggests normal T cell function. Reaction to x-ray contrast media is not mediated by any of these mechanisms.

361-364. The answers are: 361-A, 362-C, 363-C, 364-E. *(Hoekelman, pp 924, 1670-1672. Vaughan, ed 11. pp 714, 716, 720. DHEW, Morbidity and Mortality Weekly Report 28:277-279, 1979.)* In children from age four months to adolescence, *Hemophilus influenzae* is the most common cause of bacterial meningitis, followed by *Neisseria meningitidis* and *Streptococcus (Diplococcus) pneumoniae.* Infants between 6 and 18 months of age are those at greatest risk for meningitis due to *H. influenzae.*

Staphylococcal species are the most common cause of hematogenous osteomyelitis in infants and children. *H. influenzae* and streptococcal species are less frequent causes. *S. aureus* is the infecting organism in over 75 percent of cases. However, in patients with sickle-cell disease, *Salmonella* species are isolated most frequently.

In children greater than two years of age, *Staphylococcus aureus* is the most common cause of septic arthritis, followed by streptococcal species, *H. influenzae,* and *Neisseria gonorrhea.* In children under two years of age, *H. influenzae* is the predominant organism. Treatment with antibiotics has decreased the mortality rate from this disease markedly since the 1940s. However, diagnosis and treatment must be accomplished early to prevent severe and permanent musculoskeletal deformities.

In children under two months of age, the group B streptococcus is the most common cause of bacterial meningitis in many parts of the United States. Until recently, gram-negative organisms were the most common. The incidence of bacterial meningitis due to both *H. influenzae* and *Listeria monocytogenes* has increased in recent years.

365-367. The answers are: 365-A, 366-B, 367-D. *(Hoekelman, p 1228, 1233-1235. Vaughan, ed 11. pp 964-970, 1014-1016.)* The fungus *Histoplasma capsulatum* is endemic in the Mississippi Valley and may cause both widespread pulmonary and extrathoracic disease. All of its manifestations are similar to tuberculosis. A patient with the pulmonary findings of calcification and mediastinal lymph nodes who is nonreactive to standard tuberculin testing and who is from the endemic area may well have healed primary histoplasmosis lesions.

Coccidioides immitis is a fungus that may cause a chronic pulmonary disease and may spread to extrapulmonary sites. The endemic areas are the southwestern United States, California, and South America. It also may cause an acute "valley fever" syndrome with night sweats, chest pain, a rash (which may progress to erythema nodosum), pneumonitis, and arthralgia.

Entamoeba histolytica often produces an acute dysentery syndrome. It may also cause an amebic abscess of the liver, which may manifest as a febrile illness with right upper quadrant pain, hepatic tenderness, and abnormal liver tests.

Dermatology and Connective Tissue Diseases

DIRECTIONS: Each question below contains five suggested answers. Choose the **one best** response to each question.

368. The 3,400 g (7 lb, 8 oz) infant shown below was born at 37.5 weeks gestation to a 37-year-old mother. Rupture of membranes occurred 21 hours prior to a caesarean section because of variable decelerations noted on fetal heart rate monitoring. Apgar scores were 4 at one minute and 8 at five minutes. At birth, the infant appeared as shown in the figure below. Evaluation and treatment of this infant should include

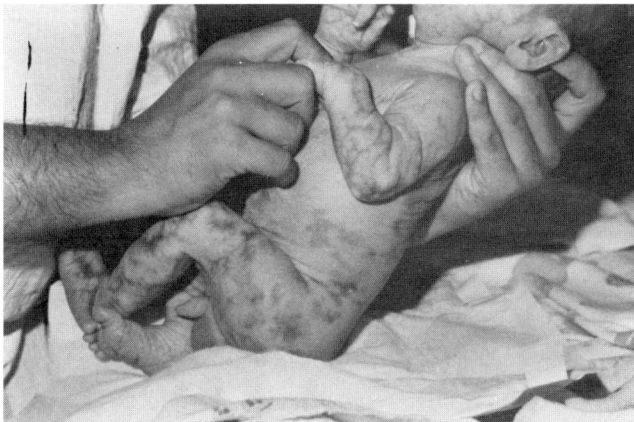

(A) intravenous penicillin (100,000 IU/kg) after a blood, urine, and cerebrospinal fluid culture
(B) a platelet count and administration of dexamethasone
(C) occlusive dressings applied to the legs and arms
✓(D) observation and reassurance to the parents
(E) continuous blood pressure recordings and volume expanders

369. The toxic effects of gamma benzene hexachloride (Kwell) have been documented to involve which of the following organ systems?

(A) Gastrointestinal system
(B) Cardiovascular system
(C) Pulmonary system
(D) Genitourinary system
✓(E) Central nervous system

370. A newborn infant presents with linear, bullous skin lesions. These lesions soon progress to a swirling "marble cake-like" hyperpigmentation. The most likely diagnosis would be

(A) bullous impetigo
(B) neonatal acne
(C) nevus sebaceous
✓(D) incontinentia pigmenti
(E) ichthyosis vulgaris

371. Which of the following substances is deficient in patients with acrodermatitis enteropathica and, when given orally, abolishes all signs and symptoms of that disorder?

(A) Copper
✓(B) Zinc
(C) Thiamine
(D) Vitamin E
(E) None of the above

372. Crops of lesions that have bright erythematous peripheries and central cyanosis, which appear "target" or "iris" shaped, are most characteristic of

(A) acne rosacea
(B) pityriasis rosea
(C) blue nevi
(D) erythropoietic protoporphyria
✓(E) erythema multiforme

373. Hyperstretchability of skin associated with hyperextensibility of joints is suggestive of

(A) scleroderma
(B) dermatomyositis
(C) neurofibromatosis
(D) dyskeratosis congenita
✓(E) Ehlers-Danlos syndrome

374. The bacterium most frequently associated with the impetigo of childhood shown in the figure below is

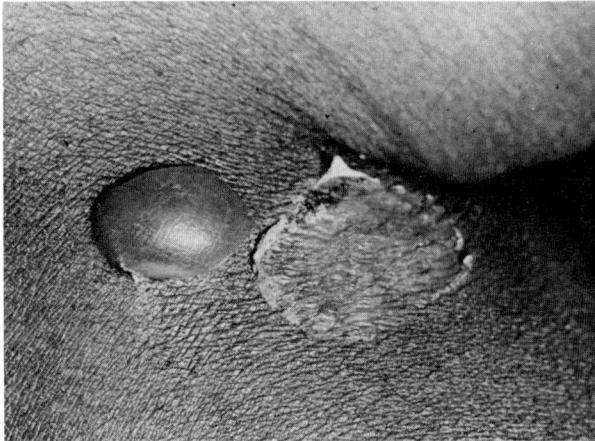

Used with permission of McGraw-Hill Book Company, from *Principles of Pediatrics: Health Care of the Young* (p 1372), by Hoekelman RA et al, ©1978 McGraw-Hill Inc.

(A) group A β-hemolytic streptococcus
(B) *Escherichia coli*
(C) *Streptococcus (Diplococcus) pneumoniae*
(D) *Staphylococcus aureus*
(E) *Hemophilus influenzae*

375. The clinical form of juvenile rheumatoid arthritis most likely to be complicated by chronic iridocyclitis is

(A) acute-systemic-onset juvenile rheumatoid arthritis
(B) pauciarticular juvenile rheumatoid arthritis
(C) polyarticular juvenile rheumatoid arthritis-rheumatoid factor negative
(D) Still's triad of polyarthritis, splenomegaly, and lymphadenopathy
(E) none of the above

376. All of the following statements concerning the management of atopic dermatitis are true EXCEPT

(A) therapy of the acute phase includes the use of moist, cooling compresses
(B) sedative or antipruritic agents may prove to be useful
(C) for the recalcitrant case, a short course of systemic steroids may be indicated
(D) food and inhalant allergens are frequently causative factors
(E) the avoidance of frequent bathing with drying soaps should be stressed

377. Scaling, macular, slightly pruritic lesions distributed as shown in the figure below are seen in which one of the following skin conditions?

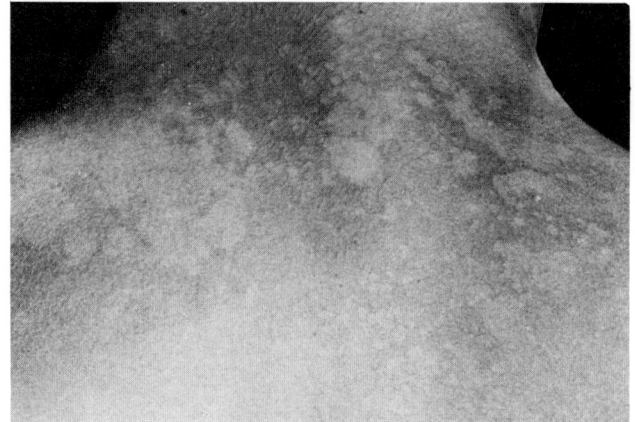

Used with permission of McGraw-Hill Book Company, from *Principles of Pediatrics: Health Care of the Young* (p 1389), by Hoekelman RA et al, ©1978 McGraw-Hill, Inc.

(A) Molluscum contagiosum
(B) Candidiasis
(C) Dermatomyositis
(D) Tinea versicolor
(E) Pediculosis corporis

378. Psoriasis in childhood has features correctly described by all of the following statements EXCEPT that

(A) the epidermal turnover time is accelerated markedly in psoriatic lesions as compared with normal epidermis
(B) there appears to be an association between childhood psoriasis and streptococcal respiratory infections
(C) the fingernails and toenails rarely present with pitting and detachment of the nail plate
(D) psoriatic lesions are found on the elbows, knees, scalp, and presacral regions
(E) untreated lesions develop scales, which yield pinpoint bleeding on removal

379. The incidence of transformation of congenital giant hairy nevi into malignant melanoma is

(A) less than 1 percent
(B) about 10 percent
(C) about 50 percent
(D) about 75 percent
(E) greater than 90 percent

380. Photophobia is commonly found in serious eye disorders in association with all of the following physical signs EXCEPT

(A) dendritic ulcer on the cornea
(B) increased intraocular pressure
(C) inflammation of the iris and ciliary body
(D) injection of the scleral conjunctival vessels predominantly in the periphery
(E) clouding of the cornea

381. Hyperpigmentation of the palmar creases, buccal mucosa, linea alba, and scrotum may be a sign of

(A) adrenal insufficiency
(B) Henoch-Schönlein purpura
(C) tuberous sclerosis
(D) scurvy
(E) syphilis

382. The scalp lesion shown in the figure below is best treated with

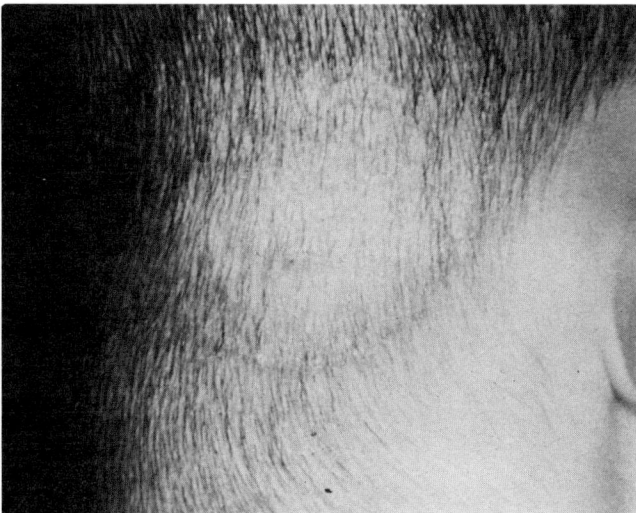

(A) oral griseofulvin
(B) topical nystatin
(C) systemic penicillin
(D) topical bacitracin
(E) none of the above

383. All of the following statements regarding different mechanisms in the development of alopecia are correct EXCEPT that

(A) regrowth is relatively rapid when alopecia is due to traumatic avulsion of hair follicles
(B) alopecia areata produces sharply defined round patches of complete hair loss
(C) current hair styles are an important determinant of alopecia prevalence
(D) trichotillomania produces irregular patches of incomplete hair loss
(E) there is a congenital form of alopecia in which hair is totally absent

384. An 18-month-old child presents with a one-day history of irritability, fever, a bright red rash, and peeling skin (see figure below). The child has been taking a sulfa preparation for one week for otitis media. The most likely diagnosis is

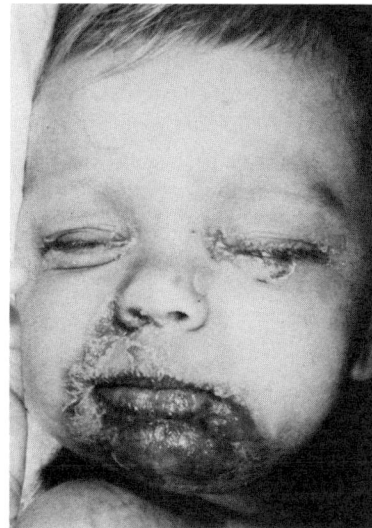

(A) primary herpes simplex
(B) Stevens-Johnson syndrome
(C) Ritter's disease
(D) staphylococcal scalded skin syndrome
(E) none of the above

385. All of the following statements concerning poison ivy dermatitis are true EXCEPT that

(A) the lesions are usually intensely pruritic
(B) involvement of the genital area is quite common
(C) the lesions often assume a vesicular nature
(D) peak involvement occurs one to three days after contact
(E) oral corticosteroids may be needed in moderate-to-severe cases

386. A six-year-old boy has a five-month history
of increasing difficulty climbing stairs, low-grade
fever, and rash. His hands appear as shown in the
figure below. All of the following laboratory
results could be expected with this diagnosis
EXCEPT for

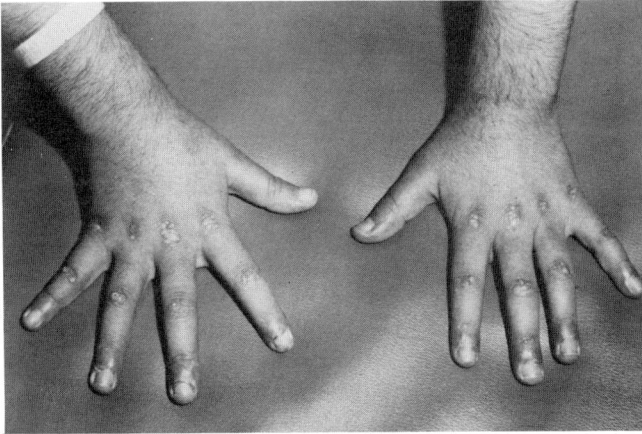

Used with permission of Virgil Hanson, M.D., Children's Hospital of
Los Angeles from *Principles of Pediatrics: Health Care of the Young*
(p 1119), by Hoekelman RA et al, © 1978 by McGraw-Hill Inc.

(A) the presence of rheumatoid factor
(B) the presence of blood in stool
(C) elevated creatine phosphokinase levels
(D) an abnormal muscle biopsy
(E) an abnormal electromyography

DIRECTIONS: Each question below contains four suggested answers of which **one** or **more** is correct. Choose the answer

A	if	**1, 2, and 3**	are correct
B	if	**1 and 3**	are correct
C	if	**2 and 4**	are correct
D	if	**4**	is correct
E	if	**1, 2, 3, and 4**	are correct

387. A neonate is found to have multiple pustular lesions on the face. Careful examination suggests a diagnosis of erythema toxicum. Laboratory studies helpful in confirming this diagnosis include

(1) Wood's lamp examination of the lesions
(2) Wright's stained smear of pustular material
(3) biopsy of skin tissue
(4) gram-stained smear of pustular material

388. Complications of neurofibromatosis (von Recklinghausen's disease) include which of the following?

(1) Scoliosis
(2) Seizures
(3) Mental retardation
(4) Pseudarthrosis

389. The application of sunscreens may be useful in the management of

(1) acne
(2) seborrheic dermatitis
(3) tinea corporis
(4) lupus erythematosus

390. Correct statements about impetigo include which of the following?

(1) It is a common cause of rheumatic fever
(2) It is highly contagious
(3) Topical therapy is sufficient treatment
(4) *Staphylococcus aureus* is the most likely pathogen

391. Features characteristic of some, but not all, of the hereditary ectodermal dysplasias include

(1) decreased numbers of eccrine sweat glands
(2) defective teeth
(3) short or dystrophic fingernails and toenails
(4) unusually thick hair (hypertrichosis)

392. Correct statements about the condition characterized by the skin lesions shown in the figure below include which of the following?

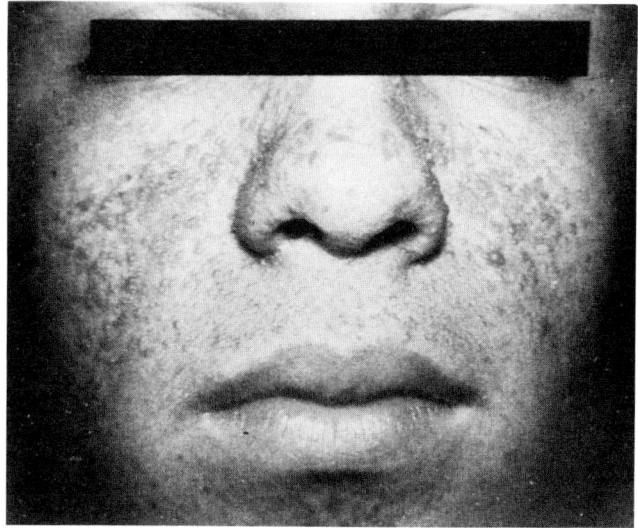

Used with permission of McGraw-Hill Book Company, from *Color Atlas of Pediatric Dermatology* (p 170), by Weinberg S et al, © 1975 McGraw-Hill Inc.

(1) Hypopigmented skin patches generally 3 to 5 cm long by 2 cm wide are common in newborns who go on to develop this condition
(2) Skin lesions, which may not be noted without the aid of Wood's light examination, are common in newborns who develop this condition
(3) Individuals with this condition may live a full, productive life
(4) Intracranial calcifications commonly develop later in childhood

393. Erythema nodosum is commonly seen in association with which of the following disorders?

(1) Streptococcal pharyngitis
(2) Leukemia
(3) Tuberculosis
(4) Ulcerative colitis

394. Accepted methods for the treatment of warts include

(1) podophyllin
(2) electrodesiccation and curettage
(3) cryocautery
(4) surgical excision

395. True statements about the lesion shown in the figure below include which of the following?

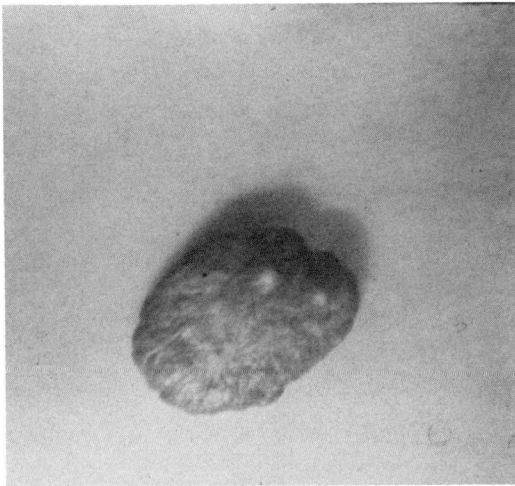

(1) It is usually not present at birth
(2) Surgical removal is usually necessary
(3) It may involute spontaneously
(4) It rarely responds to steroids

396. Characteristics of phototoxic drug photosensitization in children are described in which of the following statements?

(1) Drug photosensitization occurs in any individual in whom there is sufficient concentration of a photoactive drug and a sufficient dose of light energy delivered to the skin
(2) Photopatch testing results in eczematous eruption that extends beyond the photopatch site
(3) Skin manifestations include an enhanced sunburn response sharply limited to sun-exposed areas
(4) Drug photosensitization results from photoconversion of a drug into a hapten, which combines with skin protein to form a complete photoantigen

397. Correct statements concerning the lesion shown in the figure below include

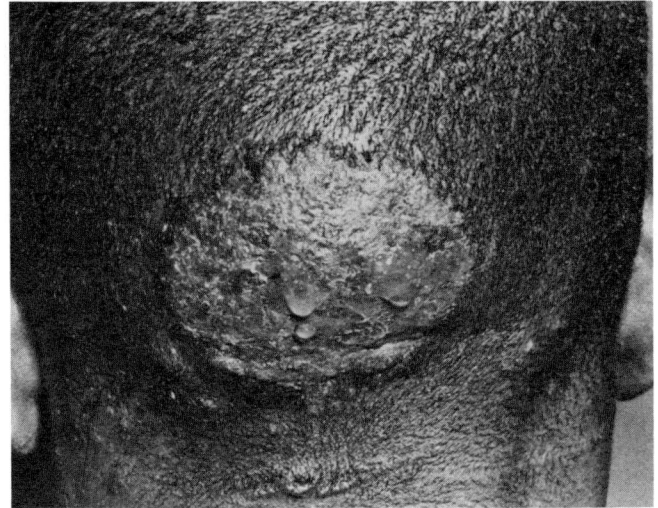

Used with permission of McGraw-Hill Book Company, from *Principles of Pediatrics: Health Care of the Young* (p 1387), by Hoekelman RA et al, ©1978 McGraw-Hill Inc.

(1) fungi are the causative agents
(2) hair loss is usually irreversible
(3) incision and drainage are not indicated
(4) antibiotics have no place in its therapy

398. Correct statements about allergic contact dermatitis include which of the following?

(1) In previously sensitized individuals, lesions may take a few hours or several weeks to develop following subsequent contact
(2) Skin lesions may be vesiculated and weeping or they may be dry, scaling, and lichenified
(3) Once primary sensitization to a substance has occurred, distribution of lesions from subsequent contact is generalized and symmetrical
(4) Substances in creams commonly used topically (e.g., for diaper dermatitis) may be potent sensitizers

399. The four major types of ichthyosis in childhood are correctly characterized by which of the following statements?

(1) Hydration and lubrication are considered to be important interventions
(2) They are hereditary disorders with well-defined patterns of inheritance, but they are not all congenital
(3) When an individual with ichthyosis is frequently exposed to an environment of low humidity, manifestations become more severe
(4) A summer climate is generally favorable for individuals with ichthyosis

400. Correct statements concerning the type of diaper dermatitis shown in the accompanying illustration include which of the following?

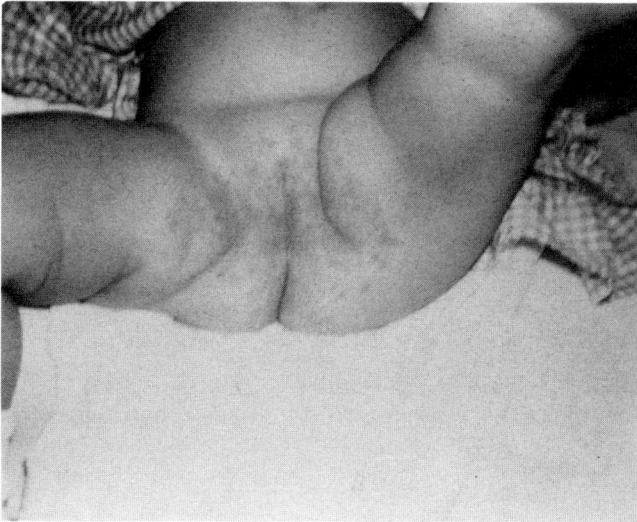

(1) Streptococci are the usual etiologic agents
(2) Warm, moist conditions favor its development
(3) Systemic antibiotics are the treatment of choice
(4) Topical nystatin is helpful

401. A 14-year-old boy presents with a two-month history of a facial rash (see the figure below) that was precipitated by a day at the beach. The patient complains of lethargy and pain in his fingers. Characteristics of this disease include

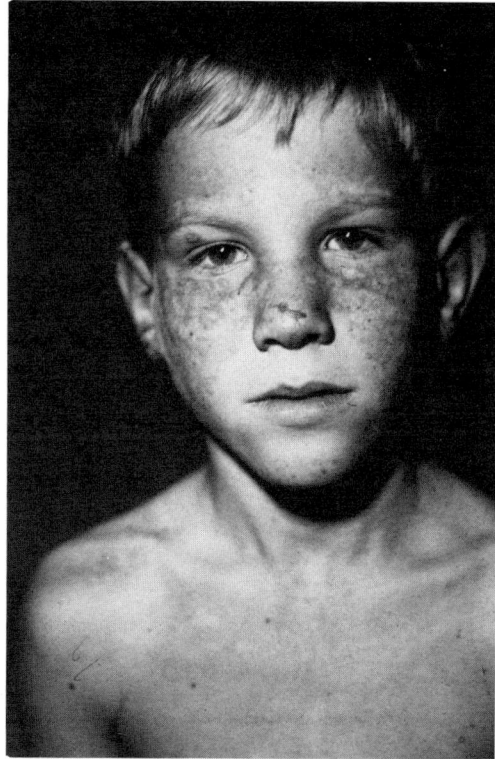

Used with permission of Virgil Hanson, M.D., Children's Hospital of Los Angeles from *Principles of Pediatrics: Health Care of the Young* (p 1114), by Hoekelman RA et al, ©1978 McGraw-Hill Inc.

(1) a female to male ratio of 10:1
(2) central nervous system involvement
(3) decreased C3 and C4 levels and an increased anti-DNA level when the disease flares up
(4) renal involvement, if any, in the first year of the disease

136   *Principles of Pediatrics*

DIRECTIONS: The groups of questions below consist of lettered choices followed by several numbered items. For each numbered item select the **one** lettered choice with which it is **most** closely associated. Each lettered choice may be used once, more than once, or not at all.

Questions 402-404

Many systemic disorders have dermatologic manifestations. For each disorder listed below, select the finding with which it is most likely to be associated.

(A) Cutaneous striae
(B) Vitiligo
(C) Lymphedema
(D) Café au lait spots
(E) None of the above

C 402. Turner's syndrome

B 403. Addison's disease

D 404. von Recklinghausen's disease (neurofibromatosis)

Questions 405-407

For each description of syndromes below, which have dermatologic manifestations, select the test which is most likely to detect an abnormality.

(A) Hematocrit
(B) Auditory screening
(C) Peripheral blood smear
(D) Visual screening
(E) Serum cholesterol and lipid level

B 405. A family in which several members have white forelocks (i.e., patches of white scalp hair over the forehead area)

C 406. A child with partial albinism and a history of recurrent skin and respiratory infections

E 407. An adolescent with xanthomas of the skin and tendon sheaths

Dermatology and Connective Tissue Diseases

Answers

368. The answer is D. *(Schaffer, ed 4. p 961.)* The infant in the figure accompanying the question has a dermatologic condition known as cutis marmorata telangiectasia congenita. This condition is a benign lesion of vascular ectasia that results in a lace-like vascular pattern involving portions of the trunk and the extremities. Observation of the infant and reassurance to the parents is the management of choice, for usually there is improvement and gradual resolution of the bluish ectasias. This infant does not have the mottling frequently associated with overwhelming infection nor the cavernous hemangioma frequently seen in the Kasabach-Merritt syndrome with associated thrombocytopenia. The excellent perfusion in nonaffected areas does not suggest neonatal shock.

369. The answer is E. *(Hoekelman, p 1450.)* Gamma benzene hexachloride (Kwell), considered by many to be the treatment of choice for scabies, has been shown to produce central nervous system toxicity when absorbed in sufficient quantity. Affected individuals often have seizures. Although, in one study, nine percent of a topically applied dose was found to be excreted in the urine, the amount absorbed in a brief treatment regimen is unknown. For this reason, some physicians avoid using this agent in infants and prescribe crotamiton (Eurax), an effective scabicide and antipruritic. There is no evidence to suggest any toxic effects on the other organ systems resulting from the use of gamma benzene hexachloride.

370. The answer is D. *(Hoekelman, pp 1344, 1411.)* The lesions of incontinentia pigmenti often are linear and bullous initially, but eventually present as hyperpigmented areas which exhibit a characteristic swirling, "marble cake" effect. Incontinentia pigmenti is a genetic disease inherited as a sex-linked dominant trait. Associated problems may include epilepsy, mental deficiency, and abnormalities of the teeth and skeletal system. Bullous impetigo is usually nonlinear, and microscopic examination of the bullous fluid will reveal neutrophils and cocci in contrast to the eosinophils seen in incontinentia pigmenti. Neonatal acne, nevus sebaceous, and ichthyosis vulgaris are nonbullous disorders.

371. The answer is B. *(Hoekelman, p 1370.)* Zinc therapy will eliminate the signs and symptoms of acrodermatitis enteropathica, a disorder characterized by vesicobullous and eczematous lesions involving perioral, acral, and perineal skin. Side effects are not known to occur with this therapy. A defect in zinc metabolism is the basic defect in this disease; however, the exact mechanism of pathogenesis is not known. Diarrhea, alopecia, stomatitis, and growth retardation can also occur in this autosomal recessive condition. Unless treated appropriately, the disorder will probably be fatal. Normal levels of copper, thiamine, and vitamin E can be expected in patients with acrodermatitis enteropathica.

372. The answer is E. *(Hoekelman, pp 1347-1349. Fitzpatrick, ed 2. pp 295-303.)* Self-limited (and occasionally recurrent) erythema multiforme is characterized by lesions that occur in crops and individually appear "target" or "iris" shaped, with bright erythematous peripheries and central cyanosis. The lesions are thought to be a manifestation of hypersensitivity to a multitude of agents, including various drugs, viruses, fungi, and occasionally to an underlying malignancy. Mucous membranes may also be involved. None of the other choices is characterized by lesions of this type.

373. The answer is E. *(Hoekelman, p 1399. Fitzpatrick, ed 2. pp 1149-1151.)* Ehlers-Danlos syndrome is characterized by hyperstretchability of the skin, hyperextensibility of joints, poor wound healing, easy bruisability, varicose veins, and in certain forms, rupture of major arteries. Scoliosis has also been observed in association with this syndrome. Depending on the type of disease, inheritance may be autosomal dominant, autosomal recessive, or X-linked recessive. None of the other choices is accompanied by looseness of the skin. Scleroderma can present with tightness of the skin.

374. The answer is D. *(Hoekelman, pp 1343, 1372.)* Cultures and smear of bullous impetigo lesions almost invariably reveal *Staphylococcus aureus.* As shown in the figure accompanying the question, the lesions of bullous impetigo are superficial bullae that often appear wrinkled and contain fluid that may be clear and straw-colored or turbid. As shown in the figure, the bulla on the right has ruptured. The use of a semisynthetic penicillin is necessary for eradication, as the organism usually produces penicillinase. Impetigo is caused by groups A, B, C, and G strains of hemolytic streptococci in over 85 percent of cases, but these cases do not present with bullous lesions. The majority of these lesions, which are initially maculopapular, are secondarily infected with staphylococci and become rounded or circinate in appearance with thick, friable, honey-colored crusts.

375. The answer is B. *(Hoekelman, pp 1101-1103.)* Chronic iridocyclitis is most commonly seen in young girls with pauciarticular arthritis, a form of juvenile rheumatoid arthritis (JRA) in which less than five joints are involved. Often there are no symptoms during the early stages, and diagnosis requires a slit-lamp examination, which should be a routine part of follow-up of patients with JRA. Band keratopathy and cataracts are sequelae of the iridocyclitis. Acute anterior uveitis is seen in boys with spondylitis and HLA-B27. In contrast to the eye involvement in young girls with pauciarticular JRA, the eye manifestations of ankylosing spondylitis are often self-limited.

376. The answer is D. *(Hoekelman, pp 1355-1360.)* Optimal management of the acute phase of atopic dermatitis includes the use of moist, cooling compresses which dry the involved areas as well as decrease the amount of pruritus. Pruritus is often so intense that sedative or antipruritic agents are also necessary. Frequent baths, particularly with drying soaps and hot water, will lead to dry skin and increased itching and thus should be limited to intertriginous regions as much as possible. Only rarely can food or inhalant allergens be implicated as causing atopic dermatitis, but in these cases removal of the specific offending agent may be helpful. Steroids may prove very helpful when given in severe, recalcitrant cases for short periods.

377. The answer is D. *(Hoekelman, p 1388.)* Scaling, macular, slightly pruritic, hypo- or hyperpigmented lesions, involving the upper portion of the trunk as well as the neck and face, are characteristic of tinea versicolor. The hyphae and spores of the causative organism, *Pityrosporon orbiculare,* can be seen with a ten percent potassium hydroxide preparation of skin scrapings. Coppery orange or blue-white fluorescence seen with Wood's light examination will also confirm the diagnosis. Selenium sulfide generally is an effective topical therapeutic agent. Each of the other choices presents a set of symptoms that differs markedly from the lesions shown and described in the question.

378. The answer is C. *(Hoekelman, pp 1362-1364.)* Nail involvement consisting of pitting of the nail plate, onycholysis, and accumulation of subungual scale is characteristic of both childhood and adult psoriasis. Guttate psoriasis is a relatively common form of psoriasis in childhood. It is differentiated, in part, from guttate parapsoriasis by the absence of nail involvement in the latter condition. Guttate psoriasis frequently seems to be precipitated by streptococcal and viral upper respiratory infections. It is one of several forms of childhood psoriasis that differs from the typical adult pattern. Markedly accelerated epidermal turnover time is also characteristic of psoriasis. Facial and intertriginous lesions are far more prominent in seborrhea than in psoriasis; scalp and extensor surface lesions of the knee and elbow are more common in psoriasis. Knee and elbow predilection in psoriasis probably reflects the fact that this condition exhibits the Koebner phenomenon—that is, the appearance of new lesions in areas where there is friction to the skin. The thick silvery or yellow-white scale of untreated psoriatic lesions may result in pinpoint bleeding (Auspitz sign) when removed.

379. The answer is B. *(Hoekelman, p 1340. Fitzpatrick, ed 2. p 634.)* Congenital giant hairy nevi vary greatly in size; 10 to 15 percent of cases may undergo transformation into malignant melanoma. At birth the appearance of the lesion is that of a fleshy brown or black mass with a cerebrate or leathery surface that may seem to "spill" into the surrounding skin area. Cosmetic reasons aside, this potential for malignancy is in itself an indication for surgical removal. In many instances the surgery must be done in stages. Occasionally, lesions occur on the neck and scalp and are associated with leptomeningeal melanocytosis. Epilepsy or focal neurologic signs may occur in association with these nevi.

380. The answer is D. *(Hoekelman, pp 1701, 1708. Miller, p 223.)* Photophobia is a symptom common to many ocular disorders, some of which pose a severe threat to vision. Other symptoms found in association with photophobia are important in the differentiation of serious eye disorders from those of a more benign nature. Vessel injection of the periphery of the scleral (bulbar) conjunctiva is characteristic of conjunctivitis, generally a mild disorder, not associated with photophobia. Keratitis (inflammation of the cornea), including the dendritic ulcer produced by herpes simplex, is characterized by injection of vessels at the limbus. Acute anterior uveitis also exhibits this characteristic. These disorders require ophthalmologic management. Increased intraocular pressure is pathognomonic for glaucoma. Clouding of the cornea usually occurs in keratitis and glaucoma. Photophobia is also a symptom of acute iridocyclitis—inflammation of the iris and ciliary body.

381. The answer is A. *(Hoekelman, pp 1294, 1398. Fitzpatrick, ed 2. pp 1249-1250.)* Hyperpigmentation of the palmar creases, buccal mucosa, linea alba, and scrotum may be seen in adrenal insufficiency. This hyperpigmentation occurs because of an increase in activity of the melanocytes in the involved areas due to their stimulation by pituitary hormones such as adrenocorticotropic hormone. Both scurvy and Henoch-Schönlein purpura can cause petechial and purpuric lesions, which discolor the skin, but these are late manifestations. While the shagreen patches of tuberous sclerosis are hyperpigmented, they are leathery in texture. Hyperpigmentation in these areas is not seen with syphilis.

382. The answer is A. *(Hoekelman, pp 1386-1387.)* Circular areas of complete or partial alopecia involving the scalp and spreading centrifugally are highly suggestive of tinea capitis. The fungus invades the hair shaft, causing it to break and crumble. As topical antifungals do not appear to reach the hair bulbs where active multiplication occurs, oral griseofulvin given for two to four weeks is considered the treatment of choice. Neither penicillin nor bacitracin is an effective antifungal agent. The causative fungus, which grows well in Sabouraud's medium, may cause hairs to fluoresce when examined under a Wood's ultraviolet light.

383. The answer is A. *(Hoekelman, pp 1400, 1403.)* Alopecia resulting from traumatic avulsion is prolonged because growing follicles forcibly avulsed require approximately three months to return to the growing phase, a fact which should be mentioned when counselling someone about this condition. A relatively common form of alopecia results from traction or avulsion applied to produce hair styles such as "cornrowing," braids, and pony tails. Hair loss from trauma is likely to be incomplete and irregular. In alopecia areata, hair loss is complete and occurs in sharply defined patches, occasionally progressing to produce total loss of scalp hair. Congenital alopecia with total absence of hair occurs rarely.

384. The answer is D. *(Hoekelman, pp 1372-1374. Vaughan, ed 11. pp 1878-1879.)* A peeling rash with yellow crusts around the mouth in an 18-month-old child should lead one to consider Stevens-Johnson syndrome and staphylococcal disease. Herpetic disease is unlikely since the lesions are not vesicular, and peeling is not found with herpes. Stevens-Johnson syndrome (erythema multiforme) usually presents with a rash and inflammatory lesions involving two mucous membranes (oral, ocular, or genital). Bullae may form on involved skin and rupture, but peeling of the skin is unusual. A hemorrhagic crusting of the lips is common. The staphylococcal scalded-skin syndrome (SSSS) includes Ritter's disease, Lyell's disease, bullous impetigo, and staphylococcal scarlet fever. All of its manifestations are caused by a toxin (exfoliatin) that produces a red rash (often with sandpaper texture), which is accentuated in the skin folds, and demonstrates Nikolsky's sign. The yellow crusting around the mouth and nostrils is very typical of this disease. Ritter's disease occurs only in infants. A skin biopsy may be useful in distinguishing between Stevens-Johnson and the staphylococcal syndromes. Blister cleavage levels within the skin are constant and therefore useful for making a diagnosis.

385. The answer is D. *(Hoekelman, p 1352.)* The antigen of poison ivy is a common cause of allergic contact dermatitis. The antigen evokes an intensely pruritic eruption, which often becomes vesicular, on areas exposed either directly or by transmission by the hand, as frequently occurs on the genitalia. This process occurs in previously sensitized individuals. Usually appearing within one to three days after initial contact, the intensity of the reaction will often increase over the next seven days before remitting. Oral corticosteroids may be used in the more severe cases.

386. The answer is A. *(Hoekelman, pp 1118-1120. Stiehm, pp 427-428.)* The mean age of onset of dermatomyositis in children is six years. It usually presents with muscle weakness, especially in the proximal leg and hip girdle muscles. The muscles are also usually tender and may be slightly edematous or indurated. A heliotrope discoloration of the upper eyelids and scaling erythematous lesions over the exterior surfaces of the joints and knuckles are characteristic. Vasculitis involving the gastrointestinal tract may result in bloody stools. Diagnosis is confirmed by elevation of creatine phosphokinase, abnormal electromyography, and abnormal muscle biopsy. Rheumatoid factor is usually absent.

387. The answer is C (2, 4). *(Hoekelman, pp 1336-1337.)* Erythema toxicum occurs in 40-60 percent of full-term infants and presents as yellow-white papulopustules on an erythematous base. They can occur anywhere, but most commonly involve the proximal limbs and trunk. The lesions usually occur on the second or third day of life and can remain for one to three days. The lesions can mimic those of infectious dermatoses, but Wright and gram-stained smears reveal an absence of bacteria and the presence of eosinophils. Wood's lamp examination is not helpful in making the diagnosis of skin lesions of the neonate. Skin biopsy is not indicated in this situation.

388. The answer is E (all). *(Hoekelman, pp 347, 1410, 1429, 1669.)* Neurofibromatosis is an autosomal dominant disorder with incomplete penetrance, characterized by the development of tumors of the nervous system. Children and adults with this disease usually have café au lait spots on the skin and may have axillary freckles. Other features include: (1) pseudarthrosis and bowing of the legs; (2) scoliosis; (3) hypertension due to narrowing of a renal artery; (4) seizures; and (5) mental retardation in approximately ten percent of the patients. People with the disease are more likely to develop malignancies such as gliomas and neurofibrosarcomas. Pheochromocytomas, schwannomas of peripheral sensory and cranial nerves, and epilepsy also occur with this disorder. Therefore, all four choices are associated with neurofibromatosis.

389. The answer is D (4). *(Hoekelman, p 1353. Fitzpatrick, ed 2. pp 983-985.)* Topical sunscreens absorb ultraviolet light and thus protect the skin against ultraviolet radiation from the sun. Para-amino benzoic acid is a very effective sunscreen. Of the disorders mentioned, only lesions of lupus erythematosus are made worse by sun exposure – indeed, acne may be improved by such exposure. Patients with lupus erythematosus should avoid direct exposure to the sun and also should apply a sunscreen to exposed areas of the skin as a preventive measure.

390. The answer is C (2, 4). *(Hoekelman, pp 1371-1372. Fitzpatrick, ed 2. pp 1428-1429.)* Impetigo is a highly contagious, superficial skin infection. The most likely pathogen associated with the condition is *Staphylococcus aureus.* However, hemolytic streptococci are often present, and it is generally prudent to treat impetigo as a streptococcal infection unless there is definite proof of the absence of hemolytic streptococci. The frequency of the possibility of streptococcal presence makes treatment with systemic antibiotics highly advisable. Hemolytic streptococci associated with impetigo are rarely implicated in rheumatic fever; however, they may cause acute nephritis.

391. The answer is A (1, 2, 3). *(Hoekelman, pp 1335, 1420, 1778.)* Features common to the hereditary ectodermal dysplasias are disorders of cutaneous appendages, particularly eccrine sweat glands, nails, hair, and teeth. Decreased numbers of sweat glands, short or dystrophic fingernails and toenails, unusually sparse hair (hypotrichosis), and defective teeth are disorders that suggest similar embryologic origins. Each of these disorders is present in several, but not all, the ectodermal dysplasias. Each of the ectodermal dysplasias has unique features in addition to the common ones mentioned.

392. The answer is E (all). *(Hoekelman, p 1340. Menkes, pp 409-410.)* Adenoma sebaceum, which is illustrated in the figure accompanying the question, is characteristic of tuberous sclerosis. Hypopigmented skin patches, often difficult to detect without Wood's light examination, are frequently the only manifestation of tuberous sclerosis in the newborn period. The reliability of these patches as a means of detecting tuberous sclerosis is high; they are present in 90 percent of infants who subsequently develop this condition. Their specificity is not known. Mental deficiency, convulsive seizures, and renal, cardiac, and other disorders commonly result from the angiofibromas present in this condition; these disorders often limit productivity and duration of life. In mildly affected individuals, however, full productive lives are possible. Normal intelligence is present in about one-third of patients. Intracranial calcifications develop eventually in approximately 50 percent of patients, although such calcifications are rare in early childhood before the age of five years.

393. The answer is E (all). *(Hoekelman, p 1349. Fitzpatrick, ed 2. pp 784-789.)* Erythema nodosum is characterized by tender, deep erythematous nodules usually localized to the anterior lower legs. It is thought to be a hypersensitivity reaction to a variety of agents. Its lesions are very tender and often require three to six weeks to resolve. Erythema nodosum is associated with the use of drugs, such as oral contraceptives and sulfonamides, infections, such as streptococcal pharyngitis and tuberculosis, and specific diseases, such as ulcerative colitis, sarcoidosis, and leukemia. It is often accompanied by malaise, polyarthralgias, and low-grade fever.

394. The answer is A (1, 2, 3). *(Hoekelman, pp 1381-1383.)* No single treatment for warts is entirely satisfactory. However, since warts affect only the epidermis and may regress spontaneously even in severe and chronic cases, under no circumstances should therapy that will lead to scarring or other changes that extend beyond this superficial layer of skin be employed. Thus, surgical excision is contraindicated as a treatment option. Podophyllin preparations, electrodesiccation and curettage, and cryocautery (liquid nitrogen) are acceptable. These treatments are less likely to result in scarring than surgery.

395. The answer is B (1, 3). *(Hoekelman, pp 1431-1434. Fitzpatrick, ed 2. pp 725-728.)* Usually bright or purplish red, the strawberry hemangioma (hemangioma simplex) is a type of capillary hemangioma that protrudes above the skin surface. It is rarely present at birth. Usually it appears within the first week following birth as a red or pink macule. The hemangioma enlarges during the first six months of life, stabilizes its rate of growth, and finally fades in color and involutes spontaneously; about 50 percent involute completely by five years of age. Excessively rapid growth, thrombocytopenia, or compromise of vital structures are indications for steroid treatment, which often hastens involution. Only occasionally is surgery necessary.

396. The answer is B (1, 3). *(Hoekelman, p 1355.)* There are two mechanisms of photosensitization—phototoxic and photoallergic. Phototoxic reactions occur in any individual in whom there is a sufficient concentration of the drug and a sufficient amount of light energy delivered to the skin. Photoallergic reactions, on the other hand, are the result of a far more complicated series of events. In photoallergic reactions, the light energy converts the drug into a hapten, which forms a bond with skin protein to form a complete photoantigen. The photoantigen is carried to regional lymph nodes where a true lymphocyte-mediated allergic sensitization takes place. Consequently the number of people who suffer from photoallergic reactions is quite small compared to the number of people who experience photosensitive drug reactions. Skin manifestations of phototoxic reactions include a noneczematous, enhanced sunburn response sharply limited to the sun-exposed areas. Photopatch testing that results in eczematous eruptions extending beyond the photopatch site is a characteristic of photoallergic reactions. Photopatch testing with a phototoxic drug causes an enhanced erythema that is sharply limited to the test site. Many drugs can cause photosensitization.

397. The answer is B (1, 3). *(Hoekelman, p 1387.)* The lesion shown is a kerion. Typically, kerions are swollen, boggy, exudative, and tender. Kerions resemble carbuncles, but are often bacterially sterile; however, fungal cultures will usually reveal the causative organism. The reason for this intense inflammatory reaction to the fungus is unknown; ordinarily fungi cause only superficial infection. Incision and drainage are not recommended, but warm compresses, debridement, epilation of the affected hairs, and tincture of iodine are very helpful in the treatment of kerions. Antibiotics are indicated for secondary bacterial infections. Permanent hair loss is unusual.

398. The answer is C (2,4). *(Hoekelman, pp 1351-1353. Esterly, Pediatr Rev 1:85-90, 1979.)* Allergic contact dermatitis should be distinguished from the contact dermatitis caused by simple physical or chemical irritation of the skin. In the latter disorder, depending on the potency of the irritant and the pre-exposure skin condition, development time may vary from a few hours to several weeks. Lesions due to irritants will develop more rapidly in dry, fissured skin or wet, macerated skin because such damaged skin provides a less effective barrier. Once sensitization has occurred in allergic contact dermatitis, a reaction will develop in 12 to 24 hours following contact. Distribution of allergic contact dermatitis is irregular and asymmetrical, corresponding directly to the contact of antigen with the skin. Specifically sensitized lymphocytes responsible for the allergic reaction are distributed generally; the release of inflammatory lymphokines, however, occurs only in areas where antigens are deposited on the skin surface. Skin lesions may be either vesicular and weeping, as exemplified by rhus dermatitis, or dry and scaling, which is often the case with shoe contact dermatitis. Neomycin, parabens, and ethylene-diamine are examples of substances present in creams often used to relieve diaper dermatitis that may produce allergic contact dermatitis. The "shotgun" approach of products containing these substances is unnecessary.

399. The answer is A (1, 2, 3). *(Hoekelman, pp 1342, 1421.)* Sweating may be impaired in individuals with ichthyosis due to plugging of eccrine ducts by keratotic material; consequently, marked discomfort may occur in very warm weather. Keratolytic agents may be an important part of therapy in addition to hydration and lubrication. This is particularly the case with lamellar ichthyosis and epidermolytic hyperkeratosis, which are true hyperproliferative states with an increased epidermal transit time. House humidification in winter is advised to help reduce scaling. While all are inherited, only ichthyosis vulgaris may have its onset beyond the period of infancy; the other three major types are present at birth or in infancy.

400. The answer is C (2, 4). *(Hoekelman, pp 1389-1390.)* Diaper dermatitis caused by *Candida albicans* often consists of a red plaque-like area of involvement, with very characteristic "satellite" lesions—papules, papulovesicles, or pustules located at the margin of the larger plaques. Warm, moist areas favor its development, thus the usual involvement of intertriginous areas. Topical nystatin and local cleansing are very helpful in the treatment of this type of diaper dermatitis. Systemic antibiotics might be needed only for a serious secondary bacterial infection. Streptococcal organisms are found only as secondary invaders in this and other forms of diaper dermatitis, but this is a rare occurrence.

401. The answer is E (all). *(Hoekelman, pp 1114-1117.)* This is the butterfly rash of systemic lupus erythematosus (SLE). This disease is characterized by erythematous blush, scaling, hyperkeratosis, and atrophy. The dermatologic manifestations of SLE include alopecia, periungual telangiectasia, palmar erythema, gangrenous lesions, and mucosal ulcers. The disease is more common in females than males. Neurologic system involvement may manifest as organic brain disease, functional psychosis, depression, seizures, strokes, and cranial or peripheral nerve involvement. Between 70 and 80 percent of these children develop renal disease, which usually manifests early in the course. The renal disease may vary from mild lesions with slight proteinuria or hematuria to the nephrotic syndrome or renal insufficiency. Laboratory studies that correlate with episodes of active disease may include decreased C3 and C4 levels and an increased anti-DNA level. An acute exacerbation of the disease may indicate the necessity for more aggressive therapy.

402-404. The answers are: 402-C, 403-B, 404-D. *(Hoekelman, pp 347, 1338, 1398. Rudolph, ed 16. p 286.)* Lymphedema, the result of lymphatic stasis, can be a complication of hemangiomas or lymphangiomas. When seen over the dorsum of the hands and feet, however, it is suggestive of Turner's syndrome. Congenital lymphedema usually recedes spontaneously during infancy.

Adrenal insufficiency (Addison's disease) may have varied skin manifestations. Areas of vitiligo can occur as well as the characteristic hyperpigmentation of scars, palmar creases, and linea alba. Hypotension and weakness are associated findings.

Neurofibromatosis (von Recklinghausen's disease), one of the phakomatoses, is inherited as an autosomal dominant condition. Characteristic findings include café au lait macules and multiple firm subcutaneous tumors. Scoliosis, mental retardation, seizures, and pheochromocytomas may also occur.

405-407. The answers are: 405-B, 406-C, 407-E. *(Hoekelman, pp 1036, 1405, 1426.)* White forelocks in several family members suggests the possibility of Waardenburg syndrome, an autosomal dominant disorder associated with lateral displacement of the medial canthi, a broad nasal base, and perceptive deafness. Clinical recognition of this syndrome should lead to audiological evaluation and management of any hearing loss detected.

Chediak-Higashi syndrome is characterized by partial albinism, lymphadenopathy, recurrent pyogenic infection, and giant blue-to-green cytoplasmic granules in granulocytes and lymphocytes that can be seen on a Wright's stain blood smear.

Xanthomas are fatty-yellow tumors of the skin, tendons, and tendon sheaths. Composed of lipid-laden cells, they almost always indicate the presence of a disorder of lipid metabolism when seen in older children or adults. They can also be seen in familial hyperlipoproteinemias, diabetes, and nephrosis. In these disorders, serum cholesterol and lipids may be elevated.

Otolaryngology and Ophthalmology

DIRECTIONS: Each question below contains five suggested answers. Choose the **one best** response to each question.

408. A three-year-old child is brought to the emergency room at 6 P.M. because he is having "difficulty breathing." No one in the immediate family has been ill recently, and everyone has been fully immunized. The morning before presentation, the child complained of a sore throat and for the last few hours, has had a change in his voice. His breathing has become progressively labored. The child is febrile and appears ill with dyspnea, intercostal retractions, and inspiratory stridor. He also keeps his chin elevated. The most likely diagnosis of this child's condition is

(A) foreign body aspiration
(B) croup
(C) diphtheria
(D) peritonsillar abscess
(E) epiglottitis

409. Laryngeal papillomas are correctly described by which one of the following statements?

(A) The larynx is the only site in the upper respiratory tract in which these neoplasms are found
(B) They are among the least common neoplasms of the larynx in children
(C) Endoscopic removal generally is not a satisfactory intervention
(D) Dyspnea and stridor are the most frequent presenting symptoms
(E) None of the above statements

410. All of the following statements about the thyroglossal duct remnant are correct EXCEPT that

(A) it may remain silent for many years following birth
(B) the distal end ascends with swallowing
(C) its embryonic origin is a branchial cleft
(D) it may develop into a cyst that contains thyroid tissue
(E) the treatment of choice is excision

411. Which of the tympanometric curves in the graph shown below is compatible with normal middle ear function?

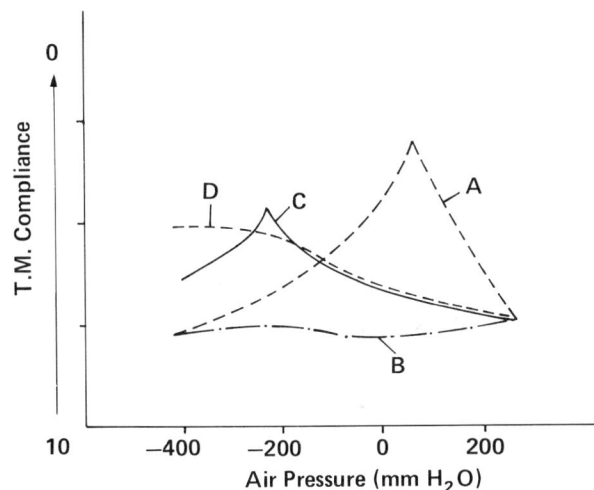

(A) Curve **A**
(B) Curve **B**
(C) Curve **C**
(D) Curve **D**
(E) None of the above curves

412. The recommended therapy for neonatal gonococcal ophthalmia is

(A) silver nitrate ophthalmic drops instilled four times a day for seven days
(B) one dose of 50 mg of amoxicillin per kg of body weight plus probenecid
(C) procaine penicillin, 10,000 units per kg of body weight for seven days
(D) one dose of 50,000 units per kg of benzathine penicillin
(E) aqueous penicillin G, 100,000 units per kg of body weight for seven days

145

413. A two-year-old child presents with a recent history of high fever, irritability, and anorexia. Examination reveals numerous small white plaques and shallow ulcers surrounded by erythema on the tongue, palate, and buccal mucosa. The anterior cervical lymph nodes are enlarged. The most likely diagnosis of this child's condition is a

(A) viral infection that will resolve in 24 hours
(B) viral infection that will further manifest itself with a generalized rash within one to two days
(C) viral infection that will improve in a week to ten days
(D) bacterial infection that should respond to penicillin therapy within 48 hours
(E) yeast infection that will respond to topical medication within five days

414. Although the tooth eruption process is not completely understood, all of the following statements are generally considered to be true EXCEPT that

(A) tooth eruption usually begins at six months of age
(B) delayed tooth eruption may be caused by hyperthyroidism
(C) girls' teeth tend to erupt earlier than boys' teeth
(D) exfoliation will be completed by age 12 in most instances
(E) the mandibular teeth usually erupt before the corresponding maxillary teeth

415. The best method to confirm the diagnosis of epiglottitis is to

(A) examine the posterior pharynx with tongue blade and light
(B) obtain lateral and posteroanterior x-ray views of the neck
(C) identify the pathogen with a throat culture
(D) identify the pathogen with a blood culture
(E) perform a laryngoscopy with a flexible laryngoscope

416. Brownish yellow discoloration of the teeth and hypoplasia of the enamel are associated with

(A) erythroblastosis fetalis
(B) congenital syphilis
(C) vitamin D-resistant rickets
(D) treatment with tetracyclines
(E) treatment with sulfonamides

417. A 16-year-old boy presents with a history of rhinitis every June for the past two years. It is worse when he mows the lawn and on windy days. Speculum examination of the nose would most probably reveal

(A) a small foreign body
(B) boggy, pale mucosa
(C) purulent drainage exiting below the nasal turbinates
(D) erythematous friable mucosa
(E) nasal polyps

418. A seven-year-old child presents with a "droopy" eyelid. All of the following should be considered as part of the differential diagnosis EXCEPT

(A) a congenital anomaly
(B) impaired sympathetic nervous system function
(C) a lesion of the third cranial nerve
(D) a lesion of the fourth cranial nerve
(E) myasthenia gravis

419. Tympanometry is helpful in evaluating young children with suspected hearing loss. The tympanogram provides information on all the following EXCEPT the

(A) degree of hearing loss
(B) mobility of the tympanic membrane
(C) middle ear pressure
(D) perforation of the tympanic membrane
(E) eustachian tube function

420. A two-day-old infant presents with a purulent eye discharge. Which of the following is the most likely diagnosis?

(A) Gonorrheal conjunctivitis
(B) *Chlamydia trachomatis* conjunctivitis
(C) Chemical irritation
(D) Inclusion blennorrhea
(E) Dacryostenosis

421. All of the following conditions may be associated with a cataract EXCEPT for

(A) a penetrating eye injury
(B) maternal rubella
(C) a cytomegalovirus infection
(D) galactosemia
(E) hypocalcemia

422. Approximately 50 percent of all children in the United States have some dental caries by the age of

(A) 2 years
(B) 3 years
(C) 4 years
(D) 5 years
(E) 6 years

DIRECTIONS: Each question below contains four suggested answers of which **one or more** is correct. Choose the answer

A	if	1, 2, and 3	are correct
B	if	1 and 3	are correct
C	if	2 and 4	are correct
D	if	4	is correct
E	if	1, 2, 3, and 4	are correct

423. Sensorineural hearing loss is associated with which of the following conditions?

(1) Pathology of the eighth cranial nerve
(2) Chickenpox
(3) Maternal rubella
(4) Visible abnormality of the tympanic membrane

424. Correct statements about choanal atresia include which of the following?

(1) Passage of an oral airway may be a life-saving measure
(2) Passage of a nasal catheter may constitute definitive treatment
(3) It may not be recognized for several years
(4) Management in the neonate generally includes gavage feeding over the first several weeks

425. Management of the child with cleft lip and cleft palate generally involves

(1) treatment of problems secondary to weakness of the tensor veli palatini muscle
(2) surgical cleft palate repair between 6 and 12 months of age
(3) services provided by an orthodontist and a speech pathologist
(4) adenoidectomy for treatment of recurrent serous and suppurative otitis media

426. Correct statements about tonsillectomy and adenoidectomy include which of the following?

(1) Of all surgical procedures requiring anesthesia, they are the most frequently performed in the United States
(2) There are approximately 150 deaths in the United States each year from these procedures
(3) They are frequently performed before the age at which the frequency of upper respiratory illness naturally tends to diminish
(4) Persistent nasal obstruction, mouth breathing, and hyponasal speech in children are considered reasonable indications for these procedures

427. Fundoscopic examination of a patient's retina reveals yellowish areas with poorly defined margins; in addition, there are some whitish areas with pigmented margins. The differential diagnosis should include

(1) toxoplasmosis
(2) syphilis
(3) cytomegalovirus infection
(4) tuberculosis

428. A four-year-old child is suspected of having a moderate hearing loss. Initial diagnostic testing reveals a normal bone-conduction threshold, but there is an increase in the air-conduction hearing threshold. After the initial testing, it would be appropriate to make which of the following statements?

(1) Serous otitis media is a common cause of this condition
(2) The child's hearing level may fluctuate
(3) The child may have a cholesteatoma
(4) The child may have a reduced ability to understand speech sounds

429. Correct statements about serous otitis media include which of the following?

(1) Approximately 20 percent of children with acute otitis media subsequently develop serous otitis media
(2) The malleus typically shifts from its normal central position to the upper anterior quadrant of the tympanic membrane
(3) The major morbidity is chronic, fluctuating hearing loss
(4) Audiometry serves as a sensitive screening test for the presence of serous otitis media

430. An eight-year-old boy is brought to the emergency room complaining of pain in his right eye and blurred vision. Physical examination reveals a cloudy cornea and diminished vision. Diagnostic procedures that should help in the differential diagnosis of this problem include

(1) measurement of intraocular pressure
(2) measurement of visual acuity
(3) fluorescein staining of cornea
(4) cover-uncover test

431. Unilateral exophthalmos in children has a variety of etiologies, including

(1) metastatic neuroblastoma
(2) periorbital cellulitis
(3) Hans-Schüller-Christian disease
(4) hyperthyroidism

432. Hearing evaluation is difficult with many children because of their inability to cooperate. Tests of hearing that are useful in these children include

(1) measurement of acoustic impedance
(2) auditory-evoked responses
(3) electrocochleography
(4) pure-tone audiometry

433. Physical examination of a patient with trauma to the left eye reveals a hyphema. True statements about this condition include which of the following?

(1) It may lead to blindness
(2) Sedation is an important aspect of its treatment
(3) Hospitalization should be undertaken in all cases
(4) Secondary bleeding may occur within three to five days

434. Altered tooth development is characteristic of which of the following inheritable disorders?

(1) Dentinogenesis imperfecta
(2) Hypophosphatasia
(3) Amelogenesis imperfecta
(4) Dysautonomia

435. Which of the following diagnoses should be considered in a child with epistaxis?

(1) The presence of a foreign body
(2) An upper respiratory infection
(3) Thrombocytopenia
(4) Whooping cough

436. The mother of the six-month-old girl shown in the figure below is concerned that her child always "keeps a cold." The cold appears to be a mild one manifested primarily by a clear nasal discharge. The mother reports that on one occasion there was a cough as well. She is also concerned because the child closes her eyes when in a room with a lot of light or when outdoors. Further evaluation is likely to reveal

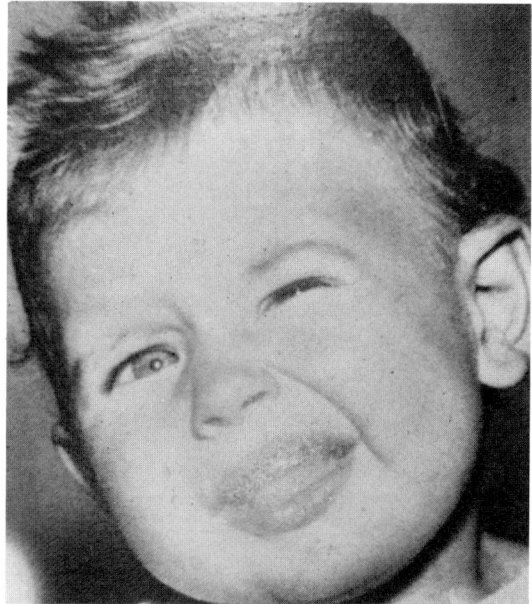

Used with permission of Henry S. Metz, M.D., University of Rochester Medical Center.

(1) a consistent avoidance response to the light from a flashlight
(2) a family history of asthma
(3) tearing of only one eye and clear nasal discharge from the homolateral nostril only
(4) a mother, who has recently separated, with few social supports and "tight" finances

437. A mother of an eight-month-old child complains that her child's eyes are "crossed." True statements about this condition include which of the following?

(1) This child may have an intraocular disease
(2) Strabismus may be a normal finding during the first four months of life
(3) Strabismus is one of the leading causes of monocular blindness
(4) Strabismus could be due to a difference in refractive error between the two eyes

DIRECTIONS: The groups of questions below consist of lettered choices followed by several numbered items. For each numbered item select the **one** lettered choice with which it is **most** closely associated. Each lettered choice may be used once, more than once, or not at all.

Questions 438-441

For each description that follows, select the diagnosis which most appropriately applies.

    (A) Acute sinusitis
    (B) Chronic sinusitis
    (C) Peritonsillar abscess
    (D) Serous otitis media
    (E) Mastoiditis

438. Periorbital cellulitis is a relatively common complication

439. Complications do not include lung or intracranial infection

440. This occurs concurrently with virtually all episodes of acute suppurative otitis media

441. Current evidence suggests that a period of "watchful waiting" is appropriate following diagnosis

Questions 442-445

For each of the ophthalmologic defects below, select the inherited metabolic disease with which it is most likely to be associated.

    (A) Tay-Sachs disease
    (B) Menkes' kinky hair syndrome
    (C) Galactosemia
    (D) Homocystinuria
    (E) Hartnup's syndrome

442. Blindness

443. Ectopia lentis

444. Cherry-red macula

445. Cataract

Otolaryngology and Ophthalmology

Answers

408. The answer is E. *(Hoekelman, pp 1751-1754.)* A three-year-old who rapidly develops an upper airway obstruction syndrome with toxicity and fever, without a cough, and who keeps his chin elevated, is most likely to have epiglottitis. Diphtheria is unlikely in an immunized child, aspiration of a foreign body should not be accompanied by fever, and a peritonsillar abscess is usually more insidious in its onset. Croup (viral laryngotracheobronchitis) is not likely in this child who has no cough and who is remarkably toxic. Epiglottitis is an acute, potentially fatal infection. The cause is almost exclusively *Hemophilus influenzae* type B. The potential fatal outcome of this disease makes early clinical recognition essential.

409. The answer is E. *(Hoekelman, p 1722.)* The most common neoplasms of the larynx in children are the multiple verrucose-appearing, benign, squamous cell neoplasms of juvenile laryngeal papillomatosis. Arising from the vocal cords, the presenting symptom is hoarseness. These same lesions may appear coincidentally or solely in the nasal or oral cavities. Endoscopic removal is the usual treatment, although repeated removal may be necessary because of the tendency for recurrence.

410. The answer is C. *(Hoekelman, p 1714.)* The thyroglossal duct cyst represents the remnant of the migration of the thyroid anlage from the base of the tongue to the neck. Consequently, this cyst lies in the midline, an important differential diagnostic point between the thyroglossal duct cyst and branchial cleft cysts which are located in the lateral neck along the anterior border of the sternocleidomastoid muscle. It is common for the thyroglossal duct cyst to present no signs or symptoms until it becomes filled with fluid. Many years may pass before this occurs. A point useful in differentiation from other midline neck lesions is that anatomical relationships cause the cyst to ascend with swallowing. Surgical excision is generally the treatment of choice because of the common complication of infection and abscess formation. Occasionally, all of the patient's functioning thyroid tissue may be found in the cyst. For this reason, a thyroid scan should be performed before surgery. If all the functioning thyroid tissue is in the cyst, surgery should not be performed.

411. The answer is A. *(Hoekelman, pp 198-201. Paradise, Pediatrics 58:198-210, 1976.)* A normal tympanogram (curve A) will have the point of maximal compliance at or near normal atmospheric pressure (zero mm H_2O air pressure). Curves B and D demonstrate tympanograms with low relative compliance without definite peak points and are typically seen with acute otitis media or tympanic membrane perforation. With a retracted tympanic membrane, there is relatively normal compliance, but the point of maximum compliance occurs at a negative pressure value, as seen in curve C.

412. The answer is E. *(Hoekelman, pp 463-464.)* Current recommendations from the Center for Disease Control and the American Academy of Pediatrics for treatment of neonatal gonococcal ophthalmia include 100,000 units per kg of body weight of aqueous penicillin given daily intramuscularly for seven days. Silver nitrate ophthalmic drops are used for prophylaxis not therapy. The serum levels of penicillin achieved with this dosage of penicillin G will be higher than those reached with the other forms and dosages listed in the other choices.

413. The answer is C. *(Hoekelman, p 1170.)* There are many conditions that cause fever, anorexia, and irritability in young children. The lesions described are characteristic of herpetic gingivostomatitis. This viral infection commonly lasts from seven to ten days and if severe, will require hospitalization for intravenous fluid therapy. Coxsackie viral infections are sometimes associated with vesicles that ulcerate and have the appearance of herpetic lesions, but these are limited to the soft palate and the posterior pharyngeal wall, and the patients are not as ill as those with herpetic gingivostomatitis. The oral lesions of moniliasis do not ulcerate nor do those of rubeola (Koplik's spots), which are limited to the buccal mucosa. Palatal petechiae and cervical adenitis accompany streptococcal pharyngitis, but ulcerative lesions are not found in this condition.

414. The answer is B. *(Hoekelman, p 1779.)* Much about the process of tooth eruption is unknown. However, it is known that: (1) in most instances, girls begin this process earlier than do boys; (2) mandibular teeth erupt first; and (3) the process usually begins at six months of age. Exfoliation, or loss of the deciduous teeth, is usually completed in both sexes by the age of 12 years. There are many causes of delayed tooth eruption, including Down's syndrome, hypopituitarism, and hypothyroidism. Alternatively, hyperthyroidism will not affect the eruption process.

415. The answer is B. *(Hoekelman, pp 1752-1753.)* The diagnosis of epiglottitis rests on the finding of the inflamed obstructing epiglottis. However, attempts at direct visualization with a light and tongue blade or with direct laryngoscopy may lead to laryngeal spasm and sudden, complete obstruction; therefore, direct visual examination should be attempted only by physicians with the necessary expertise and equipment for establishing an airway in case a sudden upper airway obstruction should occur. If the child is not severely distressed, radiologic examination will confirm the diagnosis. Following this, a planned orotracheal intubation or a tracheostomy can be performed. Throat and blood cultures, which may help in establishing the organism causing the epiglottitis (almost always type B *Hemophilus influenzae*), and concomitant antibiotic treatment are not included in the acute diagnostic maneuvers.

416. The answer is D. *(Hoekelman, pp 1781-1783.)* Discoloration of the teeth secondary to erythroblastosis fetalis is usually a blue-to-black discoloration. Medication with tetracyclines, however, usually leads to the brownish-yellowish discoloration described. Both congenital syphilis and rickets may cause an abnormality of the tooth-shaping process rather than a change in the tooth color. Sulfonamides are not known to cause any change in tooth coloration.

417. The answer is B. *(Hoekelman, pp 52, 56, 1724, 1741.)* Airborne pollen allergy is the most probable etiology of this patient's rhinitis because of its seasonal recurrence and the relationship to mowing the lawn and windy weather. The nasal mucosa is typically boggy and pale in allergic rhinitis. An erythematous friable mucosa is seen in viral rhinitis. Nasal polyps are very rare in children, except in those with cystic fibrosis. A nasal foreign body would present with a purulent discharge. Purulent drainage would also be more suggestive of an infectious rhinitis or sinusitis.

418. The answer is D. *(Rudolph, ed 16. p 1736.)* Ptosis may be congenital or acquired. Unilateral ptosis is frequently seen in myasthenia gravis, lesions of the third cranial nerve (oculomotor), and Horner's syndrome. Miosis and enophthalmos are associated with Horner's syndrome, a disease that is a manifestation of impaired sympathetic function. The fourth cranial nerve (trochlear) does not supply the muscles of the upper eyelid.

419. The answer is A. *(Hoekelman, pp 198-201.)* Tympanometry, one of the acoustic-impedance tests, measures the intactness and mobility of the tympanic membrane and the middle ear pressure; it indicates whether the eustachian tube is functioning normally. The technique does not provide information on hearing per se, and it cannot take the place of pure-tone audiometry. The stapedial muscle reflex may be evaluated by an apparatus similar to that used for tympanometry, and it can be useful in detecting sensorineural hearing loss. This technique is particularly appropriate for use with young, uncooperative patients.

420. The answer is C. *(Vaughan, ed 11. p 479.)* All of the conditions listed may present during the neonatal period. However, only silver nitrate irritation will present within six to twelve hours of age. Irritations secondary to gonorrhea are seen two to five days after birth; inclusion blennorrhea and chlamydial infections are not seen until five to fourteen days after birth. Dacryostenosis will usually not lead to a purulent discharge.

421. The answer is C. *(Hoekelman, p 1707. Vaughan, ed 11. p 1970.)* Cataracts can be either congenital or acquired. A frequent cause of congenital cataracts is maternal rubella. Galactosemia and hypocalcemia are among the frequent causes of acquired cataracts. Acquired cataracts secondary to trauma may be from either direct trauma to the eye or from a penetrating injury. A cytomegalovirus infection can cause chorioretinitis but not cataracts.

422. The answer is A. *(Hoekelman, p 173.)* Approximately 50 percent of all children in the United States show evidence of dental caries as early as two years of age. All children should be referred to a dentist before they reach the age of two and one-half to three years to prevent carious lesions from becoming extensive. Referral for such care should be made even if no dental problems are evident. Preventive dental care is particularly important for children with chronic illness, especially hematologic disorders.

423. The answer is A (1, 2, 3). *(Hoekelman, p 1758.)* Sensorineural hearing loss results from damage to the sensory end organ or cochlear hair cells. It may also be secondary to central or peripheral damage to the eighth cranial nerve. It has been associated with a number of congenital infections, including syphilis, rubella, and chickenpox. Abnormalities of the tympanic membrane are not seen in sensorineural hearing loss. For this reason, sensorineural hearing loss, which is usually irreversible, frequently escapes detection in the course of a routine ear examination.

424. The answer is E (all). *(Hoekelman, p 1715. Schaffer, ed 4. p 96.)* Choanal atresia, a stricture or total stenosis of the posterior nasal apertures, may be membranous or bony, bilateral or unilateral. Because most neonates are obligate nose breathers, bilateral atresia produces life-threatening respiratory distress in the newborn. Satisfactory immediate treatment for this condition is insertion of an oral airway or a rubber nipple with a large hole. Most infants with this condition will learn to mouth-breathe by about three weeks of age. When breathing by mouth is accomplished, it also becomes possible to coordinate sucking and breathing, and gavage feeding is usually no longer necessary. Inability to pass a nasal catheter in a neonate with respiratory distress is suggestive of choanal atresia. If the atresia is membranous, this procedure frequently will rupture the membrane; subsequent dilatation, however, may be necessary. If the atresia is unilateral, signs consist only of persistent mucous rhinorrhea; consequently, recognition often is delayed for several years.

425. The answer is B (1, 3). *(Hoekelman, pp 1717-1718.)* The adenoids are generally important to velopharyngeal closure in individuals with cleft lip and palate, because congenital weakness of the tensor veli palatini muscle is part of the cleft lip and palate syndrome. This muscle weakness precludes adequate velopharyngeal closure **unless** adenoids are present to facilitate this process. Although weakness of the tensor veli palatini muscle results in a high incidence of both serous and suppurative otitis media, adenoidectomy to correct this situation is contraindicated. Tensor veli palatini weakness is also present with submucosal cleft palate; consequently, adenoidectomy should be avoided in this condition as well. Current surgical practice is generally to repair a cleft palate between 18 and 24 months of age. Malpositioned teeth are part of this condition and require orthodontic care. Speech problems as a result of the cleft and associated hearing difficulties caused by otitis media are also common in this condition.

426. The answer is A (1, 2, 3). *(Hoekelman, pp 1754-1757. Green, ed 2. pp 47-48.)* Of all surgical procedures requiring anesthesia, tonsillectomy and adenoidectomy remain the surgical procedures most commonly performed in the United States; of the one million such procedures performed annually, it is estimated that approximately 150 deaths occur. In addition, a 1956 survey revealed a serious complication rate of 15.6 per 1000 procedures. Persistent nasal obstruction, mouth breathing, and hyponasal speech should be considered reasonable indications for surgery **only** after evaluation has shown that they are not due to allergy and there is clinical and x-ray evidence of adenoid hypertrophy. Much of the anecdotal evidence supporting the efficacy of tonsillectomy and adenoidectomy undoubtedly is due to this procedure usually being performed shortly before the time at which the frequency of upper respiratory illnesses naturally declines.

427. The answer is E (all). *(Hoekelman, pp 1698-1699, 1702. Vaughan, ed 11. pp 846, 884-885, 1011, 1971.)* The condition of the retina described in the question is chorioretinitis. It has been associated with toxoplasmosis, syphilis, cytomegalovirus infection, as well as tuberculosis. Other conditions that may lead to chorioretinitis include histoplasmosis, fungal infections, and nematode infestation. When the retina and posterior portion of the uveal tract (choroiditis) are inflamed (the two usually go hand in hand), the condition is called chorioretinitis. One of the more common causes of posterior uveitis is tuberculosis. Chorioretinitis has been associated with acquired cytomegalovirus infection in immunosuppressed patients, but toxoplasmosis is more likely to be associated with this inflammation. Chorioretinitis is an early manifestation of congenital syphilis, as is iritis.

428. The answer is A (1, 2, 3). *(Hoekelman, p 1758.)* The condition described in the question is a conductive hearing loss. It is most frequently caused in children by serous otitis media. The hearing level is not constant and may fluctuate. As there are other causes for this condition (e.g., cholesteatoma), a myringotomy with placement of ventilation tubes may not resolve the problem. Reduced ability to understand or discriminate speech sounds is a symptom of sensorineural hearing loss rather than conductive hearing loss.

429. The answer is A (1, 2, 3). *(Hoekelman, pp 198-201, 1737-1739.)* Data obtained from follow-up examinations indicate that approximately 20 percent of acute otitis media (AOM) patients, who have received appropriate management, will subsequently develop serous otitis media (SOM). Otoscopic examinations show that a shift in the position of the malleus from its normally central position to the upper anterior quadrant of the tympanic membrane is a relatively sensitive and specific finding for SOM. Otalgia often occurs in association with this condition, but it is usually mild. Tympanometry is a fairly useful tool for the evaluation of

SOM; it provides valid results, correlating well with tympanocentesis findings that are the diagnostic standard for AOM. Only 60 percent of children with SOM, detected by tympanocentesis, are found to have any hearing deficit as measured by audiometry. Therefore, audiometry cannot be considered a sensitive screening test for SOM. The rate at which children with SOM, who have normal audiometric results, subsequently develop hearing loss is not known. Most questions regarding the natural history of serous otitis media remain unanswered.

430. The answer is B (1, 3). *(Hoekelman, pp 1697, 1703.)* The most common causes of eye pain and cloudy cornea in children are acute glaucoma, keratitis, and corneal trauma. In order to differentiate these disorders, it is necessary to test for evidence of injury to the cornea from trauma or infection with fluorescein dye. This test is positive with keratitis and corneal trauma. A measurement of the intraocular pressure should also be done. High intraocular pressure is indicative of acute glaucoma. A test for strabismus—for example, the cover-uncover test—will not aid in the differential diagnosis.

431. The answer is E (all). *(Hoekelman, p 1706. Rudolph, ed 16. pp 1970-1972. Ziai, ed 2. pp 718-719.)* Exophthalmos associated with hyperthyroidism is not always bilateral. On occasion, particularly early in the disease, unilateral exophthalmos is observed. Neoplasm of any of the orbital contents can also lead to exophthalmos. Neuroblastoma metastasizing to the orbital bones is the most frequent cause of exophthalmos due to malignancy. Periorbital cellulitis and orbital abscess are also associated with unilateral exophthalmos, as is the deposition of xanthomatous materials in the orbital tissues as seen in Hans-Schüller-Christian disease. Hyperthyroidism is less frequent in children than in adults. When exophthalmos does occur in children, it is often accompanied by upper lid retraction and a feeling that there is a foreign body in the eye. The exophthalmos usually subsides with treatment for hyperthyroidism.

432. The answer is A (1, 2, 3). *(Hoekelman, pp 195-202. Rudolph, ed 16. p 965.)* Puretone audiometry is the most frequently used hearing test; however, it is a behavioral test requiring cooperation from the patient. The other hearing tests included in the question are physiologic tests requiring specialized equipment. These tests are particularly appropriate for use with infants and young children in situations where a behavioral test is difficult or impossible to use.

433. The answer is E (all). *(Hoekelman, pp 1704-1705.)* A hyphema (blood in the anterior chamber of the eye) is usually secondary to ocular contusion. The prognosis is usually good when appropriate treatment is given. This treatment includes hospitalization with strict bed rest and elevation of the head at 30°, sedation, and binocular dressings. More bleeding may occur without further trauma within three to five days following the original injury and may result in blindness.

434. The answer is E (all). *(Hoekelman, p 1779. Rudolph, ed 16. pp 937-939.)* All of the listed conditions affect tooth development. Dentinogenesis imperfecta and amelogenesis imperfecta lead to abnormal dentin and enamel formation, respectively. The former condition is probably the most frequently encountered genetic disorder affecting the formation of the teeth. Hypophosphatasia disturbs bone formation and results in small teeth with early root resorption. Dysautonomia is characterized by autonomic malfunctions. One of the symptoms, excessive grinding of the teeth, can be so excessive that the primary teeth are loosened and lost. This symptom occurs most frequently in patients two to three years of age.

435. The answer is E (all). *(Hoekelman, p 1765.)* Nosebleeds occur in all of the conditions included in the question. The incidence of epistaxis is increased with upper respiratory infections and any condition that leads to an elevated venous pressure, such as whooping cough, mitral stenosis, or superior vena cava syndrome. A foreign body in the nasal cavity may be a cause of recurrent epistaxis, especially in the young toddler. As with any unusual bleeding, thrombocytopenia should be considered with sudden, unexplainable epistaxis.

436. The answer is B (1, 3). *(Hoekelman, pp 1701, 1767. Harley, pp 390-394.)* The child shown in the picture has congenital glaucoma. The incidence of this disease is about 0.05 percent. Usual early findings are tearing of the affected eye and consequent clear nasal discharge, photophobia, and blepharospasm. Corneal enlargement develops gradually and often is not present in newborn infants. Corneal clouding results from corneal edema and is present in over 25 percent of cases at birth and over 60 percent of cases beyond the age of six months. Allergic conjunctivitis and tear-duct blockage are common mistaken diagnoses. The lack of nasal discharge in the latter condition should enable ready distinction from congenital glaucoma. In light of the knowledge that a stressful life situation correlates with increased utilization of health services, the busy health care provider might be inclined to overlook the early, subtle findings of congenital glaucoma. Blindness is the usual outcome in untreated cases of congenital glaucoma.

437. The answer is E (all). *(Rudolph, ed 16. pp 1967-1968.)* Transient strabismus, which is found in many infants in the first four months of life, is considered normal and will most likely resolve spontaneously. However, strabismus that occurs after that time should be referred to an ophthalmologist for evaluation and treatment. Strabismus is sometimes a symptom of conditions, such as retrolental fibroplasia, congenital cataracts, toxocariasis, and retinoblastoma. The most common cause is a disturbance in innervation of the extraocular muscles. If not corrected early in life, monocular blindness will result. Strabismus may sometimes be due to anisometropia, a condition characterized by a difference in refractive error between the two eyes.

438-441. The answers are: 438-A, 439-D, 440-E, 441-D. *(Hoekelman, pp 1730, 1735-1736, 1746, 1756. Paradise, Pediatrics 60:87-89, 1977.)* Periorbital cellulitis is a relatively frequent complication of acute sinusitis; it is most frequently a sequela of ethmoid sinusitis. The lateral wall of the ethmoid sinus constitutes the medial wall of the orbit. This wall, termed the lamina papyracea, is thin in children and forms a relatively poor barrier to contiguous spread of infection. Chronic bacterial infection of the sinuses is rare in children and periorbital cellulitis as a complication is even more so. Infection in the anatomic domain of the other conditions listed does not offer channels for periorbital spread.

Except for serous otitis media, all of the diagnostic labels included in the question are used to describe bacterial infections. Because of anatomic relationships, these infections, if untreated, may lead to serious complications within the respiratory tract or the central nervous system. For instance, lateral sinus thrombophlebitis may be the result of contiguous erosion from mastoiditis. Peritonsillar abscess may lead to lung infection either by rupture and aspiration or by extension to the pharyngomaxillary space and then to the internal jugular vein where thrombophlebitis leads to pulmonary septic emboli.

The mucosa of the middle ear is continuous with the mastoid air cells. For this reason, infection of the mastoid occurs in association with virtually all episodes of acute suppurative otitis media. In one to five percent of **untreated** episodes of acute otitis media, obstruction of drainage from the mastoid to the tympanic cavity develops. This obstruction may be followed by a destructive and chronic form of mastoiditis. Obstruction of mastoid drainage occurs very rarely in acute otitis media patients who have received appropriate treatment. Serous otitis media (in the other ear) often occurs concurrently with acute otitis media. Concurrence between acute otitis media and the other conditions listed is unusual.

About 80 percent of children in whom serous otitis media is diagnosed will have regained normal hearing six to eight weeks following the diagnosis. Most but not all of those with normal hearing will have **no** remaining evidence of the serous otitis media. There is no evidence that antihistamines or sympathomimetic decongestants increase the speed of resolution. If serous otitis media persists beyond eight weeks, consideration of myringotomy, with or without placement of a tympanostomy tube, is warranted. Delay in instituting active intervention has a significant chance of increasing morbidity in all of the other conditions listed in the question.

442-445. The answers are: 442-B, 443-D, 444-A, 445-C. *(Hoekelman, pp 901-903, 940, 943, 1402-1403. Rudolph, pp 1910-1911.)* Inability of the eyes to follow light by two months of age may be the presenting symptom of blindness in children with Menkes' kinky hair syndrome. A copper deficiency is the cause of this syndrome in which the hair is white and the texture of steel wool. The disease progresses rapidly and is fatal due to progressive cerebral degeneration.

Although it may not present in infancy, homocystinuric children eventually develop ectopia lentis. A careful eye examination will reveal iridodonesis or shimmering of the iris. About 50 percent of patients with homocystinuria are mentally retarded.

The macula is often red in children with Tay-Sachs disease; they may also have nystagmus or other eye movement abnormalities. Tay-Sachs victims eventually become functionally blind. No therapy is available and death is due to infection, usually pneumonia.

Cataracts may be present in young infants who have galactosemia. These cataracts can be well formed and impair the vision. The lens of the eye characteristically has a bubbly appearance. If cataracts are observed, highest priority should be given to determining the presence of a reducing substance in the urine and also assaying for the galactose transferase enzyme. There are no specific ophthalmologic disorders associated with Hartnup's disease.

Nephrology and Musculoskeletal Diseases

DIRECTIONS: Each question below contains five suggested answers. Choose the **one best** response to each question.

446. Which of the following data would be LEAST useful in the evaluation of a seven-year-old black male with a history of primary enuresis?

(A) Record of school performance
(B) Urinalysis
(C) Test for anal reflex
(D) Test for sickle cell anemia
(E) X-ray of the spine

447. A septic and dehydrated infant of a diabetic mother suddenly develops an abdominal mass. Which of the following statements is compatible with these symptoms?

(A) Urine output may be normal if the most likely etiology is unilateral
(B) Hematuria is likely to be present
(C) The nephrotic syndrome is likely to develop
(D) Anticoagulation with heparin will generally not be effective in this case
(E) The definitive diagnostic test is a renal scan

448. A premature, low-birth-weight baby girl presents with severe respiratory distress. Examination reveals low-set ears, poor pinna development, hypertelorism, a beak-like nose, and facial asymmetry. The infant has been in acute renal failure since birth, manifested by complete anuria and kidneys that cannot be palpated. The most likely diagnosis is
(A) infantile polycystic kidney disease
(B) Potter's syndrome
(C) newborn respiratory distress syndrome
(D) oculocerebrorenal syndrome of Lowe
(E) none of the above

449. The condition represented in the x-ray shown below

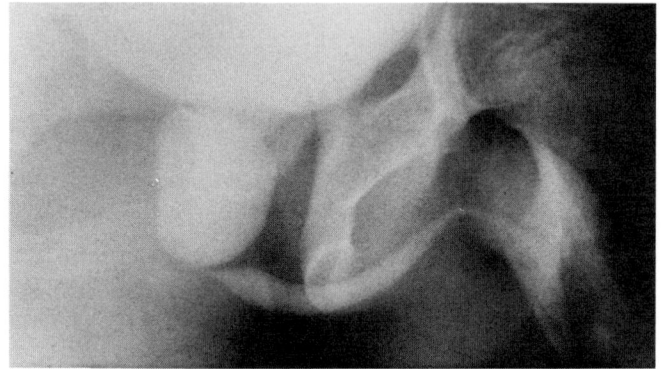

(A) is most commonly seen in females
(B) almost always is associated with ureteral reflux
(C) most often presents as a urinary tract infection
(D) usually becomes apparent clinically in the newborn period
(E) none of the above

450. Which of the following statements concerning the determination of the source of blood found in the urine is correct?

(A) Extraglomerular renal bleeding produces clots but no red cell casts in the urine
(B) A diagnosis of hydronephrosis is indicative of glomerular bleeding
(C) Glomerular bleeding usually is painful
(D) Renal calculi usually cause hematuria and proteinuria
(E) None of the above

451. At birth, the premature infant (33 weeks gestation) shown in the figure below is noted to have respiratory difficulties and to suffer a right pneumothorax soon after positive pressure ventilation is administered. There are two arteries and one vein in the umbilical cord. The lower abdominal defect is leaking a yellow fluid. In the total management of this child, which of the following sequences represents optimal neonatal management?

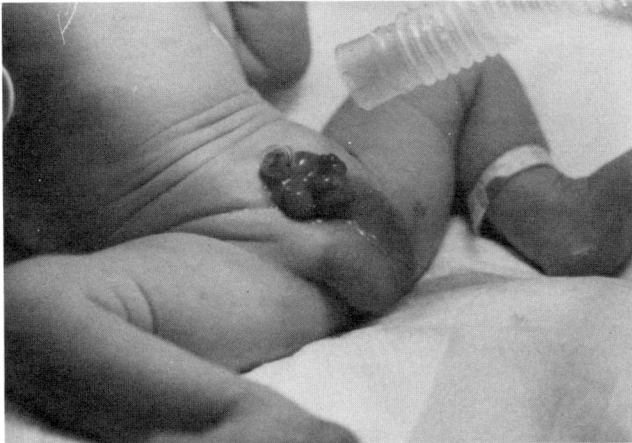

(A) Stabilize ventilation after chest tube insertion, increase intravenous fluids to 120 ml/kg/day to account for fluid losses, and catheterize the bladder

(B) Stabilize ventilation and vital signs after chest tube insertion, inspect for other abnormalities, arrange for an intravenous pyelogram along with a urologic surgical consultation, and monitor hydration according to weight and electrolyte changes

(C) Stabilize ventilation and chest tube insertion, inform both parents of the undetermined sex of the infant, request chromosome studies, and begin intravenous saline and deoxycorticosterone acetate injections

(D) Stabilize ventilation after chest tube insertion, evaluate with a 24-hour 17-hydroxy-ketosteroid pregnanediol urinary excretion test, and administer 50 mg/kg hydrocortisone immediately

(E) Consult with urologic surgeon to close the abdominal defect immediately, arrange for an intravenous pyelogram and a barium enema, and begin appropriate antibiotic prophylaxis

452. High bilateral renal masses are discovered in a newborn infant. The results of an intravenous pyelogram performed are shown below in figure A. Subsequently, the infant develops progressive uremia and hypertension and succumbs. The pathological specimen of the kidneys is shown below in figure B. The most probable diagnosis is

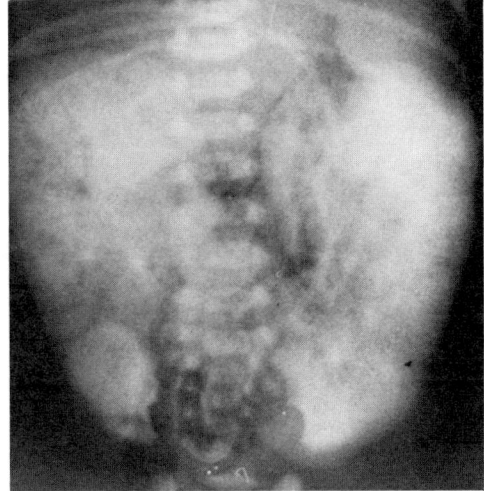

A

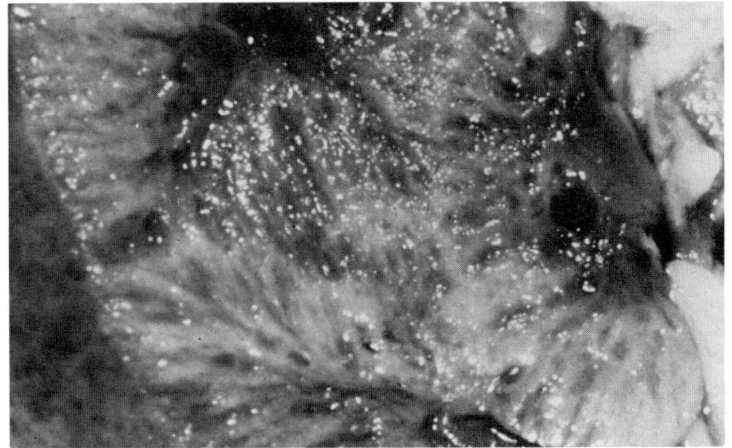

B

(A) Potter's syndrome
(B) medullary sponge kidney
(C) infantile polycystic kidney disease
(D) medullary cystic disease
(E) none of the above

453. Which of the following diseases causes proteinuria combined with hematuria?

(A) Renal neoplasm
✓(B) Membranoproliferative glomerulonephritis
(C) Hydronephrosis
(D) Nephrotic syndrome
(E) Nephroptosis

454. Which of the following statements concerning the condition shown in the picture below is correct?

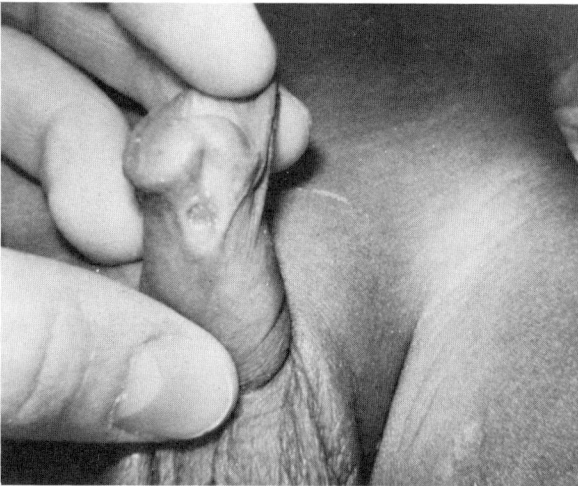

(A) There is usually no family history of this condition
(B) This abnormality represents third degree hypospadias
✓(C) Circumcision is contraindicated
(D) Cryptorchidism is associated with this finding in 25-30 percent of cases
(E) This condition can progress to a paraphimosis requiring immediate surgical intervention

455. Which of the following characteristics is most suggestive of osteoid osteoma?

(A) An x-ray appearance similar to Ewing's sarcoma
(B) A juxta-articular location
(C) Relief of pain with aspirin
(D) A moderate risk of malignant degeneration
(E) Strong familial occurrence

456. A two-week-old infant has been fussy and feeding poorly for three days. The parents brought the child in because it feels warm. Examination reveals a rectal temperature of 39.2°C (102.5°F). There is some tenderness in the left knee. The rest of the examination is unremarkable. The child is observed to kick less with the left leg than the right leg. The x-ray of the left knee is shown in the figure below. The next most important step in establishing the diagnosis is to obtain

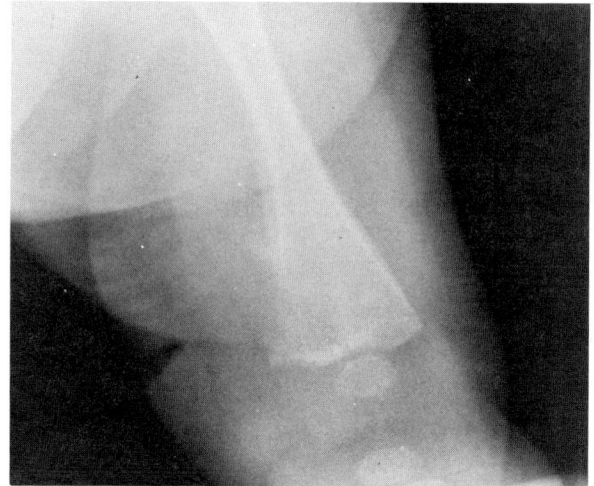

(A) two blood cultures
(B) an erythrocyte sedimentation rate
(C) a white blood cell count
✓(D) pus for culture
(E) a radionuclide scan of the affected area

457. There are several anatomical structures that make up a **stable** knee joint. Which of the following lists of components best describes these structures?

(A) Anterior and posterior cruciate ligaments, quadriceps, hamstrings, and medial and lateral menisci
(B) Anterior and posterior cruciate ligaments, quadriceps, and medial and lateral collateral ligaments
(C) Medial and lateral collateral ligaments, quadriceps, and hamstrings
(D) Medial and lateral collateral ligaments, medial and lateral menisci, quadriceps, and hamstrings
(E) Medial and lateral collateral ligaments, quadriceps, medial and lateral menisci, and patella

458. A ten-year-old boy presents for evaluation of a limp. On examination of his gait, it is found that during the midstance phase of his right lower extremity, he tends to lurch to the right (see figure below). During the toe-off and swing phase, the limb is carried normally. Through all phases of gait, the left lower extremity appears normal. The loss of function of which muscle group would cause such a gait?

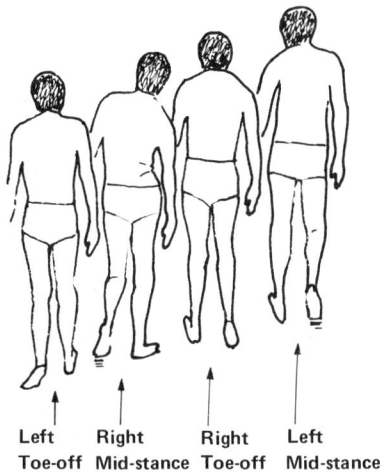

Left	Right	Right	Left
Toe-off	Mid-stance	Toe-off	Mid-stance

(A) Right hip abductors
(B) Left hip abductors
(C) Right hip adductors
(D) Left hip adductors
(E) Left paraspinal muscles

459. There is a strong association between neuro-muscular disorders of the lower extremity and

(A) pes cavus
(B) pes planus
(C) metatarsus adductus
(D) hallux valgus
(E) Köhler's disease

460. All of the following are characteristic of talipes equinovarus (congenital clubfoot) EXCEPT for

(A) a prominent transverse crease in the sole of the foot
(B) an inversion of the entire foot
(C) a plantar flexion of the foot
(D) a fusion of the talus and calcaneus
(E) an association with proximal neurologic deficits

461. The x-ray shown below is from a six-year-old girl who has pain and swelling at the site of the lesion. After the x-ray has been reviewed, initial treatment should include

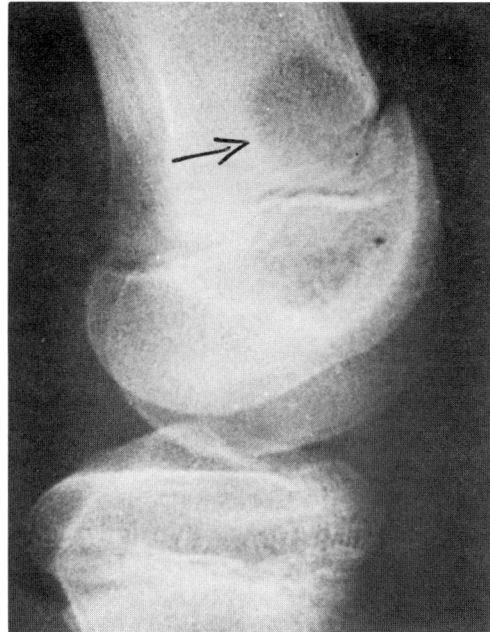

Used with permission of McGraw-Hill Book Company, from *Principles of Pediatrics: Health Care of the Young* (p 1673), by Hoekelman RA et al, ©McGraw-Hill Inc.

(A) observation without therapy for three weeks
(B) immobilization of the extremity
(C) a biopsy
(D) a needle aspiration for culture
(E) determination of the immunoreactive parathyroid hormone level

462. A two-year-old boy is brought to the emergency room at night because he began to cry when his mother removed his T-shirt at bedtime. When he was first seen, he was holding his left elbow with his right hand. The family had been to the State Fair that evening and the child did not want to leave; his parents literally had to drag him to the car. When the child is approached, he runs to his mother with his arms up asking to be picked up. The most likely diagnosis is a

(A) fracture of the left proximal radius
(B) fracture of the right clavicle
(C) radial head subluxation on the left
(D) humeral head dislocation on the left
(E) behavior problem

463. A patient presents with growth retardation, an enlarged head, depressed nasal bridge, and shortening of the proximal portions of the extremities. All of the following statements regarding this condition are true EXCEPT that

(A) broad, short hands and feet are a common feature

(B) it is inherited as an autosomal recessive disorder

(C) x-rays of the extremities show a "ball-in-socket" appearance of the epiphysis-metaphyseal interface

(D) there is a high incidence of obstructive hydrocephalus

(E) though dwarfed, these patients usually mature normally and lead productive lives

464. The findings in the x-ray of the three-year-old black child that is shown below are diagnostic of

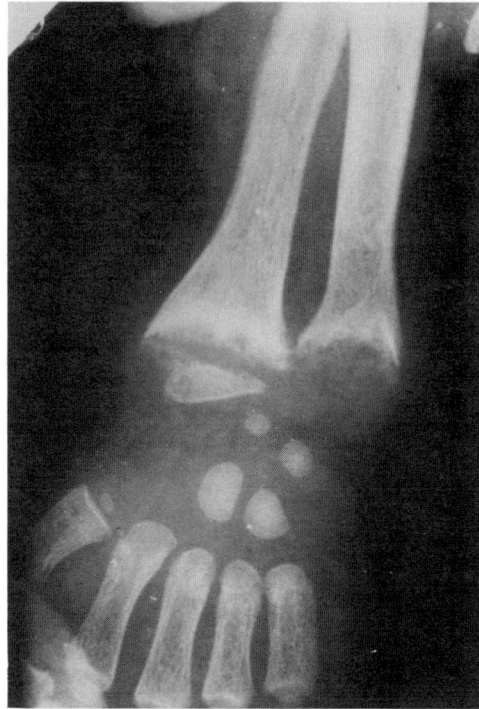

(A) rickets
(B) scurvy
(C) child abuse
(D) lead poisoning
(E) delayed bone age

DIRECTIONS: Each question below contains four suggested answers of which **one** or **more** is correct. Choose the answer

A	if	**1, 2, and 3**	are correct
B	if	**1 and 3**	are correct
C	if	**2 and 4**	are correct
D	if	**4**	is correct
E	if	**1, 2, 3, and 4**	are correct

465. Factors that contribute to the growth failure in children with chronic renal failure include

(1) chronic anemia
(2) chronic acidosis
(3) osteodystrophy
(4) recurrent infections

466. Which of the following statements characterizes methicillin nephritis?

(1) It is dose-related
(2) It is generally reversible
(3) It is frequently associated with eosinophilia
(4) It is associated with hepatic insufficiency

467. A routine urinalysis usually includes visual examination, determination of specific gravity and pH, a screening dipstick test for abnormal substances, and a microscopic examination. Therefore, routine urinalysis may be helpful in

(1) determining the presence of tyrosinemia by demonstration of homogentisic acid in the urine
(2) differentiating proximal from distal renal tubular acidosis
(3) determining the presence of hydroxybutyrate, a common ketone found in the urine
(4) diagnosing urate cystaluria, a common cause of "red" urine

468. The idiopathic nephrotic syndrome of childhood is characterized by

(1) proteinuria, hypoproteinemia, and hypolipidemia
(2) a predominance in children less than five years of age
(3) hypertension
(4) a benign urinary sediment

469. An eight-month-old white male presents with a history of abdominal pain, diarrhea, and vomiting of two weeks duration. Examination reveals pallor, extensive bruising, and oliguria of several days duration. Which of the following statements would be consistent with your suspected diagnosis?

(1) This child is likely to have hemolytic anemia as evidenced by burr cells and red cell fragments on smear
(2) Immunologic investigations are likely to be unrevealing
(3) Macroscopic hematuria and proteinuria are likely to be present
(4) Thrombocytopenia due to a hypoplastic bone marrow is likely to be found

470. Inability to concentrate the urine is a finding associated with which of the following disease states?

(1) Sickle cell hemoglobinopathy
(2) Diabetes insipidus
(3) Chronic pyelonephritis
(4) Medullary cystic disease

471. A six-year-old child presents with a complaint of general malaise. On examination periorbital edema and mild hypertension are observed. A urine sample is "coke-colored" and reveals proteinuria. The serum complement level (C3) is depressed. The differential diagnosis should include

(1) acute poststreptococcal glomerulonephritis
(2) Henoch-Schönlein purpura with nephritis
(3) membranoproliferative glomerulonephritis
(4) rapidly progressive (nonstreptococcal) glomerulonephritis

472. Correct statements about urinary tract infections in children include which of the following?

(1) They are usually caused by bacteria, and the organisms most frequently implicated are *Escherichia coli, Klebsiella pneumoniae,* and enteric streptococci

(2) They can be diagnosed by a midstream clean catch specimen revealing 10,000 organisms/ml on culture

(3) They usually can be treated effectively with a sulfonamide or ampicillin given orally for a ten-day period

(4) Approximately 35 percent of girls five-to-nine years of age with urinary tract infections demonstrate grade IV vesicoureteral reflux

473. Which of the following diagnostic studies could provide data useful in determining the etiology of asymptomatic hematuria?

(1) Urine culture
(2) Tuberculin test
(3) Total complement level
(4) Hemoglobin electrophoresis

474. Findings associated with acute renal failure include

(1) Kussmaul's breathing
(2) hypocalcemia
(3) hypertensive encephalopathy
(4) a urine/plasma osmolality ratio of > 2

475. Infection of the intervertebral disc is characterized by which of the following statements?

(1) Staphylococci are the usual etiologic agents
(2) If untreated, meningitis will result in most cases
(3) In childhood, this infection results from hematogenous spread
(4) Spiking fevers, usually greater than 38.8°C (101.8°F), are typical

476. Werdnig-Hoffman disease involves the loss of anterior horn cells in the spinal cord. True statements concerning this disorder include which of the following?

(1) It represents the most common cause of "floppy infant"
(2) A biopsy would show individual muscle fibers to be randomly affected
(3) It is transmitted as an X-linked recessive genetic trait
(4) The patient characteristically presents with alert facies

477. Which of the following statements characterizes idiopathic scoliosis?

(1) The spinal curve will progress most rapidly as the patient experiences the peak height growth velocity
(2) There is an associated rib rotation that is often severe
(3) It is more likely to occur in females than in males
(4) The Milwaukee brace should be used early to try to correct the curve

478. Myasthenia gravis is characterized by

(1) a transient course in neonates born to symptomatic mothers
(2) responsiveness to edrophonium chloride
(3) the need for surgical treatment, if the disease is intractable
(4) electromyogram findings that differentiate it easily from neonatal botulism

479. Congenital dislocation of the hip is characterized by which of the following statements?

(1) It occurs more frequently in females than males
(2) It is demonstrated by Ortolani's sign
(3) It is seen frequently in patients with meningomyelocele
(4) Double diapering is an accepted therapy

480. Correct statements concerning osteogenesis imperfecta include which of the following?

(1) The prognosis after infancy is excellent
(2) In the tarda form, the incidence of fractures increases dramatically after puberty
(3) A common complication after adolescence is otosclerosis
(4) Mental retardation is a common problem

DIRECTIONS: The groups of questions below consist of lettered choices followed by several numbered items. For each numbered item select the **one** lettered choice with which it is **most** closely associated. Each lettered choice may be used once, more than once, or not at all.

Questions 481-483

For each of the orthopedic situations below, select the disease with which it is likely to be associated.

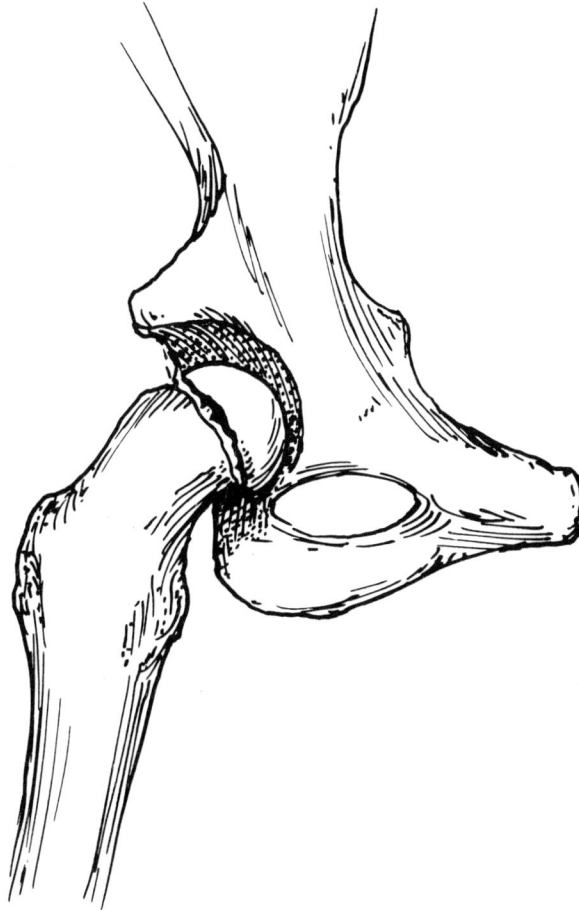

Used with permission of McGraw-Hill Book Company, from *Principles of Pediatrics: Health Care of the Young* (p 1651), by Hoekelman RA et al, © 1978 by McGraw-Hill Inc.

(A) Legg-Calvé-Perthes disease
(B) Slipped femoral capital epiphysis
(C) Blount's disease
(D) Köhler's disease
(E) None of the above diseases

481. Orthopedic emergency in an adolescent

482. Lateral view of the hip shown above

483. Bowed legs in a two-year-old child

Questions 484-486

For each of the synovial fluid analyses below, select the most compatible diagnosis.

(A) Juvenile rheumatoid arthritis
(B) Rheumatic fever
(C) Septic arthritis
(D) Osteoarthritis
(E) None of the above

	WBC	Polymorphonuclear Leukocytes (%)	Protein	Complement	Glucose Blood-Synovial Difference (mg/100 ml)
484.	15,000	75%	Increased	Decreased	30
485.	100,000	75%	Increased	Increased	91
486.	10,000	50%	Normal	Increased	6

Nephrology and Musculoskeletal Diseases

Answers

446. The answer is E. *(Hoekelman, pp 595-596.)* Enuresis has been associated with a large number of factors, including: (1) developmental delays, such as that seen with mental retardation, for which a history of school performance would be useful; (2) family history of enuresis; (3) urologic problems, such as urinary tract infection; and (4) obstructive lesions of the distal outflow tract, such as posturethral valves. Disorders affecting the amount of urine flow or the ability to concentrate urine, such as diabetes mellitus, diabetes insipidus, sickle cell anemia, and ingestion of medications, have also been indicated as infrequent causes of enuresis. Malformation of the sacral nerves (especially S2, S3, and S4) occurring in true myelodysplastic disorders may affect bladder function. The presence of an anal wink gives evidence that at least some of the function of these nerves is intact. Furthermore, the finding of spina bifida occulta on spine films has not been shown to be causally related to enuresis.

447. The answer is A. *(Hoekelman, p 1625.)* Renal vein thrombosis can occur during the newborn period as a sudden complication of sepsis or dehydration. This condition is more likely to be seen in infants of diabetic mothers than in those of nondiabetic mothers. Urine output may be normal if the thrombus is unilateral. Hematuria is usually present while proteinuria is less constant. The nephrotic syndrome is not seen in association with renal vein thrombosis. The best diagnostic test for renal vein thrombosis is epinephrine-assisted vena-cavography with renal venography. Although anticoagulants have been used, their value in the treatment of this condition has not been proved.

448. The answer is B. *(Hoekelman, pp 1584-1586.)* Bilateral renal agenesis or Potter's syndrome is usually seen in small premature infants. These infants also have characteristic facial features, pulmonary hypoplasia, and genital abnormalities. The syndrome is invariably fatal, and attempts at assisted ventilation are futile. Infantile polycystic kidney disease can also present with pulmonary insufficiency in the newborn period and the physiognomy of Potter's syndrome; however, this syndrome can be differentiated from Potter's syndrome by kidneys that generally are quite enlarged and easily palpated. The respiratory distress syndrome of the newborn does not present with the anomalies noted in this infant. The oculo-cerebrorenal syndrome of Lowe occurs only in males and is not usually associated with renal failure.

449. The answer is C. *(Hoekelman, p 1588.)* Congenital posterior urethral valves (shown on the x-ray) is a common cause of lower urinary tract obstruction in males. The condition is characterized by hypertrophy of the mucosal folds on the posterior urethra. The urethra proximal to the valves is dilated, and the bladder is enlarged. Approximately one-third of these patients will have ureteral reflux. The condition usually presents as a urinary tract infection in early or late childhood. It is diagnosed by voiding cystourethrography.

450. The answer is A. *(West, J Pediatr 89:173-182, 1976.)* In extraglomerular bleeding, clots may be found in the urine, but red cell casts are not. Although pain commonly is associated with renal calculi, and not often with glomerular bleeding, the presence of pain with hematuria cannot be used to differentiate the bleeding source. The presence of proteinuria with hematuria generally suggests glomerular disease. Proteinuria ordinarily is not found in association with renal calculi. When hematuria is present in hydronephrosis, the source of bleeding is extraglomerular.

451. The answer is B. *(Schaffer, ed 4. pp 428-430.)* This preterm infant has respiratory distress that remains undiagnosed, but the infant developed a right pneumothorax after assisted ventilation was started. In addition, the infant has exstrophy of the bladder. Thus, key decisions and management plans include: (1) relieving the right pneumothorax by chest tube placement and stabilizing the infant's ventilatory status; and (2) carefully evaluating the infant for associated anomalies, including a detailed assessment of the genitalia, associated pelvic skeletal dysplasias, and inguinal hernias frequently found in these infants. Evaluation of the abdominal defect requires the joint approach of the pediatric urologist, neonatologist, and orthopedist. This defect represents a maldevelopment of the lower abdominal wall closure. In addition to the abdominal wall and bladder, the resultant fissure involves the urethra and penis or clitoris and labia. The bladder is everted outward and is incompletely closed. The trigone and ureteral orifices are exposed, permitting urine to issue freely. Genital abnormalities are frequently associated with this abdominal defect, and the pubic rami may be widely separated. Therapy should center on maintaining hydration and adjusting electrolyte balance to prepare for surgical intervention. The defect should remain moist and protected from irritation prior to surgery.

452. The answer is C. *(Hoekelman, pp 1585-1587.)* Infantile polycystic kidney disease usually is evident at birth when physical examination reveals the presence of huge renal masses. However, the disease may present in adolescents. Pulmonary hypoplasia usually is also present and, therefore, severe respiratory insufficiency is a prominent feature of this syndrome. Few infants with this condition survive beyond the neonatal period. Medullary sponge kidney involves a cystic ectasia of the collecting ducts, while the kidney parenchyma is normal. Potter's syndrome is associated with renal agenesis. Medullary cystic disease has an insidious onset, usually presenting as a picture of chronic renal failure in late childhood or early adolescence.

453. The answer is B. *(West, J Pediatr 89:173-182, 1976.)* The glomerulonephritides generally cause proteinuria and hematuria simultaneously. Wilm's tumor and hydronephrosis can cause extraglomerular renal bleeding but usually are not associated with proteinuria. The nephrotic syndrome is the most frequent cause of asymptomatic proteinuria without hematuria. Neither proteinuria nor hematuria are found with nephroptosis. Foreign bodies in the structures of the urinary system produce a bleeding that may be mistaken for hematuria.

454. The answer is C. *(Hoekelman, p 1303. Smith, J Urol 40:239-247, 1938.)* Hypospadias is the most common congenital deformity of the penis. The tendency of the condition to occur more often in certain families strongly suggests a genetic influence. First degree hypospadias is characterized by the urethra opening in the distal one-third of the penis, second degree hypospadias in the middle third, and third degree hypospadias in the proximal third. The condition shown in the figure accompanying the question is first degree hypospadias. Hypospadias is a contraindication to circumcision because the foreskin can be used in the surgical correction of the defect. Cryptorchidism is seen in about five percent of cases of hypospadias. Paraphimosis never occurs in cases of second and third degree hypospadias and is extremely rare in cases of first degree hypospadias.

455. The answer is C. *(Hoekelman, p 1664. Hoppenfeld, Pediatr Clin North Am 24:884, 1977.)* Osteoid osteoma is found most commonly in the long bones, in the metaphysis or diaphysis, and occasionally in the vertebrae, but not in a juxta-articular location. Osteoid osteoma does not undergo malignant degeneration, but removal may be required because of pain. However, pain is so regularly relieved by aspirin that some consider this the treatment of choice. Osteoid osteoma resembles osteoblastoma in the sclerosis that often surrounds a lytic center (the "donut" seen on x-ray). It in no way resembles Ewing's sarcoma except for its location. Ewing's sarcoma is more likely to present with systemic symptoms of fever and leukocytosis, and to show mottled areas of rarefaction on x-ray, often with periosteal new bone being laid down in an "onion-skin" or "sun-ray" appearance.

456. The answer is D. *(Hoekelman, pp 1672-1673.)* With the history of irritability and fever in a young child and an x-ray that reveals bone rarefaction in an area of tenderness, osteomyelitis is the most likely diagnosis. Effective therapy is possible only if the infecting organism is known; therefore, the most important maneuver is to obtain pus for culture. The best approach is to carry out a needle aspiration at the point of tenderness. Therapy is then directed by Gram stain and culture results. Blood cultures are not as likely to reveal the infecting organism. The other tests included in the question do not supply data that would be useful in determining the identity of the infecting organism.

457. The answer is B. *(Staheli, Pediatr Clin North Am 24:841, 1977.)* Although numerous structures are involved in the function of the knee joint, the ligamentous structures are those mainly responsible for stability. The cartilaginous structures (including the fibrocartilage menisci) are more important to smooth gliding and cushioning than to stability. Of the muscular components, only the quadriceps mechanism plays an important role in stability; the hamstrings are relatively unimportant in that function.

458. The answer is A. *(Hoekelman, pp 69, 1654. Tachdjian, pp 10-11.)* This is the classic description of Trendelenburg gait, characteristic of weak hip abductors (gluteus medius), in this case only on the right side. Thus, when standing on the right leg, the weight of the trunk acts on the pelvis at the pivot joint of the right hip, lowering it on the left side. Normally, the right-sided abductors would counter this effect and keep the pelvis level. However, when these muscles are weak, this torque cannot be counteracted sufficiently, and the only way to prevent falling is to distribute the weight directly over the affected joint, which causes a lurch to the right side. This gait, often bilateral, is often seen in patients who have had poliomyelitis.

459. The answer is A. *(Hoekelman, pp 1636-1637.)* Pes cavus is so frequently associated with neuromuscular disease that its presence requires consideration of disorders such as cerebral palsy, meningomyelocele, Charcot-Marie-Tooth disease, or Friedreich's ataxia. If pes planus, or flatfoot, truly is present, it is usually associated with a structural rather than a neuromuscular abnormality, although rarely one may find the so-called peroneal spastic flatfoot in late childhood or adolescence. Hallux valgus is another structural deformity that is frequently a manifestation of a familial condition. It is usually not present prior to adolescence. Metatarsus adductus, on the other hand, is a congenital condition in which the forefoot is adducted but can be brought back passively to the neutral position. Köhler's disease is an osteochondrosis of the tarsal navicular and causes no deformity.

460. The answer is D. *(Hoekelman, pp 1632-1633. Settle, J Bone Joint Surg 45-A:1341-1354, 1963.)* Congenital clubfoot is a descriptive term for a group of deformities of which talipes equinovarus is the most common and severe type. **Talipes** is formed from the union of the words **talus** ("ankle") and **pes** ("foot"), which describes the way in which a patient will walk — that is, on the lateral aspect of the ankle — if the condition is left untreated. **Equinus** ("horse") describes the plantar flexion, while the **varus** ("angulation toward midline") refers to the inversion of the foot. The addition of forefoot adduction leads to a prominent medial ankle crease as well as a transverse sole crease. There is no fusion of the talus and calcaneus, although associated neurologic, muscular, and skeletal anomalies are common.

461. The answer is C. *(Hoekelman, pp 1279, 1673.)* The lesion shown in the figure accompanying the question is a Brodie's abscess, a form of chronic osteomyelitis. There is usually a lack of systemic symptoms; the chief complaint is localized pain and swelling. Because there is a possibility of malignancy, a biopsy is necessary for definitive diagnosis, and temporizing measures, such as observation and immobilization, are contraindicated. Organisms are rarely isolated from the lesion; therefore, needle aspiration is not likely to be useful. Hyperparathyroidism may produce areas of rarefaction, but it is usually accompanied by demineralization and more widespread destructive changes in areas of growth.

462. The answer is C. *(Hoekelman, p 1643. Tachdjian, pp 1619-1624.)* The set of symptoms in the question represents the "nursemaid elbow" of radial head subluxation that most likely occurred when the child was dragged to the car. Fractures of the proximal radius are uncommon and would be associated with an episode of moderate trauma, as are fractures of the clavicle and humeral head dislocation. The observation that the patient raised his arms when he wanted to be picked up eliminates these latter two diagnoses. A patient with persistent radial head subluxation may or may not be able to raise the affected arm. Spontaneous relocation of the radial head occurs with sufficient frequency so that patients sometimes exhibit no findings other than a disinclination to use the affected elbow. Although an underlying behavior problem may exist, the history indicates an organic pathology.

463. The answer is B. *(Hoekelman, pp 1688-1689.)* The condition described is achondroplasia, which is inherited as an autosomal dominant trait. Because of the narrowed base of the skull and small foramen magnum, there is an increased incidence of obstructive hydrocephalus in these patients. X-rays show normal epiphyses and diaphyses, but there is a ball-in-socket appearance to the epiphysis-metaphyseal interface. Broad, short hands commonly are seen. Most of these patients have normal intellectual development and lead productive lives.

464. The answer is A. *(Hoekelman, pp 883, 1690. Isselbacher, ed 9. p 1857.)* The abnormalities of the wrist x-ray are typical of rickets. The metaphyses are flared with cupping, and there is increased radiolucency. Because of the widespread fortification of foods with vitamin D in this country, rickets is only rarely due to a dietary deficiency of vitamin D. In the absence of vitamin D in the diet, it must be formed in the skin through ultraviolet irradiation of its precursor 7-dehydrocholesterol. Ultraviolet irradiation is decreased in black persons due to their increased melanin pigmentation, in northern states where ultraviolet rays are oblique, in winter months, and under smog conditions. Therefore, black children living in northern cities are most susceptible to rickets if their diet is deficient in vitamin D.

465. The answer is E (all). *(Hoekelman, pp 1609, 1611-1616.)* Chronic anemia, chronic acidosis, renal osteodystrophy, and recurrent infections are manifestations of chronic renal failure and are factors that contribute to growth failure in children. Acidosis occurs when the kidney fails to excrete hydrogen ions and reabsorbs bicarbonate. In addition, uremic toxins affect the gastrointestinal tract producing anorexia, nausea, and diarrhea, with resultant malnutrition. Protein losses in the urine and chronic corticosteroid administration also contribute to growth retardation.

466. The answer is A (1, 2, 3). *(Hoekelman, p 295. Rudolph, ed 16. p 1291.)* Methicillin is not an infrequent cause of drug-induced interstitial nephritis. This type of nephritis usually is associated with hematuria, proteinuria, red cell casts, eosinophilia, and fever. Fortunately, it is reversible with a decreased dose or discontinuation of the methicillin. However, since the majority of methicillin is excreted unchanged in the urine, hepatic insufficiency does not alter the serum levels or increase the incidence of nephritis.

467. The answer is C (2, 4). *(Hoekelman, pp 1577-1579, 1592. Kreisberg, Ann Intern Med 88:681-695, 1978.)* Homogentisic acid is excreted in the urine of patients with alkaptonuria and produces a dark or black urine upon standing. However, in tyrosinemia, homogentisic acid production is blocked, and it is not excreted in the urine. The clinical differentiation of distal and proximal renal tubular acidosis can be based on several parameters, including urine pH ($>$ 6 in distal type), age (usually less than two years of age in the proximal type), sex (usually female in the distal type), and the presence of bone disease with hypercalciuria (frequently seen in the distal type). A red color to urine does not necessarily mean that blood is present; therefore, it is important to perform a microscopic examination to determine whether red blood cells are present or whether there is another cause for the red urine such as urate crystals, which are easily seen under the microscope. Of the ketoacids produced during ketogenesis, as seen in diabetic ketoacidosis, during salicylate poisoning, and during starvation, acetoacetic acid is the only ketone that reacts with the nitroprusside reagent present on dipsticks and in ketone test tablets. It is important to know this because the amount of acetoacetic acid in the urine may not always reflect the degree of ketonemia present.

468. The answer is C (2, 4). *(Hoekelman, pp 1603-1608.)* Patients affected with the idiopathic nephrotic syndrome of childhood are generally under five years of age. Proteinuria is the hallmark of the disease and usually leads to hypoproteinemia and edema. Periorbital edema on waking up in the morning, followed by edema in the ankles and feet later in the day are frequently the first symptoms noticed by the parents. Hyperlipidemia is a constant finding, but the mechanism for its occurrence in the nephrotic syndrome is not understood. Other than malaise and the discomfort caused by the marked edema, there are few complaints. Hypertension rarely develops. Although hematuria is present in rare instances, the urinary sediment usually is benign.

469. The answer is A (1, 2, 3). *(Hoekelman, pp 1624-1625. Kaplan, Pediatr Clin North Am 23:761-767, 1976.)* The hemolytic-uremic syndrome can be diagnosed where there is a sudden hemolysis with an associated fall in hemoglobin level, thrombocytopenia, and acute renal failure. The thrombocytopenia is due to increased platelet consumption rather than decreased production. The syndrome is usually seen in children less than two years of age and more frequently in whites than blacks. Often, a prodrome of gastroenteritis lasting one to ten days is reported. The renal failure is characterized by a high BUN and severe oliguria; hematuria and proteinuria are often present, and the nephrotic syndrome may occur. No specific immunologic abnormality has been demonstrated in children with the hemolytic-uremic syndrome. Treatment is supportive, and the prognosis varies with the duration of renal failure. Prolonged renal failure is associated with a more guarded prognosis.

470. The answer is E (all). *(Hoekelman, pp 1586-1587, 1592, 1620, 1625.)* Sickle cell patients frequently are unable to concentrate their urine, usually as a result of infarcts involving the vasa recta. Similar infarcts result from lack of or unresponsiveness to vasopressin, as seen in central and nephrogenic diabetes insipidus, respectively. Patients with chronic pyelonephritis may have interstitial tubular damage, and those with medullary cystic disease (juvenile nephrophthisis) have cysts in the medullary region of their kidneys. Both of these conditions, therefore, can be associated with an inability to concentrate the urine.

471. The answer is B (1, 3). *(Hoekelman, pp 1594-1603.)* Acute poststreptococcal glomerulonephritis is the most common form of glomerulonephritis in children. Most patients present with an acute nephritic syndrome. The proteinuria present usually parallels the degree of hematuria. A reduction in serum C3 is seen in more than 80 percent of patients with this disease. The nephritis of Henoch-Schönlein purpura usually becomes evident one to four weeks following the onset of the nonrenal manifestations, and the serum complement levels usually are normal. Membranoproliferative glomerulonephritis occurs most commonly in older children and young adults, but can become manifest in younger children. Also called chronic hypocomplementemic glomerulonephritis, the disease can present as a nephritic or a nephrotic syndrome. Rapidly progressive glomerulonephritis is characterized by the development of acute renal failure. The clinical presentation and urinalysis findings are similar for other acute nephritis syndromes, but the complement values are normal.

472. The answer is B (1, 3). *(Hoekelman, pp 1616-1621. Kunin, Hosp Prac II:91-98, 1976.)* Symptomatic urinary tract infections (UTI) of viral etiology, such as hemorrhagic cystitis, are rare compared to urinary tract infections caused by bacterial organisms. Uncontaminated clean-catch specimens are difficult to obtain and therefore must be interpreted with caution. At least 100,000 organisms/ml of a single bacterial species should be present to diagnose a UTI. Specimens of urine obtained by catheter or by direct aspiration of the bladder through aseptic suprapubic skin are preferable for culture. Although successful treatment has been reported with a single parenteral injection of an aminoglycoside, oral sulfonamides or ampicillin given for ten days remains the standard treatment. Girls five-to-nine years of age are at highest risk for UTI, and many of these may demonstrate ureteral reflux. However, grade IV reflux, which extends to the kidney and is associated with renal parenchymal loss, is an uncommon finding.

473. The answer is E (all). *(West, J Pediatr 89:173-182, 1976.)* There are many causes of asymptomatic hematuria. Some authors suggest that urinary tract infection is the most frequent cause. Renal tuberculosis is unusual in the United States; however, the screening tine test is simple and it should be included in the workup of any child with hematuria. The various glomerulonephritis syndromes can be partially differentiated on the basis of the serum complement level. Sickle cell trait and sickle cell-hemoglobin C disease predispose to episodic hematuria; however, it is an uncommon complication of sickle cell disease per se. Therefore, all of the above studies might be valuable in determining the etiology.

474. The answer is A (1, 2, 3). *(Hoekelman, pp 1609-1611.)* Acute renal failure is a syndrome that must be recognized early, since delay in making the diagnosis can result in serious consequences. The biochemical abnormalities are complex and interrelated. Hyperkalemia, a hallmark of the condition, can lead to cardiac arrhythmia. Metabolic acidosis results from the inability of the kidney to excrete acids and reabsorb bases. The acidosis promotes hyperkalemia. Respiratory compensation for the acidosis is reflected clinically with Kussmaul's breathing. Failure of phosphate excretion produces concomitant hypocalcemia, which can lead to convulsions. Other causes of seizures in acute renal failure include hypertensive encephalopathy, uremia, and water intoxication. Intrinsic renal oliguria can be differentiated from prerenal oliguria by several clinical tests including, among others, an increase in the urine sodium content (> 20 mEq/L) and a urine/plasma osmolality ratio of ≤ 1.

475. The answer is B (1, 3). *(Hoekelman, pp 1662-1663. Tachdjian, pp 1250-1252.)* Intervertebral disc space infection (discitis) may present with few findings. The history usually includes one-to-two weeks of generally mild back pain, often producing a limp. Physical examination reveals mild fever rarely above 38°C (100.4°F), paravertebral muscle spasm, and local tenderness but little else of significance. Similarly, the laboratory evaluation may reveal only an elevated erythrocyte sedimentation rate, with or without leukocytosis. When an infectious agent is recovered, it is most often a staphylococcus organism. These gain access to the disc space by the hematogenous route in childhood. In the adult, there is relatively little blood supply to this area, so that infection usually spreads from contiguous structures. Treatment consists of rest, with or without antibiotics. Meningitis is not recognized as a complication.

476. The answer is D (4). *(Hoekelman, pp 1675-1676, 1679.)* Although Werdnig-Hoffman disease (infantile spinal muscular atrophy) represents the most common **neuromuscular** cause of the "floppy infant," overall central nervous system disorders account for the overwhelming majority of cases. Infantile spinal muscular atrophy is transmitted as an autosomal recessive trait. Because the loss of anterior horn cells results in loss of motor units, there tends to be atrophy of fascicles of muscle fibers rather than atrophy of individual fibers at random. Since the brain is unaffected in these infants, intellect is normal, and the patients appear alert but weak.

477. The answer is A (1, 2, 3). *(Hoekelman, pp 1655-1661.)* Idiopathic scoliosis, as the name implies, has no structural abnormality discernible initially, but with progression, there is always wedging of the vertebrae that results in rotation of the vertebrae and the attached ribs. Sixty to seventy percent of idiopathic scoliosis patients are female. The most prevalent curve pattern is right thoracic. Evidence now points to an incomplete penetrant mode of autosomal dominant inheritance, although the genetic mode of inheritance may vary widely. The Milwaukee brace is used only to **prevent progression** of the curve, not to correct it. Because the curve tends to progress the most during the peak height velocity of the adolescent growth spurt, patients should be followed closely at this time.

478. The answer is A (1, 2, 3). *(Hoekelman, p 1681. Vaughan, ed 11. pp 1801-1802.)* Myasthenia gravis is a disorder of neuromuscular transmission wherein acetylcholine is blocked from acting at the receptor sites of muscle membrane, probably by a circulating antibody that can cross the placenta. Thus, the course frequently is transient in neonates born to affected mothers if the infants can be supported in their ventilatory efforts. This form of the disease is generally recognized as transient neonatal myasthenia gravis. When these same symptoms are present in the infant but not in the mother, the disease is termed persistent neonatal myasthenia gravis. A third form, juvenile myasthenia gravis, usually has its onset after the age of ten. Occurring about six times more often in girls than in boys, this form of the disease is characterized by (1) ptosis and double vision, (2) weakness of facial, neck, bulbar, and intercostal muscles, and (3) relief of symptoms after rest and exacerbation after activity. Myasthenic crises, sudden life-threatening attacks, may occur during periods of stress such as infections. Edrophonium chloride (Tensilon) is an anticholinesterase that increases the local concentration of acetylcholine, allowing for increased neuromuscular transmission and marked improvement in muscle strength. However, intractable myasthenia in childhood may require surgical removal of the thymus gland, the supposed source of antibodies. Because the pathophysiologic mechanism in both botulism and myasthenia gravis is a blockage of neuromuscular transmission, the electromyogram findings are identical.

479. The answer is A (1, 2, 3). *(Hoekelman, pp 1650-1653.)* Congenital dislocation (or dysplasia) of the hip joint occurs in 1-2 per 1000 live births. Females are afflicted four times more frequently than males, and monozygotic twins are affected more often than dizygotic twins. There is a familial incidence in 20-30 percent of cases, and both hip joints are involved in 25 percent of cases. Hip instability can be demonstrated by the Ortolani sign by placing the fingers on the greater trochanter of the femur as the thumbs grip the inner aspect of the thigh. The femur is then lifted forward as the thighs are adducted. If hip dysplasia is present, the head of the femur can be felt to slip into the acetabulum with a "click." The thighs are adducted, and, if the head dislocates, it will be felt again as a "click" and seen as it suddenly jerks over the anterior rim of the acetabulum. Congenital hip dysplasia is associated with: (1) first pregnancies, (2) premature rupture of fetal membranes, (3) oligohydramnios, (4) breech presentations, and (5) infants with meningomyelocele. The blood supply to the head of the femur or to the acetabulum has not been shown to be compromised in congenital hip dysplasia. Clinically, the neonate with congenital hip dysplasia does not have adduction tightness or contracture but may develop these signs by two-to-three months of age. Extra diapering is not an effective mode of therapy. Treatment from birth to the walking stage is geared at preventing adduction and extension of the hips while still allowing freedom of hip movement. Closed reduction of the hips in flexion and adduction may also be required to maintain femoral head and acetabular alignment. Infrequently, surgically releasing the inferior capsule and placing the femoral head in the acetabulum is required.

480. The answer is B (1, 3). *(Hoekelman, pp 347-348. Smith, 1976. pp 286-289.)* Osteogenesis imperfecta (brittle bone disease) is an inherited disease of mesenchymal tissue (sclera, bones, and ligaments). The autosomal recessive form (congenita) presents prenatally and usually results in perinatal death. Children affected with the congenita form have short limbs, blue sclera, poor mineralization of the skull, and multiple fractures at birth. If, however, the autosomal dominant type (tarda) is present, the outlook may be significantly better. Although bronchopneumonia takes its toll of infants, the long-term survivors primarily have orthopedic and otologic (otosclerosis) problems. Other problems of those with the tarda form of the disease include translucent, discolored teeth in association with hypoplasia of the dentitia and pulp. For unknown reasons, the incidence of fractures is reduced markedly after puberty. No intellectual deficits have been related to these diseases.

481-483. The answers are: 481-B, 482-B, 483-C. *(Hoekelman, pp 1644-1649, 1684.)* The illustration in the question depicts the classical findings of a slipped femoral capital epiphysis with posterior and inferior displacement of the femoral capital epiphysis relative to the femoral neck. This disorder is usually seen in tall, obese, adolescent males and is bilateral in 25 percent of cases. It is an orthopedic emergency that requires bed rest, traction, and usually surgery.

Legg-Calvé-Perthes disease (coxa plana) occurs five times more often in boys. Usually occurring between the ages of four and seven, it has been noted as early as three and as late as eleven years of age. The most commonly accepted theory of the etiology of the disease is the occurrence of avascular necrosis of the ossific nucleus of the femoral head. The result is fragmentation and revascularization of the femoral head. In adults, avascular necrosis does not result in healing and the restoration of the spherical shape of the femoral head. The characteristic physiology of growth in children, however, may contribute significantly to the healing process. A less accepted theory is that the disease is an osteochondritis of the cartilage and ossific nucleus of the femoral head. Surgical intervention is much less likely to be required as compared to slipped capital femoral epiphysis. Bed rest with traction followed by orthotic devices to prevent weightbearing is the only therapy required.

Blount's disease involves a growth disturbance of the medial proximal tibia, which can progress from an almost imperceptible condition to various degrees of "beaking," epiphyseal depression, and medial metaphyseal fragmentation, all of which can lead to marked bowing. The disease usually begins in the toddler years; osteotomy may be required for its correction.

Kohler's disease is found more frequently in children three to eight years of age. Its symptoms are not severe, although pain is produced over the dorsum of the foot, which may swell. Treatment consists of restricted activity or, if the case is severe, casting.

484-486. The answers are: 484-A, 485-C, 486-B. *(Hoekelman, p 1099. Grossman, Curr Probl Pediatr 5:25-28, 1975.)* Analysis of joint aspirates may be helpful in differentiating monoarticular juvenile rheumatoid arthritis (JRA) from a septic joint. The normal joint has less than 2000 white blood cells per cubic millimeter with less than 40 percent of these being polymorphonuclear leukocytes. The protein is usually one-third that of the serum protein level. The septic joint has a greater number of white blood cells and polymorphonuclear leukocytes than usually found in the joint affected by JRA or rheumatic fever.

The joint fluid of osteoarthritis usually has less than 2000 white blood cells per cubic millimeter. A normal difference in blood and synovial glucose levels (10) would suggest rheumatic fever or osteoarthritis. The difference is increased in the septic joint or rheumatoid arthritis.

The synovial fluid in rheumatic fever usually has a normal protein and mucin clot, but the synovial fluid of rheumatoid arthritis and of a septic joint has an increased protein and abnormal mucin clot. Synovial fluid complement may be decreased in juvenile rheumatoid arthritis.

Health Supervision and Psychosocial Pediatrics

DIRECTIONS: Each question below contains five suggested answers. Choose the **one best** response to each question.

487. All of the following statements about tuberculin testing are true EXCEPT that

(A) the Mantoux method is most definitive
(B) "second strength" purified protein derivative will elicit nonspecific sensitivity to any mycobacterial antigen
(C) vesiculation at the site of a tine test warrants institution of therapy without further testing
(D) routine screening of children should begin at 24 months of age
(E) doubtful reactions may signify sensitivity to either *Mycobacterium tuberculosis* or atypical mycobacteria

488. According to the most widely accepted estimates, the daily protein requirement for infants (grams per kg of body weight) in the first few months of life is about

(A) 0.5 g/kg
(B) 1 g/kg
(C) 2 g/kg
(D) 4 g/kg
(E) 5 g/kg

489. All of the following statements about breath-holding spells in children are true EXCEPT that

(A) the electroencephalograms of affected children are normal
(B) there is often a positive family history
(C) they can occur in children as old as five years
(D) the pallid variety is sometimes treated with atropine
(E) the pallid variety is more likely to lead to significant sequelae

490. Which of the following statements about somnambulism in children is correct?

(A) Somnambulating children rarely hurt themselves
(B) Somnambulating children may be engaged in meaningful conversations
(C) Somnambulism occurs as morning approaches
(D) Somnambulators often have serious psychiatric disturbances
(E) None of the above

491. Excluding children who reside in central areas of large cities, what percentage of children one to four years of age in the United States are immunized against measles?

(A) 60 percent
(B) 70 percent
(C) 80 percent
(D) 90 percent
(E) 95 percent

492. Which of the following statements about childhood phobias is true?

(A) They are most common in the 10- to 12-year-old age group
(B) They are usually accompanied by serious psychopathology
(C) They are not always pathological conditions
(D) They generally present with headache or other somatic complaints
(E) The prognosis is considered to be excellent

493. Premature infants are at risk for developing vitamin E deficiency. All of the following are associated with or contribute to the development of this entity EXCEPT for

(A) a high intake of iron
(B) a low intake of polyunsaturated fatty acids
(C) low α-tocopherol blood levels
(D) anemia
(E) increased fragility of the red blood cells

176

494. All of the following statements about adolescent suicide are true EXCEPT that

(A) the rate is higher in the 10-14 age group than in the 15-19 age group
(B) suicide gestures are seen more often in adolescent girls than boys
(C) more adolescent boys than girls are reported to commit suicide
(D) there is usually a long-standing history of multiple problems
(E) most adolescents have thought about committing suicide

495. The most important factor in the etiology of kwashiorkor is

(A) an overall reduction in calories
(B) a reduction in calories derived from carbohydrates
(C) a reduction in calories derived from protein
(D) a reduction in vitamin A intake
(E) a reduction in calories obtained from fatty acids

496. In general, the best approach to the management of a runaway teenager is

(A) individual psychotherapy
(B) referral to a developmental disabilities program
(C) a community-based program that deals with runaway youth
(D) consultation with a social worker
(E) consultation with the primary care physician

497. All of the following statements about incest are true EXCEPT that

(A) other family members are usually aware of the situation
(B) incest between a mother and a son usually is associated with severe psychopathology in at least one of them
(C) incest between siblings is the most common variety
(D) it seldom occurs in families that are emotionally sound
(E) it usually presents clinically with a physical complaint concerning the genitals

DIRECTIONS: Each question below contains four suggested answers of which **one** or **more** is correct. Choose the answer

A	if	**1, 2, and 3**	are correct
B	if	**1 and 3**	are correct
C	if	**2 and 4**	are correct
D	if	**4**	is correct
E	if	**1, 2, 3, and 4**	are correct

498. Comparisons between the protein composition of breast milk and of the most commonly used infant formulas based on cow's milk reveal that

(1) the protein concentration in human milk is the same as that found in formula
(2) human milk and formula contain the same type of whey proteins
(3) the whey protein-to-casein ratio is similar for both human milk and formula
(4) casein represents 80 percent of the protein in formula but only 40 percent in human milk

499. Breast-feeding is contraindicated if the mother is receiving

(1) metronidazole
(2) lithium
(3) thiouracil
(4) radioactive iodine

500. Newborn infants may be fed a formula that can be prepared in the home. One quart of formula should be prepared according to which of the following proportions in order to provide the caloric needs of a neonate?

(1) 23 ounces of whole milk plus 9 ounces of water plus 3 tablespoons of corn syrup
(2) 25 ounces of whole milk plus 7 ounces of water plus 4 tablespoons of sugar
(3) 13 ounces of evaporated milk plus 19 ounces of water plus 3 tablespoons of Dextrimaltose
(4) 10 ounces of evaporated milk plus 22 ounces of water plus 2 tablespoons of corn syrup

501. A three-year-old child, who is brought to the emergency room with contusions on the back, elbows, knees, and shoulders, seems reluctant to move his right arm. The parents report that the child fell down the stairs a few hours earlier. A diagnosis of child abuse would be strongly suggested by which of the following observations?

(1) Some of the contusions appear to be several days old
(2) The child has had several previous visits to the emergency room with similar complaints
(3) X-rays show a chip fracture of the right distal radial metaphysis without callus formation
(4) X-rays show a transverse fracture of the right distal radial shaft without callus formation

502. A five-year-old child is brought to the physician for evaluation of temper tantrums, an aversion to change, and a regression in speaking skills of recent onset. Previously the child had shown normal development. The differential diagnosis should include

(1) childhood schizophrenia
(2) olivopontocerebellar atrophy
(3) subacute sclerosing panencephalitis
(4) Friedreich's disease

503. Depression in middle childhood often presents with

(1) grief and mourning
(2) aggressive behavior
(3) somatic complaints
(4) overeating

504. The management of a seven-year-old boy with a recent onset of a tic involving the blinking of both eyes should include

(1) reassurance that the tic will most likely improve as adolescence approaches
(2) follow-up of the child to watch for the onset of vocal symptomatology
(3) positive reinforcement of tic-free intervals
(4) attempts to discover and ameliorate stress in the child's life

505. A mother is concerned about the temper tantrums of her two-year-old child. Effective maternal counseling should include which of the following ideas and suggestions?

(1) Temper tantrums are part of the normal negativistic behavior in children of this age
(2) Temper tantrums generally subside by four years of age
(3) Children of this age need help learning to verbalize their feelings
(4) Physical punishment for temper tantrums often makes the problem worse

506. School phobia occurring in the young school-age child has which of the following characteristics?

(1) It generally presents to the physician as a complaint from the parents that the child refuses to go to school
(2) It can rarely be prevented, because the population at risk is not easily identified
(3) It is unlikely in the presence of normal or above normal intelligence
(4) It is less likely to be a sign of serious psychopathology than it is in the adolescent

507. Correct statements about child abuse and neglect include which of the following?

(1) Child abuse and neglect seldom occur in middle class families
(2) Premature infants are more likely to be abused or neglected than infants born at term
(3) Severe psychopathology is present in at least one of the parents
(4) Parents who abuse or neglect their children often were abused or neglected themselves

508. Conversion symptoms in teenagers are diagnosed on the basis of which of the following criteria?

(1) The ability to cope with the environment through secondary gain
(2) Development of a symptom for which there is no medical explanation
(3) Reduction of anxiety through primary gain
(4) A conversion reaction that occurs during non-stressful times

509. Differential diagnosis of anorexia nervosa includes

(1) hypopituitarism
(2) malabsorption syndrome
(3) primary ovarian dysfunction
(4) chronic infection

510. An acute depressive reaction in adolescence is characterized by

(1) an attempt to mask the depressive feelings
(2) a short-lived depression which seldom interferes with sleeping and eating
(3) an impairment of reality testing
(4) a transient grief response to the death or separation of a loved one

511. Neurotic delinquency is characterized by

(1) the sudden onset of illegal acts in childhood
(2) a need to be caught in the delinquent act
(3) an association with underlying depression
(4) a failure to respond to counseling by a primary care physician

DIRECTIONS: The groups of questions below consist of lettered choices followed by several numbered items. For each numbered item select the **one** lettered choice with which it is **most** closely associated. Each lettered choice may be used once, more than once, or not at all.

Questions 512-514

Screening tests are used to detect potentially preventable or treatable diseases in presymptomatic individuals. For each definition that follows, select the term that best describes the validity or results of a screening test.

(A) False positive
(B) False negative
(C) Sensitivity
(D) Specificity
(E) None of the above

512. Correct identification of **all** those who have the disease

513. Correct identification of **only** those who have the disease

514. Well people labeled as having the disease

Questions 515-518

For each of the complications or side effects that follow, select the immunizing agent most likely to be associated with it.

(A) Diphtheria toxoid
(B) Pertussis vaccine
(C) Measles vaccine
(D) Mumps vaccine
(E) None of the above

515. Fever 7-10 days following immunization

516. Local erythema and swelling

517. Arthritis

518. Neurological complications

Questions 519-523

For each of the following vaccines, select the appropriate description of the organism used in its preparation.

(A) Bacterial—killed, whole organism
(B) Bacterial—toxoid
(C) Bacterial—live, attenuated
(D) Viral—killed
(E) Viral—live, attenuated

519. Diphtheria vaccine

520. Pertussis vaccine

521. Oral polio vaccine

522. Measles vaccine

523. Influenza vaccine

Questions 524-528

For each vitamin listed below, select the diet for which it is recommended as a supplement for a full-term infant.

(A) Breast milk
(B) Proprietary formulas in common use
(C) Evaporated milk formula
(D) Goat's milk formula
(E) None of the above

524. Vitamin A

525. Vitamin C

526. Vitamin D

527. Folic acid and vitamins C and D

528. Vitamin E

Health Supervision and Psychosocial Pediatrics

Answers

487. The answer is D. *(Hoekelman, pp 189-191. Gellis, ed 9. pp 563-568.)* The Committee on Infectious Diseases of the American Academy of Pediatrics recommends that all children be screened for tuberculosis at one year of age. Thereafter, screening programs for tuberculosis should reflect local prevalence rates. Surveillance programs must be coupled with adequate public health follow-up to ensure that infected individuals and their contacts receive appropriate treatment or prophylaxis. Isoniazid, at a dose of 10 mg/kg/day to a maximum of 300 mg/day in a single dose is the therapy of choice for chemoprophylaxis. All members of the household of a patient with active disease should be treated for at least three months regardless of reactivity to purified protein derivative (PPD) testing. Individuals with a positive tuberculin test, but no evidence of disease, should be treated for one year. The Mantoux or intradermal method, using 5 tuberculin units in 0.1 ml of solution, is the preferred screening test. Induration of 10 mm or more at the application site is considered diagnostic for past or current *Mycobacterium tuberculosis* infection. Induration of 5-9 mm is considered a doubtful reaction and may signify sensitivity to *M. tuberculosis* or atypical mycobacterium. Intradermal inoculation with "second strength" (250 unit PPD) tuberculin may elicit nonspecific sensitivity to a variety of mycobacterial antigens and is not recommended. A positive tine test (multiple puncture method) usually is confirmed by the Mantoux method. An exception is made when vesiculation occurs at the tine test puncture sites, which is indicative of disease.

488. The answer is C. *(Hoekelman, p 133.)* The precise protein requirement for any age group is difficult to determine. Protein also varies in quality. Estimates of protein needs for the first few months of life are based on the average milk intake of thriving infants. The most widely accepted estimates are those of the National Academy of Sciences (NAS) (1974) and the Food and Agricultural Organization of the World (FAO,1973). The NAS and FAO estimates for the first few months of life are similar, that is, about 2 g/kg/day. Protein needs for older children are somewhat less (0.5 to 1 g/kg/day). A protein intake of more than 5 g/kg/day may result in toxicity manifested by a rising BUN, albuminuria, and fever.

489. The answer is E. *(Hoekelman, pp 587, 951.)* The diagnosis of a breath-holding spell can usually be made on the basis of a careful history. This history often reveals that a family member had breath-holding spells. The spells are most common at about one year of age but may occur as early as six months and as late as five years. Frequently, repeated episodes of the pallid variety, which is thought to be vasovagal in nature, are sometimes treated with atropine-like drugs. Neither the pallid nor the cyanotic variety is associated with an abnormal electroencephalogram or with pathologic sequelae.

490. The answer is E. *(Hoekelman, pp 601-602.)* Somnambulation usually occurs about 90 to 100 minutes after the child has fallen asleep and frequently leads to injury. Purposeful activity and meaningful conversation during an episode suggest a psychiatric disorder rather than somnambulism. Somnambulism itself is not indicative of psychopathology. Sleepwalking affects more males than females. Sleepwalkers are not carrying out any purposeful activity, nor is somnambulating the acting out of a dream. Attempts to talk to a somnambulist elicit, if anything, incoherent, monosyllabic utterances.

491. The answer is B. *(Hoekelman, p 125.)* In 1974, almost 70 percent of one- to four-year-old children in the United States were immunized against rubeola. This figure excludes children from the central cities for whom the immunization rate was 63 percent. Live attenuated measles vaccine has been in use for over 15 years, and the immunity conferred is long lasting. Hence, eradication of the disease is conceivable if all individuals at risk were to be immunized. Preliminary data for 1978 (unpublished) indicate a 90 percent rubeola immunization rate for children in the United States upon entry to public school.

492. The answer is E. *(Hoekelman, p 605.)* Phobias are most common in early childhood. The prognosis for affected children, who generally function very well outside the phobic sphere, is excellent. Some fears are so common that they are not classified as phobias. These include the fear of the dark in the young child, the fear of animals in the preschooler, and the fear of death in seven- to eight-year-old children. These fears generally occur in a predictable sequence and are related to the stages of intellectual (cognitive) development. Childhood phobias usually are not accompanied by somatic symptoms.

493. The answer is B. *(Hoekelman, p 884.)* Premature infants often develop vitamin E deficiency manifested by a hemolytic anemia resulting from increased red blood cell fragility. Blood levels of α-tocopherol (vitamin E) are decreased. The vitamin E requirement increases when the diet is high in polyunsaturated fatty acids or iron. It is often reasonable to supplement the infant's diet with this vitamin in order to prevent the development of the anemia.

494. The answer is A. *(Hoekelman, pp 665-668. Hofmann, Med Clin North Am 59:1429-1437, 1975.)* Violent means of suicide and successful suicide attempts are usually noted in adolescent boys rather than girls. However, most suicide gestures are noted in girls between the ages of 16 and 17. A common example is a drug overdose as an hysterical reaction to the end of a love relationship. Sometimes the gesture is a means of obtaining attention or is a cry for help. There is often a history of childhood and adolescent psychosocial problems prior to the actual gesture or suicide attempt, including suicide attempts among the parents or close relatives, a chaotic home, and other evidence of significant environmental change. Also, most adolescents have some periods of mild mood swings that are frequently accompanied by depression and thoughts of suicide.

495. The answer is C. *(Hoekelman, pp 876-877.)* Kwashiokor is a form of severe malnutrition characterized by organomegaly, edema, peeling skin, moon facies, and reddish color of the hair. It is caused by a very low protein intake. Marasmus, another form of severe malnutrition, results from an overall reduction of both calories and proteins. Vitamin A deficiency often is seen concurrently in children with kwashiorkor, but it is not an etiologic factor. A selective reduction of carbohydrate intake occurs infrequently. An excessive intake of carbohydrates contributes to obesity. Although impairment of fat absorption is associated with disease, a reduction of fatty acid calorie intake is not a cause.

496. The answer is C. *(Hoekelman, pp 677-678. Reilly, Clin Pediatr 17:886-892, 1978.)* Successful intervention for runaway teenagers is very difficult to achieve. It is a problem in which many factors are involved, including disrupted family relationships, intense mid-adolescent conflicts, and sexual concerns. Mental retardation or psychosis usually is not observed in such individuals. Many demonstrate a marked self-destructive behavior. Treatment must be directed to establishing a relationship between the adolescent and a community program that deals with this problem. Treatment of the whole family may be necessary. Individual counseling by physicians or other health care professionals is usually not successful.

497. The answer is E. *(Hoekelman, pp 511-513.)* Although a physical complaint concerning the genitals is one way in which incest is brought to the attention of the physician, it is more common for incest to present with somatic complaints concerning other parts of the body, such as, fatigue, school difficulties, or depression, including suicidal behavior. Incest is usually an indication that a serious breakdown in the family's function has occurred. The taboo against mother-son incest is very strong, and this variety is usually associated with major mental illness in one or another of the partners. The most frequently reported incest is father-daughter. However, incest between siblings appears to be the most common variety, but is not brought to the attention of authorities as frequently as father-daughter incidents.

498. The answer is D (4). *(Hoekelman, p 144-145. Hambraeus, Pediatr Clin North Am 24:17-36, 1977.)* Casein represents 80 percent of the protein both in whole cow's milk and in formula, compared with 40 percent in human milk. The total protein concentration is 3.5 g/100 ml in whole cow's milk, 1.5 g/100 ml in formula, and approximately 1 g/100 ml in human milk. Casein causes higher curd tension, which results in decreased digestibility, a problem that is ameliorated to some extent by special treatment of the infant formulas. The whey proteins are different in human milk and cow's milk, as are the whey protein-to-casein protein ratios. Breast milk has a lower protein content than cow's milk. However, almost all the protein in breast milk is digested and absorbed, while about half the protein in cow's milk passes out in the stool.

499. The answer is E (all). *(Medical Letter 21:21-24, 1979.)* Breast-feeding is contraindicated if the mother is receiving any of the substances listed in the question. Systemic metronidazole should not be given to a mother who is breast-feeding because of potential harmful effects in the infant. The drug has been shown to be carcinogenic in rodents. Lithium is excreted in breast milk and has been shown to cause neurologic symptoms in infants. The breast milk concentration of thiouracil is high enough to suppress the infant's thyroid function. Radioactive iodine ^{131}I occurring in breast milk may destroy the infant's thyroid gland.

500. The answer is B (1, 3). *(Hoekelman, p 151.)* An infant formula may be prepared in the home using evaporated milk (or whole cow's milk), water, and a source of carbohydrate. The goal is to produce a formula that provides approximately 20 calories/ounce, but with a lower protein concentration than whole cow's milk. Whole milk provides 20 calories/ounce and evaporated milk, 44 calories/ounce. Commonly used carbohydrate sources are sugar (60 calories/tablespoon), corn syrup (60 calories/tablespoon), and Dextrimaltose (30 calories/tablespoon). Formula choices 1 and 3 would produce approximately 20 calories/ounce, while choice 2 is too concentrated (23 calories/ounce), and choice 4 is too diluted (17½ calories/ounce).

501. The answer is A (1, 2, 3). *(Hoekelman, pp 69, 614-622, 881-882, 1417, 1424. Schmitt, Curr Probl Pediatr 5:15-17, 1975.)* Repeated episodes of suspicious trauma strongly suggest the possibility of child abuse, as does a history inconsistent with the physical findings, such as the reported timing of injury and the appearance of bruises and contusions. A metaphyseal chip fracture generally results from a wrenching or jerking force applied to the limb and therefore strongly suggests child abuse. A transverse fracture of the distal radius would be consistent with a history of falling downstairs and would therefore not be strong evidence for child abuse.

502. The answer is B (1, 3). *(Hoekelman, pp 626-627, 942-943, 1187.)* The onset of temper tantrums, aversion to change, and regression of speaking skills in a five-year-old child strongly suggest childhood schizophrenia, which can begin as early as two-to-five years of age following an infancy that was considered normal. In this situation many of the symptoms can mimic those of infantile autism, such as a lack of tolerance for change; strange, garbled speech patterns or a total loss of previously achieved language skills; ritualistic, repetitive behavior; poor grasp of body integrity even to the point of loss of identity of being a separate person; aloofness and a tendency to regard people as inanimate objects; and periods of severe anxiety. Subacute sclerosing panencephalitis could also cause these symptoms. Ataxia, not dementia, is the predominate feature of olivopontocerebellar atrophy and Friedreich's disease, both of which are characterized by signs and symptoms of spinocerebellar degeneration.

503. The answer is E (all). *(Hoekelman, pp 610-612.)* Depression in middle childhood may present openly with grief and mourning, or it may be masked, presenting with somatic complaints, behavior problems, or overeating. Masked depression generally is chronic, is frequently the result of such problems as child neglect or marital discord, and is far more difficult to treat than the open variety. Masked depression is also difficult to diagnose, often escaping the attention of both the physician and the family. Episodes of behavior, such as clowning, belligerence, bravado, and occasional running away and delinquent acts alternating with periods of boredom, fatigue, and feelings of despair may be indicative of masked depression.

504. The answer is C (2, 4). *(Hoekelman, pp 603-605. Golden, Am J Dis Child 131:531-534, 1977.)* Tics are generally a symptom of prolonged psychological stress without adequate outlet. Therapy aimed at the tic rather than at the stress is likely to make the situation worse. The tic may also get worse with the approach of adolescence. An eye-blinking tic involving both eyes is the most common presenting symptom of the Gilles de la Tourette syndrome, which then progresses to include vocal symptoms such as throat-clearing, inarticulate sounds, or coprolalia (profuse swearing). Haloperidol has been shown to be an effective therapeutic agent. Misdiagnosis of the Gilles de la Tourette syndrome sometimes leads to inappropriate therapies, such as antihistamines, decongestants, antibiotics, and tonsillectomies.

505. The answer is E (all). *(Hoekelman, pp 169, 585-588.)* Temper tantrums are a normal expression of the negativism of a two-year-old child who is striving for autonomy. By encouraging a child to express his feelings in words, parents can help him to develop better control. Frequent temper tantrums after the age of four are unusual. Physical punishment for temper tantrums causes many children to become more negativistic, which leads to even greater conflict with their parents. Tantrums are best handled by ignoring them (except in instances where the child's behavior is destructive to himself, others, or property), by offering nurturance after the episode is over and by helping the child learn to express his feelings verbally.

506. The answer is D. *(Hoekelman, pp 558-560. Schmitt, Pediatrics 48:440, 1971.)* School phobia usually presents with a somatic complaint not suggestive of the true problem. A child who (1) is seen as being vulnerable, (2) has overprotective parents or parents who are separating, or (3) has been slow in achieving independence is at high risk for developing school phobia. Appropriate counseling will often prevent its occurrence. Affected children are usually of average or better intellectual abilities. While school phobia in a young child generally is a symptom of difficulties in separating from the parents, in an adolescent it is commonly an expression of more global kinds of problems. Unless the adolescent's school phobia is of recent onset or is related to an obvious cause, the adolescent patient is likely to be schizophrenic or seriously depressed and will probably need long-term psychotherapy.

507. The answer is C (2, 4). *(Hoekelman, pp 615, 621-622.)* Child abuse and neglect occur in all strata of society. Premature, retarded, handicapped, or "special" infants are more likely to be the victims. Low birth-weight infants are often separated from the parents, which can hinder the development of positive parental feelings toward the child. Unplanned births, multiple births, or unwanted children are also at risk. Severe psychopathology is rare in parents who abuse or neglect, but many of these parents were themselves mistreated children.

508. The answer is A (1, 2, 3). *(Hoekelman, pp 687-693. Friedman, Pediatr Clin North Am 20:873-882, 1973.)* Criteria for making the diagnosis of conversion symptoms in adolescents include the development of a symptom that has symbolic meaning for the patient and that does not fit any known medical explanation. Conversion symptoms are often seen in patients with an "hysterical" personality accompanied by an apparent lack of anxiety over their problem ("la belle indifference"). Their reaction often reduces overall anxiety (primary gain) and helps the individual cope with his or her environment (secondary gain). Conversion symptoms usually occur during times of stress and often are based on a model set of symptoms noted beforehand in other individuals.

509. The answer is E (all). *(Hoekelman, pp 669-676.)* Many medical disorders must be excluded before the diagnosis of anorexia nervosa can be made, including all of those listed for this question. A careful history, including the prior occurrence of menarche, and a thorough physical examination are essential in making these exclusions, as is the presence of a normal bone age and normal levels of gonadotropins, pituitary hormones, and estrogens. Hypopituitarism can result in symptoms similar to those of anorexia nervosa. These include amenorrhea, cachexia, decreased excretion of urinary 17-ketosteroids, and a general hypometabolic state. Occasionally a supracellar cyst may cause anorexia nervosa-like symptoms. Malabsorption syndromes can cause severe weight loss and are usually accompanied by bloating, steatorrhea, and hypoproteinuria. Prior menarche and generally normal development of secondary sexual characteristics can usually rule out primary ovarian dysfunction. Inflammatory bowel disease or chronic infection sometimes may mimic anorexia nervosa. An elevated erythrocyte sedimentation rate may provide a clue to the presence of these other disorders.

510. The answer is D (4). *(Hoekelman, p 666. Malmquist, N Engl J Med 284:958-960, 1971.)* There are several types of depression in teenagers. Acute depressive reactions refer to an adaptive state of depression that occurs in response to the loss of a loved one such as a family member or a friend. It is a reaction that can interfere with daily activities for weeks or months. An attempt by a youth to mask or hide depressive feelings is called masked depression of adolescents—a subgroup of the neurotic depressive disorders. When reality testing is impaired with depression, the condition is termed the psychotic depressive disorder. Finally, transient depressive mood swings are normal in adolescents and do not interfere with daily function.

511. The answer is A (1, 2, 3). *(Hoekelman, pp 674-677. Weiner, Pediatr Clin North Am 22:673-684, 1975.)* Juvenile delinquency is often divided into three basic types: sociological, characterological, and neurotic. Sociological delinquency is often manifested as part of a group or gang activity to merit praise from the general peer group. Neighborhood rehabilitation programs work best for these individuals. Characterological delinquency is based on an asocial personality, in which the individual has no regard for the rights of others. This is a serious form of psychopathology, requiring intense psychotherapy. Acts are committed, but guilt is not felt by these youths, who tend to be "loners." Neurotic delinquency usually is sudden in onset and is a manifestation of an underlying depression. The neurotic delinquent has a need to be caught in the antisocial act. Neurotic delinquency is the type of juvenile delinquency that may respond to counseling by interested pediatricians.

512-514. The answers are: 512-C, 513-D, 514-A. *(Hoekelman, p 182.)* **False positive** results label well individuals as having the disease. **False negative** results fail to identify some people who have the disease. The **sensitivity** of a test is its ability to label correctly **all** those who have the disease. The **specificity** reflects the ability of the test to identify **only** those who have the disease. An inverse relationship frequently exists between the sensitivity and the specificity of a test. For some tests, a high degree of sensitivity (few false negatives) may only be attainable if the specificity is low (many false positives). Many factors determine which screening test to use in the detection of a particular disease. Among these are the severity of the disease and the cost of working up those with false positive screening tests.

515-518. The answers are: 515-C, 516-B, 517-E, 518-B. *(Hoekelman, pp 162-165. Koplan, N Engl J Med 301:906-912, 1979.)* Pertussis vaccine is usually given in conjunction with diphtheria and tetanus toxoid in a combined preparation (DPT). Pertussis vaccine causes more side effects than any of the other commonly used vaccines. It has not been possible to identify and produce an antigen responsible for immunity to pertussis. The pertussis portion of DPT is a crude preparation of killed bacteria. Local erythema and swelling are seen frequently at the injection site. Fever within 48 hours of administration is also common. These local and systemic reactions are diminished if the dose of DPT is reduced by half. If this is done, the lower dose should be given at intervals of six weeks until the total cumulative amount is administered. Neurological complications, ranging from seizures to coma, have been associated with pertussis vaccine. Several cases of fatal central nervous system impairment have been documented, and permanent brain damage may also ensue. The overall incidence of severe reactions is approximately 1 per 34,000 vaccine doses administered. Persistent, uncontrollable crying for 6-24 hours following immunization is also sometimes considered a central nervous system side effect of the pertussis vaccine. This reaction occurs in approximately 1 per 3500 vaccine doses administered. Diphtheria and tetanus toxoids cause few side effects.

Administration of the measles vaccine is often followed by a fever seven-to-ten days later. A rash and general malaise may accompany the fever. Arthritis is not a complication of any of the vaccines discussed above. It has, however, been seen following rubella vaccination.

519-523. The answers are: 519-B, 520-A, 521-E, 522-E, 523-D. *(Hoekelman, pp 162-166).* The vaccine against **diphtheria** is a purified toxoid. Antibodies induced by the toxoid protect against development of the disease caused by *Corynebacterium diphtheriae.* In older children and adults, the dose of diphtheria toxoid should be reduced in order to avoid the reactions seen with use of the larger dose given to infants. **Pertussis vaccine** is produced from whole, killed bacteria. It is a crude vaccine, since it has not been possible to identify and produce a pure substance that would induce immunity against the disease. Only 80-90 percent of infants given pertussis vaccine become immunized successfully, as compared to almost 100 percent given diphtheria toxoid. **Oral polio vaccine** (Sabin) contains live, attenuated virus. Trivalent vaccines contain types 1, 2, and 3 virus in proportions that result in immunity to all three. **Measles vaccine** also contains a live, attenuated virus; it is administered intramuscularly. **Influenza vaccine** is a killed virus. In general, toxoids and inactivated vaccines require more frequent administration to maintain immunity. Live vaccines produce immunity that more closely resembles that following natural infection, many producing long-lasting immunity. Patients receiving immunosuppressant therapy should not receive live vaccines, since they may develop serious disease similar to that seen with natural infection. Inactivated polio vaccine (Salk) may be given to children if the use of the live vaccine is contraindicated.

524-528. The answers are: 524-E, 525-C, 526-A, 527-D, 528-E. *(Hoekelman, pp 136-140. Fomon, ed 2. p 477.)* Breast milk contains adequate amounts of vitamins A and C if the mother is on a normal diet. Vitamin D has been demonstrated in the water-soluble fraction of human milk; however, the clinical significance of this finding has not been established. Hence, it is recommended that breast-fed infants receive a vitamin D supplement. Vitamin D is of particular importance for infants who live in northern climates and have pigmented skin – that is, for those with decreased exposure to sunlight.

The commonly used proprietary infant formulas are fully fortified and require no vitamin supplements. This is true both for the cow's milk-based formulas and for soy-based formulas.

Infants fed on an evaporated milk formula should receive a vitamin C supplement, since the processing of the milk destroys this vitamin. The vitamin A content of cow's milk is adequate and higher than that of human milk. Since almost all evaporated milk sold in this country is fortified with vitamin D, no supplement is necessary.

Folic acid should be given to children fed a formula based on goat's milk, which contains low concentrations of this nutrient. They should also receive vitamins C and D. Goat's milk does not contain adequate amounts of vitamin D, and any ascorbic acid in the milk would be destroyed during pasteurization. Vitamins C and D should be given to infants whose formula is based on cow's milk that has not been fortified with vitamin D. Again, the addition of vitamin C would be necessary because of its destruction during pasteurization.

Supplementation with vitamin E is not needed for the full-term infant receiving any of these diets. Only premature infants have an increased requirement for this vitamin. Vitamin A supplementation is also unnecessary for any of the infant diets mentioned.

Therapeutics

DIRECTIONS: Each question below contains five suggested answers. Choose the **one best** response to each question.

529. All of the following statements regarding fluid balance and age are correct EXCEPT that

(A) the greater percentage of interstitial fluid in children under six months of age makes the shift of potassium from cellular to extracellular fluid during acidosis clinically unimportant
(B) because of greater relative surface area, children under 18 months of age become dehydrated more rapidly than older children
(C) because of a relatively greater interstitial fluid volume, children under 18 months of age can tolerate a greater percentage of total fluid loss than can older children
(D) a one-day-old infant requires less maintenance fluid than a three-week-old infant who weighs the same as the younger infant
(E) while maintenance fluid requirements per calorie intake are constant over age, maintenance requirements per kilogram body weight vary with age

530. In the treatment of hyperkalemia, the administration of which of the following substances has an immediate protective effect on the heart?

(A) Sodium polystyrene sulfonate sodium-potassium exchange resin
(B) Glucose and insulin
(C) Calcium gluconate
(D) Sodium bicarbonate
(E) A potassium-losing diuretic

531. All of the following statements concerning chloramphenicol are true EXCEPT that

(A) it is absorbed well from the gastrointestinal tract
(B) it is metabolized in the kidney
(C) it may cause reversible bone marrow depression
(D) it is known to be present in breast milk of mothers taking the drug
(E) it should be avoided in the premature infant and the neonate

532. A hospitalized patient is given the following parenteral fluid: 200 ml lactated Ringer's solution in the first hour; 700 ml five percent dextrose in half-normal saline in the next seven hours with 20 mEq of potassium chloride added to each liter; and finally, 1100 ml of five percent dextrose in quarter-normal saline given from the 8th to the 24th hour (with 20 mEq of potassium chloride in each liter). This fluid regimen is the most appropriate management for which of the following situations?

(A) A child who weighs 10 kg (22 lb) is in heat stroke after being locked in a car on a summer day
(B) A child who weighs 10 kg (22 lb) has inappropriate antidiabetic hormone activity secondary to meningitis
(C) A child who weighs 10 kg (22 lb) suffers from 10 percent hypotonic dehydration secondary to diarrhea
(D) A child who weighs 20 kg (44 lb) suffers from 5 percent dehydration secondary to diarrhea
(E) A child who weighs 20 kg (44 lb) is recuperating from maxillary surgery and is otherwise normal

533. Hemolytic transfusion reactions are due to the

(A) presence of white cell leukoagglutinins in platelet concentrates
(B) presence of platelet antibodies in the recipient's blood
(C) presence of erythrocyte antibodies in the recipient's blood
(D) rapid infusion of whole blood
(E) infusion of outdated blood

534. An axillary temperature of 37.8°C (100°F) is equivalent to a rectal temperature of

(A) 37.2°C (99°F)
(B) 37.8°C (100°F)
(C) 38.3°C (101°F)
(D) 38.9°C (102°F)
(E) 39.4°C (103°F)

535. In the graph shown below, which area best represents the intracellular fluid concentration of sodium?

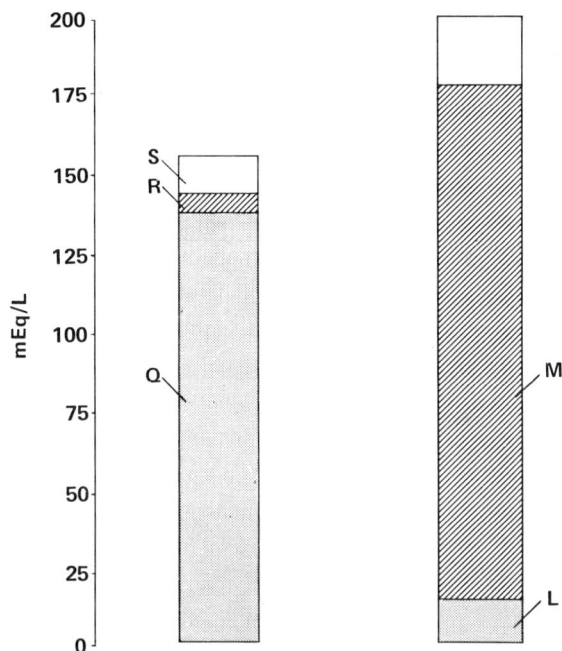

(A) Area **L**
(B) Area **M**
(C) Area **Q**
(D) Area **R**
(E) Area **S**

536. The most common cause of hypernatremic dehydration in childhood is

(A) diabetes insipidus
(B) diabetic ketoacidosis
(C) acute gastroenteritis
(D) pyloric stenosis
(E) bronchiolitis

537. In order to diagnose the syndrome of inappropriate antidiuretic hormone secretion accurately, all of the following conditions must exist EXCEPT for

(A) hyponatremia
(B) absence of intrinsic renal, cardiac, or adrenal disease
(C) normal renal function
(D) urine osmolality inappropriately higher than serum osmolality
(E) low urinary sodium concentration

538. The most common effect of a toxic dose of acetaminophen is

(A) gastrointestinal bleeding
(B) hepatocellular necrosis
(C) agranulocytosis
(D) hyperpyrexia
(E) tinnitus

539. All of the following statements concerning drug absorption are correct EXCEPT that

(A) activated charcoal is useful in the treatment of acute aspirin overdose even if given 12 hours after ingestion
(B) dairy products and antacids enhance the rate of absorption of tetracycline
(C) oral polio vaccine should not be given during an episode of gastroenteritis
(D) the addition of small amounts of suitable antacids to aspirin increases the rate of dissolution and absorption
(E) the variable rectal absorption rate of theophylline contraindicates rectal administration of this drug

DIRECTIONS: Each question below contains four suggested answers of which **one** or **more** is correct. Choose the answer

A	if	1, 2, and 3	are correct
B	if	1 and 3	are correct
C	if	2 and 4	are correct
D	if	4	is correct
E	if	1, 2, 3, and 4	are correct

540. Correct statements concerning pharmacokinetics in children include which of the following?

(1) Four to eight days of repeated doses of phenobarbital are required to achieve a steady state, regardless of the size of the maintenance dose
(2) Normograms used to correlate symptoms with drug blood levels for acute overdoses may be misleading if used in cases of toxicity from chronic drug ingestion
(3) For children on maintenance aspirin or phenytoin therapy, small dosage increases can lead to greater elevations in serum concentration than expected
(4) Infants need and tolerate more of some drugs on a milligram per square meter of body surface basis than do older children and adults

541. Aldosterone secretion will be enhanced by which of the following conditions?

(1) Hemorrhage
(2) "Third spacing" of fluids
(3) Hyponatremia
(4) Hypervolemia

542. Appropriate ways to correct severe hypernatremic dehydration include

(1) rapid infusion of normal saline at 20 ml/kg of body weight
(2) rapid infusion of D_5W at 20 ml/kg of body weight
(3) reduction of serum sodium levels over a period of 48 hours
(4) administration of a natriuretic

543. True statements concerning drug distribution include which of the following?

(1) Albumin is the protein that plays the major role in drug binding
(2) Factors that influence the concentration of a drug in a tissue include its blood flow, fat content, and mass
(3) Only a free, unbound drug can migrate into body tissues
(4) Although neonates have an increased total body water, lower doses of drugs (per kilogram of body weight) are necessary for therapeutic effect

544. A child with a ventricular septal defect is about to undergo bilateral ureteral reimplantation. Which of the following antibiotics would be acceptable to use for the prevention of bacterial endocarditis?

(1) Penicillin and gentamicin intramuscularly
(2) Ampicillin intravenously and streptomycin intramuscularly
(3) Vancomycin intravenously and streptomycin intramuscularly
(4) Penicillin intramuscularly

545. Hypovolemic shock may be secondary to which of the following conditions or situations?

(1) Blood loss
(2) Gastrointestinal infarction
(3) Withdrawal of ascitic fluid by paracentesis
(4) Ventricular fibrillation

546. Toxic effects of theophylline include

(1) emesis
(2) tachycardia
(3) convulsions
(4) diuresis

SUMMARY OF DIRECTIONS

A	B	C	D	E
1, 2, 3 only	1, 3 only	2, 4 only	4 only	All are correct

547. For which of the following drugs would the pattern of distribution, elimination, or both differ in a two-day-old term newborn from that of a two-year-old healthy child?

(1) Phenytoin (diphenylhydantoin)
(2) Theophylline
(3) Gentamicin
(4) Chloramphenicol

548. Which of the following factors would be expected to affect the maintenance water requirements for a child who is receiving parenteral fluid therapy?

(1) Body temperature
(2) Activity level
(3) Respiratory rate
(4) Body weight for height

549. Anaphylaxis due to penicillin allergy is mediated by which of the following?

(1) IgE antibodies
(2) SRS-A
(3) Histamine
(4) IgA antibodies

550. Sodium content in the extracellular fluid space is controlled by which of the following mechanisms?

(1) Aldosterone secretion
(2) Glomerular filtration rate
(3) Cortisol secretion
(4) Antidiuretic hormone secretion

551. Blood products that carry a risk of transfusion-associated homogenous serum hepatitis include

(1) fresh frozen plasma
(2) gamma globulin
(3) frozen red blood cells
(4) albumin

552. True statements concerning theophylline include which of the following?

(1) Theophylline is primarily metabolized by the kidneys
(2) Children metabolize theophylline more rapidly than adults
(3) Administration of theophylline by suppository is recommended for patients who are vomiting
(4) About 50 percent of theophylline is protein-bound

553. The curves in the graph shown below illustrate the effect of antibiotic combinations on bacterial viability. The effect demonstrated by curve 4 is produced by which of the following drug combinations?

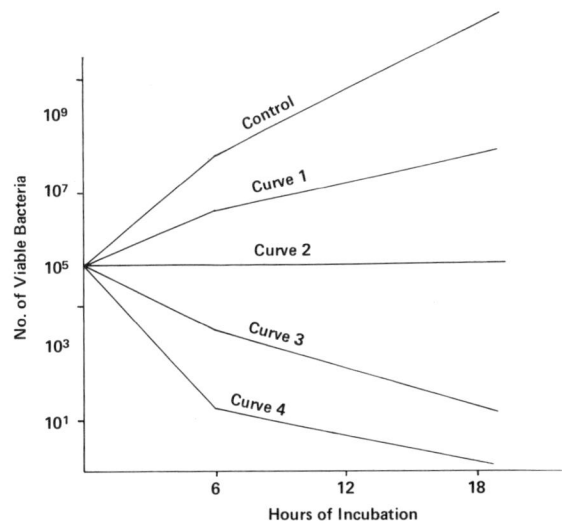

Used with permission of Williams and Wilkins Company, from *Medicine* 57(2) March 1978, (p 181) by Rahal JJ.

(1) Nafcillin and gentamicin in *Staphylococcus aureus* osteomyelitis
(2) Penicillin and tetracycline in *Streptococcus (Diplococcus) pneumoniae* meningitis
(3) Ticarcillin and tobramycin in *Pseudomonas aeruginosa* pneumonia
(4) Ampicillin and chloramphenicol in *Hemophilus influenzae* b septic arthritis

554. Chloramphenicol can produce two kinds of bone marrow suppression — idiosyncratic and dose-dependent. The idiosyncratic reaction can be differentiated from the dose-dependent reaction by which of the following features?

(1) The idiosyncratic reaction is quite rare (1/1,000,000)
(2) Dose-dependent toxicity is reversible with cessation of the drug
(3) The idiosyncratic reaction usually becomes manifest within 24-48 hours of the start of therapy
(4) The earliest dose-dependent effect of the drug on the marrow is depression of erythropoiesis

555. True statements about binding of antimicrobials to serum proteins include which of the following?

(1) Penetration of antibiotics into most tissues and inflammatory fluids is not correlated with the level of free drug in serum
(2) Only free, unbound antibiotics are active antimicrobially
(3) If an antibiotic is 50 percent bound to protein, the amount of free drug in the body is 50 percent
(4) Sulfonamides are moderately or highly protein bound, which can lead to displacement of other protein-bound molecules (e.g., bilirubin)

DIRECTIONS: The groups of questions below consist of lettered choices followed by several numbered items. For each numbered item select the **one** lettered choice with which it is **most** closely associated. Each lettered choice may be used once, more than once, or not at all.

Questions 556-558

For each reaction below, select the substance with which it is most closely associated.

(A) Aspirin
(B) Endogenous pyrogens
(C) Acetaminophen
(D) Brown fat
(E) Exogenous pyrogens

556. Increases circulating catecholamines

557. Elevates the hypothalamic set-point temperature

558. Causes peripheral vasodilation by direct action on muscle

Questions 559-563

For each antibiotic listed below, select the side-effect with which it is most commonly associated.

(A) Rash
(B) Bone marrow suppression
(C) Renal dysfunction
(D) Hepatic dysfunction
(E) Gastrointestinal dysfunction

559. Erythromycin estolate

560. Methicillin sodium

561. Amoxicillin sodium

562. Trimethoprim-sulfamethoxazole

563. Nitrofurantoin

Questions 564-567

It is recommended that passive immunity be produced against the diseases listed below under defined circumstances. For each disease, select the type of immunizing agent currently recommended.

(A) Standard human immune serum globulin
(B) Special immune serum globulin
(C) Toxoid
(D) Antitoxin
(E) Live antigen

564. Viral hepatitis, type A

565. Tetanus

566. Measles

567. Rabies

Therapeutics

Answers

529. The answer is A. *(Hoekelman, pp 256-259.)* During the growth of a normal child, a number of changes occur which affect fluid and electrolyte balance. Children under 18 months of age have a greater relative body surface area in relation to their weight and thus become dehydrated more rapidly than older children. However, because they have a relatively greater interstitial fluid volume, they can tolerate a greater percentage of total fluid loss than can the older child. Also, maintenance fluid requirements for full-term normal newborn infants during the first few days of life are less than those after the infant is a week or so of age. Therefore, even though they are of the same weight, a one-day-old infant would require less fluid than a three-week-old infant. Because fluid requirements are related to body metabolism, fluid requirements per calorie intake are constant over age. However, because caloric intake per kilogram of body weight varies with age, maintenance requirements also vary with age. Thus, while a child who weighs 4 kg (8 lb, 13 oz) would have a daily intake of 150 ml/kg, a child who weighs 30 kg (about 66 lb) would take in only 72 ml/kg (fluid requirements per body surface area, like intake per calorie, are relatively constant over age).

530. The answer is C. *(Hoekelman, p 251. Kempe, ed 4. pp 956-957.)* The administration of calcium does not alter serum levels of potassium, but does counteract depolarization of cardiac muscle and thus immediately reduces the risk of arrhythmias. This effect lasts for only a short time, however. It is imperative, therefore, that means be utilized to reduce the absolute potassium content of serum. An infusion of sodium bicarbonate will correct any acidosis that may be causing potassium to shift intracellularly. Likewise, a glucose and insulin infusion will shift potassium into cells concomitant with the transport of glucose. Finally, polystyrene sulfonate (Kayexalate) and diuretics will eliminate potassium from the body. These agents act much more slowly than calcium gluconate and will not confer any immediate protection to the heart.

531. The answer is B. *(Hoekelman, pp 287-295.)* Chloramphenicol is an excellent drug as long as it is utilized with the appropriate precautions and for the proper indications. It penetrates well into virtually all body tissues, is absorbed well from the gastrointestinal tract, provides high cerebrospinal fluid and brain tissue levels, and is metabolized in the liver. Toxic effects may be significant, however, particularly in the neonate and premature infant. Special care should be taken by the breast-feeding mother, since variable quantities may be contained in the breast milk if the mother takes the drug. High serum levels occur in these small infants (since there is a relative inability of the immature liver to conjugate the chloramphenicol) resulting occasionally in cardiovascular collapse (the "gray syndrome"). Bone marrow aplasia may occur in some patients. This reaction is unpredictable. When it does occur, it usually manifests several weeks after the drug has been discontinued. Related to dose and length of treatment, the adverse reaction is reversible. The tendency toward this side effect may be inherited.

532. The answer is C. *(Hoekelman, pp 261-267. Vaughan, ed 11. pp 286-289.)* Parenteral fluid replacement needs are determined by estimating maintenance needs and adding fluids as necessary to make up the calculated losses. Losses may be replaced in 12 to 48 hours depending on the condition of the child (with hypernatremia, losses should be corrected more slowly). The patient described in the question has received 2000 ml of fluid in a 24-hour period. This dosage would be slightly high for a child weighing 20 kg (44 lb) who is post-operative and otherwise normal (his maintenance would be approximately 1500 ml/24-hour period), especially since inappropriate antidiuretic hormone (ADH) activity may occur post-operatively and lead to hyponatremia, with or without neurologic symptoms. Since weight loss during dehydration is assumed to be all fluid, the child who weighs 20 kg with five percent dehydration would require 1000 ml to correct his dehydration and 1500 ml to supply his maintenance, totaling 2500 ml/day. The fluid lost in a child with heat stroke is hypotonic; therefore, the use of half-normal saline for seven hours would be inappropriate. (It may be necessary in these children to initiate resuscitation with normal saline or lactated Ringer's solution or even albumin or blood; however, the primary need of these patients is for water rather than electrolytes.) A child who weighs 10 kg with a ten percent hypotonic dehydration secondary to diarrhea would require approximately 2 L of fluid in a 24-hour period with a greater than maintenance amount of sodium. The regimen described in choice C, therefore, would be most appropriate for this child.

533. The answer is C. *(Hoekelman, p 283.)* There are several types of transfusion reactions, including hemolytic, allergic, febrile, and delayed. Hemolytic transfusion reactions are caused by the presence of pre-formed antibodies on the erythrocytes or the recipient's blood. These antibodies react to either the major or minor blood group determinants (antigens) on the donor's erythrocytes. Hemoglobinemia and hemoglobinuria, vomiting, fever, and back pain may occur. The immediate danger is acute renal failure due to the toxic effects of hemoglobin on the renal tubules. Simple febrile reactions frequently are associated with platelet transfusions. Platelets are usually not type-specific and contain white blood cell agglutinins as well. The rapid infusion of whole blood may cause cardiovascular overload but rarely causes hemolysis. It therefore is recommended that no more than ten percent of the blood volume be transfused at a time and that at least three hours should elapse during its administration. Outdated blood contains deteriorating red blood cells, so that the effect of the transfusion on the hematocrit will be short-lived. A classic hemolytic transfusion reaction usually does not occur with outdated blood.

534. The answer is D. *(Hoekelman, p 276.)* An axillary temperature is usually 2°F lower than a rectal temperature and 1°F lower than an oral temperature. The rectal temperature is the most accurate measurement, since it is less prone to errors due to positioning of the thermometer and to ambient influences. There is also considerable variation in the accuracy of thermometers from different manufacturers. If possible, the same thermometer should be used during an illness.

535. The answer is A. *(Hoekelman, pp 248-249.)* The electrolyte concentration of intracellular fluids is generally around 200 mEq/L, while that of serum is approximately 160 mEq/L. The sodium concentration of serum and the potassium concentration of intracellular fluids are approximately the same (140-145 mEq/L); intracellular sodium concentration is generally 10-12 mEq/L. In cellular fluid, calcium and magnesium are the other major cations, and phosphate and proteinate are the major anions.

536. The answer is C. *(Hoekelman, pp 263-264. Smith, 1977. pp 279-281.)* Acute gastroenteritis is the most common cause of hypernatremic dehydration. Patients may present with severe hypovolemia, but on physical examination may appear to be less dehydrated than they actually are. They are very irritable and are likely to have seizures because of loss of cerebral intracellular fluid to the hypertonic extracellular space. Both diabetes insipidus and bronchiolitis may cause hypertonic dehydration due to excess fluid loss through the kidneys and the respiratory tract respectively. In diabetic ketoacidosis, the serum sodium frequently is normal or low, and in pyloric stenosis there is a loss of chloride, potassium, sodium, and hydrogen ion resulting in a hypochloremic alkalosis.

537. The answer is E. *(Hoekelman, p 482. Mendoza, Pediatr Clin North Am 23:681, 1976.)* The syndrome of inappropriate antidiuretic hormone secretion (SIADH) causes an increase in water reabsorption in the distal tubules. This syndrome results in oliguria, a high urine osmolality, and an excess of total body water, causing a dilutional hyponatremia (hypomolality). Urine sodium concentration is usually high. Since renal disease with impaired renal function and intrinsic cardiac and adrenal disease may lead to similar serum and electrolyte disturbances, SIADH cannot be diagnosed if any of these conditions is present.

538. The answer is B. *(Hoekelman, pp 277-278. American Academy of Pediatrics, Pediatrics 61:108-112, 1978.)* Gastrointestinal bleeding, tinnitus, and hyperpyrexia are all toxic effects of salicylates. Hepatocellular necrosis can result from ingestion of toxic amounts of acetaminophen, appearing as late as 72 hours postingestion. N-acetylcysteine given orally is recommended to counteract this effect, but the precise mechanism of the action of this drug is unclear. Agranulocytosis has not been reported following the ingestion of acetaminophen in therapeutic or toxic doses. Toxic effects of acetaminophen on the liver can be reduced by intravenous administration of methionine or cysteamine. This treatment is effective only if started within ten hours of the overdose. However, this treatment can have a number of side-effects, such as, nausea, vomiting, severe malaise, and drowsiness, and thus should be used only when the condition of the patient makes its use imperative and only within ten hours of ingestion of the analgesic.

539. The answer is B. *(Goodman, ed 5. pp 5-7, 1185. Levy, Pediatrics 62:868, 1978.)* A number of factors may affect the absorption of a drug from the intestinal tract. These include the presence of other substances in the gastrointestinal tract, the pH, the nature of the drug being given (e.g., enteric coated tablet versus liquid), the transit time, the location in the gastrointestinal tract where absorption occurs, and the time of gastric emptying, including the presence of vomiting. Aspirin, especially in an acute overdose, may be absorbed slowly, and activated charcoal should always be given in the first 12 hours after intake. Calcium products such as antacids and dairy products bind tetracycline in the gastrointestinal tract and **decrease** its absorption. Polio vaccine is usually not given during gastroenteritis because of the presence of interferon, which would affect replication of the virus and have an adverse effect on local antibody response. The addition of antacids to aspirin increases the pH near the aspirin particles, thereby increasing the rate of absorption and dissolution of the tablet. Most medications, including theophylline, are inconsistently absorbed when given rectally, and because of the dangers of both an adequate dosage and overdosage, this method should not be used, especially for theophylline.

540. The answer is E (all). *(Hoekelman, pp 237, 239-241.)* The absorption, distribution, metabolism, and excretion of many drugs are related to the age of a child. For children on drug regimens with repeated dosing at fixed intervals, four to five half-lives are required before a steady state may be achieved, regardless of the size of the maintenance dose. A loading dose can be given to achieve a steady state concentration sooner, but this dose is larger than the usual maintenance dose and carries a risk of toxicity. The normograms used to correlate symptoms with blood levels are designed for acute intoxication, and although levels in chronic ingestions that are above the symptomatic range are useful, those below may lead the clinician to think that the drug is not responsible for the symptoms, when in fact it is. For certain medications such as aspirin, phenytoin, and ethanol, the pathways available for elimination become saturated at a certain drug concentration. They thus follow first order elimination kinetics when low doses are administered, but zero order kinetics when higher doses are administered. Once above saturation, small dosage changes will lead to greater than expected elevations in serum concentration. Finally, since infants have a greater percentage of extracellular water than do older children and adults, they therefore need and tolerate more of some drugs per surface area than do adults. Therefore, all four choices are correct.

541. The answer is A (1, 2, 3). *(Hoekelman, p 249. Pitts, ed 3. pp 247-250.)* Aldosterone, which is produced by the zona glomerulosa adrenal cortex, exerts its effect on the distal tubule of the kidney, where it enhances sodium reabsorption. Secretion of aldosterone is enhanced by any state of intravascular volume depletion such as those secondary to hemorrhage or to "third spacing" of fluids. In addition, aldosterone serves as a sodium sparing mechanism in states of body sodium depletion. ACTH is also known to increase aldosterone secretion.

542. The answer is B (1, 3). *(Hoekelman, pp 263-264. Smith, 1977. pp 279-281.)* The primary danger in the treatment of hypernatremic dehydration is the production of rapid extracellular-to-intracellular fluid shifts, which may cause cerebral edema. Since these shifts appear to be related directly to the rapid drop in extracellular sodium, careful reduction of serum sodium levels over 48 hours generally is recommended. If the state of dehydration is severe enough to cause shock, normal saline (20 ml/kg) should be administered rapidly. Normal saline still is relatively hypotonic to the high extracellular sodium, and yet not so dilute that serum sodium will fall precipitously, as would occur if a hypotonic fluid such as D_5W were administered. It is obviously inappropriate to give a natriuretic, since the underlying problem is not too much sodium, but too little fluid. In addition, a natriuresis would probably also produce an osmotic diuresis and worsen dehydration.

543. The answer is A (1, 2, 3). *(Hoekelman, pp 236-238.)* Albumin is the major protein that affects drug binding. Laboratory determinations of the total serum content of a drug can be misleading. These determinations are generally measurements of the total (free plus bound) drug concentration. Only the free unbound portion is active and can diffuse into body tissues. How much actually diffuses depends on tissue blood flow, fat content, and other factors that probably vary with the individual. The resulting concentration of drug within the tissue, therefore, is relatively variable. For instance, drug dose (per kilogram of body weight) required to achieve a certain tissue concentration would have to be higher in the neonate, since there is a higher total body water content than in older children and adults.

544. The answer is A (1, 2, 3). *(Hoekelman, p 297. Nadas, ed 3. pp 182-189. Vaughan, ed 11. pp 690-692.)* Penicillin alone may not prevent infections due to enterococci; therefore, an aminoglycoside such as streptomycin or gentamicin also is required for prophylaxis against bacterial endocarditis due to these organisms. Vancomycin is an excellent substitute for penicillin or ampicillin in those patients who have penicillin allergy. This drug penetrates well into virtually all tissues and is highly effective against *Staphylococcus aureus* as well.

545. The answer is A (1, 2, 3). *(Hoekelman, p 256.)* Hypovolemic shock is caused by loss of intravascular volume. Blood loss, then, would be an obvious cause of hypovolemic shock. In ventricular fibrillation, the etiology of the shock is pump failure **with** an adequate volume (cardiogenic shock). Shock occurring in gastrointestinal infarction, and following the withdrawal of ascitic fluid is secondary to "third spacing," with fluid shifting from the intravascular to an extravascular space—for example, to the bowel lumen and to the peritoneal cavity. Hypovolemia in the absence of overt loss of fluid from the body should be suspected in patients with gastrointestinal catastrophies. However, the sequestration of large amounts of fluid in the bowel lumen may not be clinically evident in these patients. On the other hand, accumulation of ascitic fluid or fluid in the subcutaneous spaces following clysis is usually quite evident on physical examination.

546. The answer is E (all). *(Hoekelman, p 242.)* Theophylline belongs to the class of the methylxanthines that affects the gastrointestinal, cardiovascular, and central nervous systems. There is a correlation between serum concentration of the drug and both therapeutic and toxic effects. The therapeutic concentration is considered to be 10 to 20 mg/L. Toxicity may occur at 20 mg/L, although bronchodilation continues for some patients at that level. It is not uncommon, however, to see emesis, arrhythmias, seizure activity, diuresis, and headaches with toxic blood levels, that is, greater than 20 mg/L.

547. The answer is E (all). *(Schaffer, ed 4. pp 1026-1032.)* The dose-response relationships for the newborn are often very different from those of older children. Newborns generally have a deficiency in plasma proteins that bind to drugs, leading to a higher percentage of active unbound medication in the plasma. The metabolism of drugs through oxidation and through conjugation, such as glucuronidation, sulfation, and acetylation, is also diminished in the newborn. Finally, elimination through renal excretion is also diminished. Phenytoin and theophylline both bind to protein and are metabolized by oxidation, and their patterns of metabolism and distribution in newborns differ from those of older children. Gentamicin and the other aminoglycosides are eliminated by glomerular filtration and are more likely to accumulate in a newborn than in older children. Chloramphenicol must be glucuronidated before being eliminated and tends to accumulate in newborns. If the blood levels rise significantly, the child is at risk for toxicity (the "gray baby" syndrome).

548. The answer is E (all). *(Hoekelman, pp 256-259.)* Factors which must be taken into account in the calculation of maintenance fluid requirements for a child include the child's basal caloric intake, surface area, and weight. However, the figure obtained from these calculations is a basal figure for a child of normal body habitus. An extremely obese child will require less fluid per kilogram of body weight. Those conditions that increase evaporative water losses such as fever, high activity level, and high respiratory rate must also be considered in the calculation of maintenance fluids. For example, for each 1°F rise in body temperature, an additional 50 to 100 ml per square meter of body surface should be added for maintenance; thus, all four choices are correct.

549. The answer is A (1, 2, 3). *(Hoekelman, pp 1085-1087. Lockey, Med Clin North Am 58:149, 1974. Vaughan, ed 11. pp 640-641.)* In certain individuals, penicillin induces the production of IgE antibodies, which attach themselves to the surface of mast cells. Subsequent administration of penicillin may cause a violent antigen-antibody reaction with disruption of the mast cell wall and release of histamine and of slow reacting substance of anaphylaxis (SRS-A). Histamine and SRS-A are the main determinants of the clinical symptoms. IgA antibodies are secretory antibodies and are not involved in type 1 hypersensitivity reactions.

550. The answer is A (1, 2, 3). *(Hoekelman, pp 249-250.)* Sodium content in the extracellular fluid is regulated by several mechanisms, the majority of which are mediated through the kidney. Aldosterone as well as cortisol enhances sodium reabsorption in the distal tubule by a sodium-potassium exchange mechanism. The glomerular filtration rate controls the rate and quantity of sodium presented to the tubules and so exerts an effect on reabsorption. In addition, the capillary hydrostatic and oncotic pressures influence sodium reabsorption in the proximal tubule directly. An increase in the oncotic pressure and a decrease in the hydrostatic pressure promote the reabsorption of sodium. Antidiuretic hormone may alter the **concentration** of sodium by increasing water absorption, but it has no effect on the absolute **quantity** of sodium in the extracellular fluid.

551. The answer is B (1, 3). *(Hoekelman, pp 281-283.)* Transfusions of various blood products have become a routine and accepted part of medical practice. However, transfusions are not without certain risks, such as hepatitis (or another infectious disease), hypervolemia, transfusion reactions, and hemosiderosis. The risk of hepatitis has decreased since the inception of immunologic screening methods and the use of volunteer donors, but it is still substantial. It is highest in fibrinogen and cryoprecipitate concentrates where plasma from many donors is pooled. There is no risk of hepatitis with the use of gamma globulin or albumin, as these components are heat-treated.

552. The answer is C (2, 4). *(Hoekelman, pp 242-244.)* Children metabolize theophylline significantly faster than adults; therefore, children will have lower serum levels than adults who have taken similar doses. The average theophylline dose for continual infusion is 0.9 mg/kg/hr in children and 1.1 mg/kg/hr in adults. A little over 50 percent of theophylline is bound to plasma proteins, and about 90 to 95 percent of theophylline is excreted mainly by hepatic metabolism; liver disease causes a prolonged half-life for the drug. The remainder of theophylline excretion occurs through the kidneys. In addition, there is a great deal of individual variability in theophylline metabolism, necessitating the frequent monitoring of serum levels to determine optimal dosing requirements. Administration of theophylline by rectal suppository is extremely dangerous, as rectal absorption of the drug is erratic, and overdosage by this route is common.

553. The answer is B (1, 3). *(Rahal, Medicine 57:179-195, 1978.)* Antibiotic synergy is of significant clinical relevance in several settings. Examples of synergy include the use of penicillin and aminoglycosides to treat enterococcal endocarditis, a semisynthetic penicillin such as nafcillin and an aminoglycoside (e.g., gentamicin) to treat *Staphylococcus aureus* infections, and ticarcillin and tobramycin to treat *Pseudomonas aeruginosa* infections in the neutropenic patient. Drugs can also be antagonistic. Curve 1 in the graph shows the action of drugs that are mutually antagonistic. Curve 2 shows antagonism of one drug by another, curve 3 shows drugs that are neither synergistic nor antagonistic to each other (indifferent), and curve 4 shows mutual synergism. Drug combinations are prescribed: (1) to achieve a broad range of antimicrobial activity in patients who are critically ill due to undefined bacterial infections, (2) for the treatment of mixed bacterial infections that may involve organisms that do not have a common antibiotic susceptibility, (3) to cut down on the chances that a resistant organism will emerge, and (4) to achieve an additive or synergistic effect. Though any combination of a bacteriostatic agent and a bacteriocidal agent could theoretically produce an antagonistic drug effect, this effect is rarely seen clinically. An example of an established antagonistic drug effect is seen with penicillin and tetracycline in the treatment of pneumococcal meningitis (curve 1).

554. The answer is C (2, 4). *(Yunis, Prog Hematol 4:138, 1964.)* The idiosyncratic reaction to chloramphenicol therapy results in the development of aplastic anemia in 1 out of 25,000 to 40,000 cases. It is usually irreversible and fatal, in contrast to the dose-dependent type of toxicity, which is reversible. The idiosyncratic reaction usually occurs several weeks after the cessation of therapy, although it may occur as late as several months afterwards. The earliest and most consistent pharmacologic effect of the drug is a depression of erythropoiesis, as reflected by a falling reticulocyte count.

555. The answer is C (2, 4). *(Craig, Scand J Infect Dis 14:92-99, 1978.)* Protein binding of antibiotics affects their distribution, elimination, and activity. Only free, unbound drugs can readily pass from the capillaries to tissue fluids and exert an antimicrobial effect. The effect of protein binding is buffered by the apparent volume of distribution (AVD); thus, greater than 80 percent binding of an antibiotic is required to decrease the concentration of free drug in serum by 50 percent. The clinical importance of antibiotic-protein binding is only too evident by the increased incidence of kernicterus in neonates treated with sulfonamides.

556-558. The answers are: 556-D, 557-B, 558-A. *(Hoekelman, pp 275-277.)* Endogenous pyrogens are humoral substances released from neutrophils and bone marrow-derived phagocytes. The pyrogens act directly on the hypothalamic thermoregulatory center to "reset" body temperature, an action that results in enhanced heat conservation by the body. An exogenous pyrogen (e.g., a gram-negative endotoxin or an antigen-antibody complex) activates lymphocytes to release lymphokine; then, endogenous pyrogen is released, which acts to increase the hypothalamic set-point temperature.

Both aspirin and acetaminophen counteract the endogenous pyrogens at the level of the hypothalamus. In addition, aspirin has a peripheral vasodilating effect, which enhances heat dissipation. This effect, however, may be undesirable in a dehydrated child with intravascular volume depletion.

Augmented cellular metabolism, induced by sympathetic stimulation and circulating catecholamine levels, is another way of increasing heat production. This mechanism is related to brown fat, a mitochondria-rich substance present in neonates. Brown fat is the locus for catecholamine production and thus contributes to increased cellular metabolism and heat production.

559-563. The answers are: 559-D, 560-C, 561-A, 562-A, 563-E. *(Rudolph, ed 16, pp 402-405.)* **Erythromycin** in its estolate form causes a cholestatic hepatitis manifested as jaundice and detectable through abnormal liver function tests. This reaction is particularly likely to occur if the drug is used over a long period. The other salts of this drug are not associated with this side effect; they more commonly cause gastrointestinal symptoms. **Methicillin** can cause an interstitial nephritis manifested by abnormal urinalysis. This effect is probably more common with methicillin than with the other penicillinase-resistant penicillins. **Amoxicillin**, like ampicillin, causes rashes. The incidence of gastrointestinal symptoms due to amoxicillin is lower than that caused by ampicillin. Although **trimethoprim-sulfamethoxazole** is associated with rashes, hepatic dysfunction, and gastrointestinal upset, the dermal manifestations are most common. **Nitrofurantoin** can cause (in order of decreasing frequency) nausea and vomiting, rashes, hypersensitivity, pneumonitis, and hemolytic anemia in glucose-6-phosphate dehydrogenase-deficient patients.

564-567. The answers are: 564-A, 565-B, 566-A, 567-B. *(Hoekelman, pp 158-162. Yow, ed 18. pp 17-18, 214, 284.)* Standard **human immune globulin** is effective in the prevention of viral hepatitis type A and in the prevention or modification (depending on dose) of measles. **Tetanus immune globulin** is recommended for prevention of disease in patients at risk who have not been adequately immunized. Tetanus antitoxin carries a significant risk of producing serious allergic reactions and is indicated only if tetanus immune globulin is not available. **Rabies immune globulin** is efficacious in preventing disease after exposure, and is given concurrently with active immunization (duck embryo vaccine). **Toxoids** and **live antigens** are given to produce active immunity in persons not immediately at risk for contracting the disease in question.

Miscellaneous Conditions and Diseases

DIRECTIONS: Each question below contains five suggested answers. Choose the **one best** response to each question.

568. The most frequent cause of fatal home accidents in children under six years of age is

(A) electrocution
(B) foreign body aspiration
(C) poisoning
(D) fire
(E) firearms

569. All the following statements concerning Hurler's syndrome are true EXCEPT that

(A) it is an autosomal recessive disease
(B) hydrocephalus is a frequent clinical finding
(C) life expectancy is about 25 years
(D) death usually results from cardiovascular pathology
(E) severe visual impairment is common

570. In the pediatric age range, the major source of morbidity secondary to sarcoidosis is the

(A) spleen
(B) lungs
(C) kidneys
(D) liver
(E) eyes

571. All of the following statements about obesity are true EXCEPT that

(A) most obese children have at least one obese parent
(B) more weight is gained during winter than during summer
(C) obesity is inversely proportional to social class
(D) breast-feeding appears to help prevent obesity
(E) salt and sugar cravings are usually physiologic

572. A four-year-old girl is found unconscious in a swimming pool less than ten minutes after having been seen in her home by her mother. A neighbor initiated appropriate cardiopulmonary resuscitation while the ambulance was summoned. Spontaneous respirations and heart rate returned, but in the ambulance the patient began to have generalized convulsions. The most likely etiology for these convulsions is

(A) anoxia due to laryngospasm
(B) brain ischemia due to dilutional anemia
(C) hyponatremia due to dilution
(D) hyperkalemia due to hemolysis
(E) cold stress

573. In a child who is not anemic, the most sensitive indicator of a lead burden that requires therapy is

(A) the blood lead level
(B) the blood free erythrocyte protoporphyrin level
(C) urine uroporphyrin level
(D) abdominal x-ray
(E) knee x-ray

574. An eight-year-old girl is seen because of a malodorous bloody, vaginal discharge. The most likely cause is

(A) *Neisseria gonorrhoeae*
(B) *Trichomonas vaginalis*
(C) *Candida albicans*
(D) β-hemolytic streptococci
(E) a foreign body

575. The immature, shy 15-year-old boy shown in the figure below is brought to a pediatric clinic because his parents are concerned about his slow sexual development. Physical examination reveals a Tanner stage II boy with prominent breast development and very long arms and legs. All of the following statements about this adolescent are true EXCEPT that

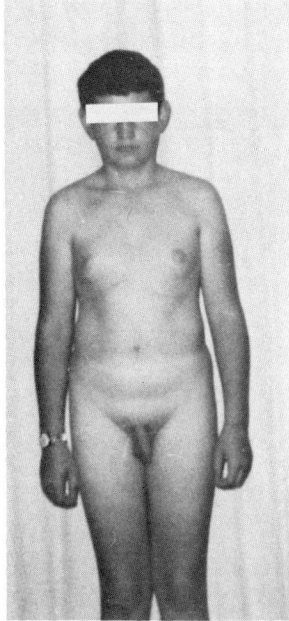

(A) he has an increased potential for diabetes mellitus
(B) testicular biopsy would probably show seminiferous tubular dysgenesis
(C) he is mentally retarded
(D) his condition is due to a maternal chromosome error
(E) he is very likely to have a behavior disorder

576. All of the following statements concerning the Treacher Collins syndrome are correct EXCEPT that

(A) mental retardation is a rare finding
(B) conductive hearing loss is present in approximately 50 percent of patients
(C) pubescence is usually delayed
(D) it is characterized by molar hypoplasia, antimongoloid palpebral fissures, and malformation of the external ears
(E) affected females are more likely to have affected offspring than are affected males

577. The "rule of nines" estimation for determination of body surface area in the initial management of burns is LEAST accurate if

(A) the burn is less than full thickness
(B) the burn is limited to a single extremity
(C) the burn involves the head and neck
(D) the patient is under one year of age
(E) the patient is older than 14 years of age

578. All the following statements concerning Cornelia de Lange's syndrome are correct EXCEPT that

(A) significant short stature is common
(B) hyperkinesis is frequent
(C) affected infants demonstrate a weak, low-pitched growl
(D) virtually all affected individuals have a small nose with anteverted nostrils
(E) the diagnosis is made strictly on clinical grounds

579. Hydroceles are commonly seen in infants and also are found occasionally in children and adolescents. Which of the following statements about hydroceles is correct?

(A) They are easily confused with hematomas
(B) They can be reduced easily
(C) They change size with crying
(D) They transilluminate easily
(E) They usually require surgical treatment

580. Sudden infant death syndrome (SIDS) has been shown to be more common among all of the following infants EXCEPT

(A) low-birth-weight infants
(B) infants with a family history of SIDS
(C) infant boys
(D) infants less than one month of age
(E) infants of low socioeconomic level

581. A 20-month-old child is found sitting in the family garage drinking from an 8-ounce soft drink bottle half-full of paint thinner. Upon arrival in the emergency room 15 minutes later, the child is alert and in no distress. The most common complication following this kind of ingestion is

(A) pneumonitis
(B) esophageal stricture
(C) renal failure
(D) encephalopathy
(E) myocardiopathy

582. All of the following statements about chronic illness in childhood and adolescence are true EXCEPT that

(A) children with visible disabilities usually receive earlier attention and intervention than children with hidden disabilities .

(B) compliance in following medical instructions usually increases in early and middle adolescence

(C) parental anger directed toward the physician often is the result of guilt

(D) healthy siblings sometimes wish that their chronically ill brothers or sisters would die

(E) feelings about being different from peers often result in low self-esteem

583. A two-year-old child presents in the emergency department with anemia, fever, and abdominal pain. Further examination reveals increased intracranial pressure. The blood workup shows basophilic stippling of the red blood cells and the presence of δ-aminolevulinic acid dehydratase in the erythrocytes. The most probable diagnosis is

(A) gastrointestinal infection
(B) chronic lead intoxication
(C) acute lead intoxication
(D) encephalopathy of unknown origin
(E) meningitis

584. A 14-month-old boy develops a persistent fever for one week accompanied by bilateral congestion of the ocular conjunctivae, reddening of the lips and oral cavity, and protuberance of the tongue papillae. His cervical lymph nodes are swollen. On the third day of illness he develops a reddening of the palms and soles, which remain swollen on day five. During the second week of illness his hands appear as shown in the picture below. All the following statements about this condition are true EXCEPT that

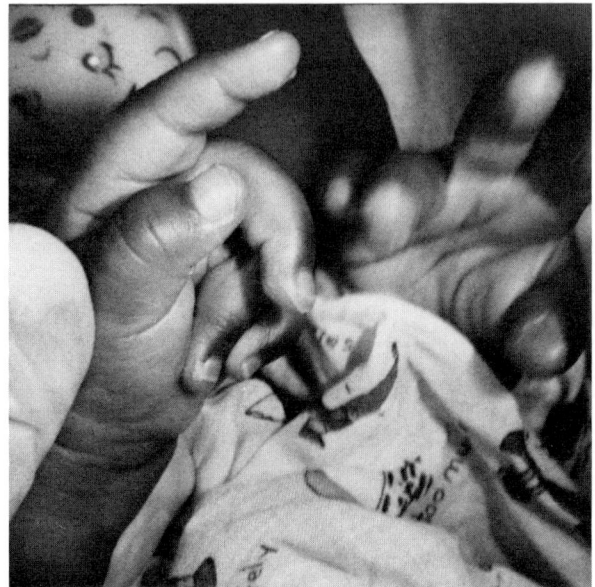

(A) it is often accompanied by arthritis and diarrhea
(B) myocarditis is a frequent symptom
(C) it is associated with aneurysms in the arteries
(D) it is associated with a positive antistreptolysin titer
(E) an increased erythrocyte sedimentation rate is characteristic

DIRECTIONS: Each question below contains four suggested answers of which **one** or **more** is correct. Choose the answer

A	if	**1, 2, and 3**	are correct
B	if	**1 and 3**	are correct
C	if	**2 and 4**	are correct
D	if	**4**	is correct
E	if	**1, 2, 3, and 4**	are correct

585. Petechiae of less than 3 mm in diameter are indicative of which of the following conditions?

(1) Liver disease
(2) Vasculopathy
(3) Coagulopathy
(4) A platelet disorder

586. A four-year-old boy has bilateral cryptorchidism. Although there are controversial aspects in the management of this problem, advice about treatment and therapy and its timing are based on the knowledge that, with cryptorchidism

(1) there is an increased risk of neoplasia
(2) infertility may result if untreated
(3) there may be psychological sequelae if untreated
(4) the best age for treatment from a developmental standpoint is four years

587. A 17-year-old boy with very thick glasses presents for a routine health maintenance visit. Physical examination reveals a height of 200.6 cm (6 ft, 7 in) and a weight of 74.9 kg (165 lb). A grade II/VI blowing, early-diastolic murmur is noted in the second right intercostal space. This young man probably

(1) is mentally retarded
(2) will not have further ophthalmologic complications
(3) is not expected to live past age 30
(4) has a lesion in the ascending aorta

588. The decision to hospitalize patients with burns must be made according to the individual case. There are certain conditions concerning burns, however, which make admission imperative. Which of the following clinical situations describe any of these conditions?

(1) A 13-month-old girl who was teething on an electrical cord and received a 1 cm third-degree burn at each of the angles of the mouth
(2) A 4-year-old boy who was playing with matches in a closet caused an explosion and fire but received no visible injuries other than singed eyebrows and a soot-covered face
(3) A 10-year-old boy who opened a steam valve received second-degree burns on the palms of both hands
(4) A 6-year-old girl who stayed too long at a swimming pool and received a first-degree sunburn over 40 percent of her body and a second-degree sunburn over 15 percent of her body

589. An adolescent boy with testicular pain that is relieved by elevating the scrotum could have

(1) epididymitis
(2) torsion of the testes
(3) orchitis
(4) torsion of the appendix testis

590. Correct statements about the cri du chat syndrome include which of the following?

(1) It results from a partial autosomal deletion
(2) It always is associated with mental retardation
(3) Patients usually have low-set ears
(4) Scoliosis is a frequent problem

591. The 14-year-old girl shown below is brought to the physician by her parents because of their concern that she shows no sign of pubescence. Although a history reveals a bilateral hearing deficit, she has done well in school. Physical examination reveals a 139.7 cm (4 ft, 7 in) white female with a low posterior hairline, a precordial systolic murmur, and diminished femoral pulse. True statements concerning this patient include which of the following?

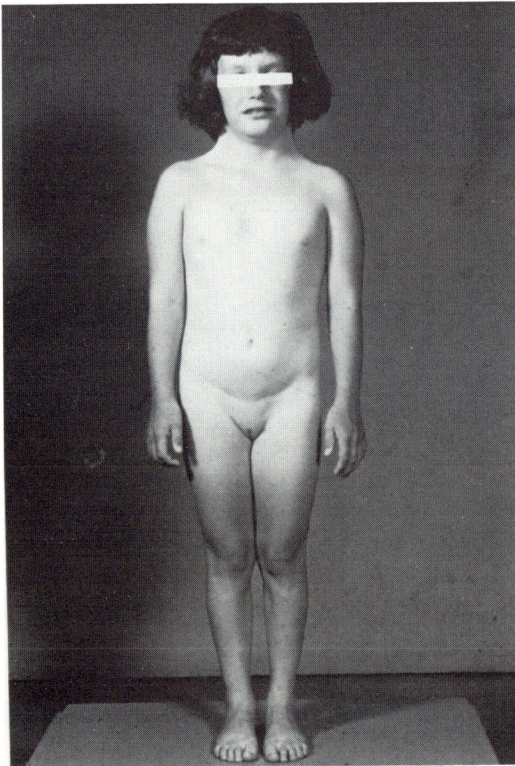

Used with permission of Gilbert B. Forbes, M.D., University of Rochester Medical Center.

(1) A renal anomaly may be present but probably will require no treatment
(2) Diagnosis of the condition could have been made at birth
(3) Barr bodies may be present on buccal smear
(4) There is no chance of her being fertile

592. Animals capable of producing and delivering venoms potent enough to cause venomous disease include

(1) sea anemones
(2) black widow spiders
(3) diamondback rattlesnakes
(4) Gila monsters

593. Correct statements concerning the Robin anomalad include which of the following?

(1) All the components are believed to be the result of a primary anomaly—early mandibular hypoplasia
(2) Aside from mental retardation of variable degree, anomalad patients do well once they pass the newborn period
(3) The anomalad may be seen in the trisomy 18 syndrome
(4) The etiology is believed to be an inherited translocation

594. A five-year-old girl is brought to the emergency room because, according to her parents, she seemed a little "funny" at dinner, had little appetite, and progressed rapidly from lethargy to coma. She had spent the afternoon "spraying for bugs" with her 17-year-old brother who reports that she was with him when he mixed the spray (spilling a little on her slacks and sneakers); however, he was sure that she had not ingested any of the insecticide. Physical examination reveals a regular pulse of 52/min, a blood pressure of 100/60, respiratory rate of 40/min, and a temperature of 38.2°C (100.7°F). She exhibits profuse sweating and salivation, and her pupils are miotic. She is responsive only to deep pain. Considering the initial history and physical examination, reasonable differential diagnostic possibilities include

(1) envenomation from a black widow spider
(2) overdose with tricyclic antidepressants
(3) conversion reaction because of incestuous relationship with brother
(4) organophosphate poisoning

595. A 12-year-old girl presents with malaise, cervical lymphadenopathy, headache, myalgia, and anorexia. Physical examination reveals a temperature of 39.2°C (102.5°F), an erythematous pharynx, and mild hepatosplenomegaly. Her family and friends have only had mild colds recently. Her blood count revealed: hemoglobin, 11.5 g; white blood count, 12,000 with 20% segmented forms, 48% lymphocytes, 15% atypical lymphocytes, 11% monocytes, and 6% basophils; a platelet count was 90,000. This syndrome may be caused by

(1) cytomegalovirus
(2) *Toxoplasma gondii*
(3) Epstein-Barr virus
(4) echovirus

596. An increased association of HLA-B27 has been found with which of the following diseases?

✓ (1) Acute anterior uveitis
✓ (2) Ankylosing spondylitis
✓ (3) Reiter's syndrome
   (4) Still's disease

DIRECTIONS: The groups of questions below consist of lettered choices followed by several numbered items. For each numbered item select the **one** lettered choice with which it is **most** closely associated. Each lettered choice may be used once, more than once, or not at all.

Questions 597-599

For each of the terms below used in defining the frequency of occurrence of a disease, select the definition with which it is most closely associated.

(A) $\dfrac{\text{Number of people who develop the disease}}{\text{Population at risk (in a given period)}}$

(B) $\dfrac{\text{Number of people with the disease}}{\text{Population at risk (in a given period)}}$

(C) $\dfrac{\text{Number of people with the disease}}{\text{Population at risk (at a given point in time)}}$

(D) $\dfrac{\text{Number of people with the disease}}{\text{Total population (at a given point in time)}}$

(E) None of the above

597. Incidence rate

598. Period prevalence rate

599. Point prevalence rate

Questions 600-603

For each characteristic below, select the drug which is most closely associated with it:

(A) Marihuana
(B) Hallucinogens
(C) Barbiturates
(D) Opiates
(E) Phencyclidine

600. 40 percent of abusers have abnormal liver function tests

601. Abrupt withdrawal often leads to grand mal seizures

602. Common cause of teenage traffic accidents

603. Diazepam or haloperidol used for complications

Questions 604-608

For each statement listed below, select the age distribution with which it is most likely to be associated.

(A) Four to six months of age
(B) Eight to ten months of age
(C) Two to four years of age
(D) Eight to ten years of age
(E) None of the above ages

604. Tetracycline given prior to this age is liable to cause cosmetically important staining of permanent teeth

605. A deaf child makes the same sounds as a normal child until this age

606. Iron deficiency anemia prior to this age is least likely to be due to inadequate dietary iron

607. After this age, patching of the better eye in a child with strabismus is not likely to improve the visual acuity in the amblyopic eye

608. Slipped femoral capital epiphysis is most likely to occur at this age

Questions 609-612

For each of the toxic substances listed below, select the antidote that would be most appropriate.

(A) Dimercaprol (BAL—British anti-Lewisite)
(B) Atropine
(C) Naloxone hydrochloride (Narcan)
(D) Methylene blue
(E) Deferoxamine mesylate (Desferal)

609. Organophosphates

610. Propoxyphene

611. Iron

612. Arsenic

Questions 613-615

For each of the clinical presentations listed below, select the drug that is most likely to be associated with it.

(A) Amphetamine abuse
(B) Phenothiazine abuse
(C) LSD abuse
(D) Barbiturate abuse
(E) Cocaine abuse

613. Vivid hallucinations, combative behavior, hyperthermia, and cardiac arrhythmias; seizures and death from respiratory failure can result from excessive doses

614. Hyperactivity, choreiform movement, hypertension, tachycardia, and tachypnea; intracerebral hemorrhage noted with intravenous use

615. Normal or wide pulse pressure with postural hypotension; respiratory depression not noted; extrapyramidal reactions are common

Miscellaneous Conditions and Diseases

Answers

568. The answer is B. *(Hoekelman, pp 1791-1812.)* Among children under six years of age, aspiration is the leading cause of accidental death in the home. Approximately 2900 deaths from suffocation due to ingested foreign objects occurred in 1974. Predisposing factors to the ingestion of foreign bodies include improper chewing of food and laughing or running with a foreign object in the mouth. Peanuts are frequently aspirated and should not be given to children until they are at least four years of age, at which point the chewing habit is well established. Certain clinical conditions, including head trauma, seizures, familial dysautonomia, and cerebral palsy also predispose the child to aspiration. Although poisonings are common among children, they are infrequently fatal. Of the more than 96,000 poisonings in children under five years of age reported to the National Clearinghouse for Poison Control Centers in 1974, only 135 were fatal. Home accidental deaths, secondary to burns and electrical accidents, are also significant considerations in this age group, although they rank behind aspiration in the number of fatalities. Firearm accidents are more significant as causes of accidental death in the older child and adolescent.

569. The answer is C. *(Hoekelman, pp 943, 1688. Rudolph, ed 16. pp 1899, 1902-1903. Vaughan, ed 11. pp 1845-1846.)* Hurler's syndrome is an autosomal recessive mucopolysaccharidosis (MPS Type I-H) caused by deficiency of α_1-iduronidase and accumulation of heparin and dermatan sulfates. Hydrocephalus associated with visual and auditory impairment characterizes the shortened life-span; death is common in the early adolescent years, usually as a result of infiltration of the heart valves and coronary arteries with the implicated mucopolysaccharides. Patients have thick lips that are widely separated, an enlarged tongue, widely separated, peg-like teeth, and hypertrophic gums. They also exhibit retarded growth and an enlarged skull.

570. The answer is E. *(Hoekelman, pp 1858-1860.)* As in adults, the most frequently involved organ in sarcoidosis is the lungs, which are involved in 72 percent of cases of childhood sarcoid. Althought the eyes are involved in only 43 percent of cases, they are a greater source of morbidity because of the frequent occurrence of anterior granulomatous uveitis, retinal periphlebitis, and retinal hemorrhage, all of which can lead to blindness. Because of the potential consequences of this condition, all diagnosed cases of pediatric sarcoidosis should be referred to an ophthalmologist. While other organ systems can be involved, the morbidity that results is usually less important than that seen in the ocular manifestations of childhood sarcoid.

571. The answer is E. *(Hoekelman, pp 155-157, 877-879. Mann, N Engl J Med 291:226-232, 1974.)* Obesity is a disorder of appetite, a learned physiologic pattern for coping with emotional, rather than nutritional, needs. A number of factors appear to be related to the development of obesity, including familial tendency, food abundance, sedentary life styles, and lower social class. Of particular interest is the finding that obesity is less common among breast-fed infants than among formula-fed infants. Endocrine abnormalities associated with obesity usually are secondary rather than causative factors. Salt and sugar cravings, for example, are learned rather than physiologic responses. Because frustration, compulsion, and anxiety also appear to be related to obesity, treatment must include psychological support as well as decreased food intake and increased activity. For those individuals for whom the emotional crutch of eating is paramount, treatment may be unsuccessful even with intensive psychotherapy.

572. The answer is A. *(Hoekelman, pp 1802-1804. Peterson, Pediatrics 59:364-370, 1977.)* Historically, electrolyte disturbances, such as hyperkalemia or hyponatremia, and dilutional complications, such as anemia, were thought to be important causes of morbidity in freshwater near drownings. It is clear that lack of oxygenation due to either laryngospasm or pulmonary edema is the prime pathophysiologic disturbance and needs to be treated aggressively. Loss of surfactant can also be a significant factor. This is especially true for submersions in cold water, since this factor seems to be protective insofar as the pulse is slowed, but often not stopped, and blood is shunted to the brain in cold water. Indeed, controlled hypothermia has been used with remarkable success in conjunction with barbiturate coma and in the management of anoxia following submersion.

573. The answer is B. *(Hoekelman, pp 192-193, 1833.)* Free erythrocyte protoporphyrin (FEP) level is the most sensitive indicator of a significant lead burden. An abnormally high FEP level in the face of only minimal elevation of the lead level usually indicates active lead exposure. Subsequent lead levels are likely to be higher. The FEP level may also be elevated in iron-deficiency anemia and in the rare genetic disorder erythropoietic protoporphyria. The level of urinary excretion of uroporphyrin is normal in children with plumbism; however, the excretion of coproporphyrin is elevated. Radiopaque material may be seen on the abdominal x-ray, suggesting recent ingestion of lead-containing material, and knee x-rays may reveal "lead lines" in the metaphyseal regions. However, the absence of either or both of these radiographic findings does not exclude the possibility of lead poisoning.

574. The answer is E. *(Hoekelman, pp 656, 1321-1323.)* In a prepubescent girl, a discharge which is both malodorous and bloody suggests the presence of a foreign body. Foreign bodies are among the more common causes of vaginal bleeding in children. Small children often insert objects into the vagina as readily as they insert them into the mouth, ear, or nose. Gonorrhea in a prepubertal girl is characterized by a profuse creamy-yellowish discharge, free of blood, and not particularly malodorous. The discharge with *Trichomonas* infections is frothy, green and foul-smelling, but not bloody. *Candida albicans* vaginitis produces a striking mucosal erythema and pruritus, and β-hemolytic streptococci cause a purulent, nonbloody discharge.

575. The answer is C. *(Hoekelman, p 355. Smith, 1976. pp 38-39.)* Gynecomastia in a relatively long-limbed adolescent boy with delayed sexual development suggests Klinefelter's syndrome. The genotype is most often XXY, and seminiferous tubular dysgenesis is the pathologic *sine qua non*. Only 15 to 20 percent demonstrate an IQ less than 80. Two-thirds of these patients inherit a maternal chromosome error, and approximately eight percent develop diabetes mellitus. Behavior problems, insecurity, and poor judgment frequently are present. Androgen replacement therapy enhances the possibility of normal adolescent development, and helps to prevent obesity in later life.

576. The answer is C. *(Hoekelman, p 356. Smith, 1976. pp 134-135.)* Treacher Collins syndrome presents clinically with molar hypoplasia, antimongoloid palpebral fissures, malformation of the pinna, colobomas, and other physical abnormalities of the head, the neck, and occasionally the extremities. Mental retardation is seen in less than five percent of cases. Conductive hearing loss with its developmental ramifications is present in approximately 50 percent of the affected individuals. Pubescence is unaffected. Although the etiology is unclear, an autosomal dominant pattern of inheritance is believed to be active in some families, although 60 percent of new cases may be due to mutations. Nongenetic (nonchromosomal) factors are involved in some cases as affected women transmit the syndrome to an excessive number of offspring, while affected males have few affected offspring.

577. The answer is D. *(Schuberth, ed 8. p 206.)* The "rule of nines" estimation for determination of body surface area for burn management is a good first approximation for the body surface area involved in patients older than 14 years of age. Using this rule, both of the upper extremities and the head are estimated to contain nine percent of the body surface area apiece; both the anterior and posterior surfaces of each of the lower extremities are also estimated to represent nine percent of the total body surface area. The anterior and posterior trunk are estimated to each represent 18 percent of the total body surface area. The genitalia make up one percent. This rule, however, is highly inaccurate in younger patients, where the head represents a relatively greater, and the lower extremities a relatively smaller, proportion of the total body surface area. The thickness of burns is not addressed by the rule of nines estimation.

578. The answer is B. *(Hoekelman, p 356. Smith, 1976. pp 56-57.)* Cornelia de Lange's syndrome is characterized by neonatal short stature which does not resolve, small noses with anteverted nostrils, and a weak, low-pitched growl. A clinical diagnosis is necessary, as no definite chromosomal abnormality or other etiologic explanation has been demonstrated. A wide spectrum of severity has been documented. Uniform mental retardation and physical sluggishness are noted. These infants do not exhibit hyperkinesis.

579. The answer is D. *(Hoekelman, p 1306.)* A hydrocele is an accumulation of fluid in a sac formed by the tunica vaginalis testis or the processus vaginalis of the spermatic cord. Hydroceles are painless masses and are not reducible. They occur most often in newborn males. They do not change size with crying, and they transilluminate readily. A scrotal hydrocele must be differentiated from a hematoma and an inguinal hernia, but this differentiation is not difficult since neither of these latter transilluminates. Hydroceles usually require no treatment and disappear over time.

580. The answer is D. *(Hoekelman, p 1850.)* Although sudden infant death syndrome accounts for approximately one-third and one-half of the infant mortality that occurs between one week and one year of age, it is relatively infrequent in the first few weeks of life, and unusual after six months of age. The highest incidence is between the fourth and sixteenth weeks of life and is inversely related to birth weight. Other factors associated with a higher incidence are: (1) being male; (2) having a low socioeconomic background; and (3) having a predisposing mild illness such as nasopharyngitis. The risk of occurrence in subsequent siblings is between 11 and 22 per 1000 siblings, in contrast to 2-3 per 1000 in the general population.

581. The answer is A. *(Hoekelman, pp 1830-1831. Vaughan, ed 11. pp 2018-2019.)* By far the most common and most rapidly occurring complication of petroleum distillate ingestion is pneumonitis. X-ray changes can appear within 30 minutes to 12 hours of the ingestion. Since the likelihood of aspiration into the tracheobronchial tree may be increased with induced emesis or gastric lavage, these treatments usually are reserved for individuals who have ingested amounts in excess of 30 ml. Steroid therapy has not been positively demonstrated to be advantageous in preventing the pneumonitis or altering its course. Antibiotic therapy usually is instituted only after signs of secondary bacterial infection have appeared. Renal toxicity, central nervous system depression, and myocardiopathy also can result from hydrocarbon ingestion but are much less frequent than pneumonitis. Esophageal stricture is a common complication following the ingestion of a strong alkali.

582. The answer is B. *(Hoekelman, pp 227-230, 641-642.)* The relationship between chronic illness and psychological health is not understood clearly. However, having a chronic illness puts some children at greater risk than their healthy peers for having an emotional problem diagnosed. Because chronically ill children are often in close contact with the health care system, there is a good chance that aggressive or hostile behavior will be discussed with a health professional, even if the "symptoms" would be considered entirely normal under other circumstances. On the other hand, the typical appearance of disregard for authority, which occurs during early to middle adolescence, can have some deleterious, if not life-endangering, consequences when it interferes with necessary treatment regimens such as daily insulin injections for the diabetic. In the young adolescent who is too immature cognitively to appreciate the consequences of his actions, it is even more difficult to distinguish between psychological health and illness. In addition, the chronically ill adolescent's wish for identification with his or her peer group is threatened by feelings of being different from friends, a feeling that may lead to low self-esteem. Children with visible disabilities usually receive earlier attention and intervention than do children with hidden disabilities. However, they are also more likely to be the objects of ridicule or unsympathetic animosity from casual acquaintances. Chronic illness is a family affair. Parental guilt may manifest itself as anger toward the impotence of the medical professional, especially the physician. Sibling rivalry may surface as death wishes toward the chronically ill brother or sister. Although such wishes are common among all siblings, they can have significant negative long-term psychological effects if the ill child does indeed die. Parental guilt may also be expressed as hostility toward the ill child or a spouse.

583. The answer is C. *(Hoekelman, pp 936-937.)* Acute lead intoxication occurs most commonly in children between the ages of one and three. Abdominal pain and fever generally are not present in chronic intoxication, but are symptoms of acute intoxication in this age group. Anemia is also a symptom of acute lead intoxication. Examination of the child may reveal a clinical picture similar to meningitis, but examination of the cerebrospinal fluid of the acutely lead-intoxicated child will reveal basophilic stippling of the red blood cells. Other encephalopathic conditions are unlikely with this pattern in the blood. A gastrointestinal infection unrelated to lead intoxication also is unlikely with these central nervous system findings.

584. The answer is D. *(Hoekelman, p 1122. Kawasaki, Pediatrics 54:271-276, 1974.)* The mucocutaneous lymph node syndrome (Kawasaki disease) is characterized by persistent fever unresponsive to routine treatment, conjunctivitis, redness of the lips and mouth, protuberance of the tongue papillae ("strawberry tongue"), redness of the palms and soles, and nonpurulent swelling of the cervical lymph nodes. During the convalescent stage, desquamation of the skin on the tips of the fingers and toes occurs, beginning at the junction of the nails. Carditis and coronary thromboarteritis with aneurysmal dilatation may precipitate myocardial infarction. Arthritis and diarrhea are not uncommon and the erythrocyte sedimentation rate is usually elevated. The antistreptolysin titer is not elevated, as it is in scarlet fever which, because of the desquamation of the hands and feet, is often considered in the differential diagnosis. Scarlet fever, however, is not characterized by reddening of the eyes, lips, or peripheral extremities.

585. The answer is C (2, 4). *(McMillan, vol 2. pp 211-212.)* Purpura and petechiae may be caused by many conditions. Petechiae do not always occur in association with purpura; for example, they are rare in purpura fulminans. However, if they occur and are less than 3 mm in diameter, the etiology is most likely a platelet disorder or vasculopathy. Liver disease or some other cause of dysfunction of the coagulation mechanism rarely causes petechiae. Vasculitic petechiae often are palpable, while thrombocytopenic petechiae are not.

586. The answer is A (1, 2, 3). *(Hoekelman, pp 1304-1305. Gardner, ed 2. pp 649-651.)* The increased risk of neoplasia in abdominal testes and the possibility of infertility are reasons for attempting to correct cryptorchidism, as is the possibility of emotional problems in adolescence relating to absent scrotal testes. Choices of types of treatment include a course of human chorionic gonadotropin (HCG) and orchiopexy. Some therapists recommend a trial of HCG followed by orchiopexy if the testes do not descend. Although most surgeons seem to favor treatment prior to school age, psychiatrists and other developmentalists cannot agree upon a developmental age that is optimal for surgery. Long-term HCG therapy does not increase the potential for success over short-term therapy; however, it does increase the risk for side effects, including testicular atrophy and precocious puberty.

587. The answer is D (4). *(Hoekelman, p 347. Smith, 1976. pp 276-277.)* An extremely tall, thin adolescent with severe myopia and a murmur suggestive of aortic regurgitation should make an astute clinician suspect Marfan's syndrome. This autosomal dominant syndrome never results in mental retardation. Ophthalmologic problems can be severe. Myopia, ectopia lentis, retinal detachment, and glaucoma are common. Skeletal abnormalities also occur. Death frequently is related to dissecting aneurysm of the ascending aorta, and secondary aortic regurgitation that may occur at any age. Scoliosis is a common problem in these adolescents.

588. The answer is A (1, 2, 3). *(Touloukian, pp 597-608.)* Electrical burns of the mouth are managed best in the hospital because they are characteristically quite deep. When the eschar falls off after seven to ten days, arterial bleeding from the underlying tissues is common. Burns of the hands, unless mild, also are best managed in the hospital to ensure maximal return of function. Steam is especially serious in the case described, because it can be much hotter than boiling water. The four-year-old child may have received no visible injuries, but the soot-covered face and singed eyebrows are indications of smoke inhalation. Serious airway obstruction due to edema can develop after such an incident; bacterial pneumonia is also a common complication. Although the six-year-old child received the most extensive burn, its nature is such that few complications would develop, and it probably could be managed on an outpatient basis.

589. The answer is B (1, 3). *(Hoekelman, pp 1305-1306.)* Testicular pain due to orchitis or epididymitis is relieved by gently elevating the scrotum. Pain caused by torsion of the testis or torsion of the appendix testis is not reduced by this maneuver. If there is no pain relief after the scrotum is raised, consultation with a urologist should be sought as soon as possible. Torsion of the testis involves venous occlusion, and if the degree of this occlusion is great, hemorrhagic necrosis of the testis can occur within 24 hours of the onset of symptoms. Pain associated with torsion of the appendix testis comes on more gradually than is the case with torsion of the testis. This condition almost always resolves spontaneously. There is, however, general agreement that if there is any doubt about the cause of testicular pain, the case should be referred to a urologist or surgeon.

590. The answer is E (all). *(Hoekelman, p 354. Smith, 1976. pp 24-25.)* The cri du chat syndrome is caused by a partial deletion of the short arm of chromosome five. The syndrome is characterized by the high-pitched cry of a hypoplastic larynx, low-set ears, scoliosis, and mental retardation. Cri du chat is French for "cat cry," an allusion to the "mew-like" crying sound made by affected infants. Hypotonia, failure to thrive, and congenital heart disease are also frequent symptoms. Cri du chat infants have microcephaly, a round face, hypertelorism, antimongoloid slant of the palpebral fissures, strabismus, and epicanthal folds.

591. The answer is A (1, 2, 3). *(Hoekelman, pp 354-355. Smith, 1976. pp 46-49.)* The clinical presentation is that of Turner's syndrome, genotype XO, a diagnosis that must be considered in early adolescent girls who fail to mature. These patients demonstrate extreme short stature, rarely reaching over 152 cm (5 ft). Other features of Turner's syndrome include a low posterior hairline and congenital heart disease, usually coarctation of the aorta. Note the wide spacial nipples on the shield-like chest of this patient. Not demonstrated in the picture is the increased carrying angle of the arms. Over 50 percent of affected individuals have significant impairment of hearing. The most frequent renal anomaly is a horseshoe kidney, which needs no treatment. Pubescence with menarche is rare without exogenous cyclic hormonal augmentation. Ovarian dysgenesis results in infertility in the vast majority of females with Turner's syndrome, but exceptions exist. Although XO genotypes give a negative buccal smear, Barr bodies may be demonstrated in cells from individuals with mosaicism or defective X chromosomes. An alert pediatrician can also diagnose Turner's syndrome in newborns or infants if they present with: (1) loose, sometimes webbed, skin folds over the nape of the neck, (2) edema of the dorsum of the hands and feet, (3) short stature, (4) low weight, and (5) prominent ears. The diagnosis can be confirmed with chromosome studies.

592. The answer is E (all). *(Hoekelman, pp 1834-1836. Vaughan, ed 11. pp 992-993, 2032-2034.)* The black widow spider, identifiable by its red ventral spots and variable red dorsal spots, is one of the few spiders that produces a venom potent enough to endanger human beings. Double fang marks found at the inoculation site help to make the proper diagnosis. Treatment consists of intramuscular antivenin, pain control, and muscle relaxants. The sea anemone, a venomous coelenterate, inflicts its sting through its tentacles. The severity of symptoms is proportional to the length of time the tentacles are in contact with the skin; thus, they should be removed promptly. Treatment consists of warm saline soaks, antihistamines, and corticosteroids. Rattlesnakes, water moccasins, and coral snakes account for about 7000 bites, but less than 20 fatalities annually, in the United States. Species-specific antivenin should be administered. Local care consists of incision, suction, and retardation of absorption of venom with the use of tourniquets. Supportive measures such as blood transfusions and intravenous infusions are helpful. The only lizard poisonous to man is the Gila monster. Local care and supportive measures as described for snakebites should be provided. No antivenin is available.

593. The answer is B (1, 3). *(Hoekelman, p 356. Smith, 1976. pp 130-131. Vaughan, ed 11. pp 1019-1020.)* The Robin anomalad is characterized by (1) micrognathia, (2) glossoptosis, and (3) cleft soft palate. The anomalad is believed to be the result of mandibular hypoplasia in the first trimester of pregnancy. Mandibular hypoplasia may be a single finding or it may be a component of a syndrome such as trisomy 18. However, no genetic basis for the Robin anomalad has been elucidated. A problem of many newborn infants with this syndrome is respiratory compromise, which may be so severe as to require a temporary tracheostomy. Children who survive the early complications can be aided by palatal correction. After the surgery, the mandible usually grows to normal proportions. Most Robin anomalad victims have normal intelligence.

594. The answer is D (4). *(Hoekelman, pp 1831-1832.)* The patient presents classic signs of overactivity of the parasympathetic nervous system, in this case due to organophosphate poisoning and its resultant inhibition of acetylcholinesterase. Tricyclic antidepressants produce the opposite effect — that is, an atropine-like effect with tachycardia, dry mouth, decreased sweating, and mydriasis. A black widow spiderbite also is associated with tachycardia but not with the other signs listed above. There usually is intense pain at the site of envenomation and also spasms of voluntary and involuntary muscles. Conversion reaction might be entertained as a diagnosis, but **only** in the absence of coma. To cause symptoms, the organophosphate in the insecticide need not be ingested, since there is rapid cutaneous absorption. Hence, the clothing should be removed and the patient bathed as soon as she is stable. Definitive treatment consists of atropine, 0.1-0.2 mg/kg intravenously, repeated at five- to ten-minute intervals until atropinization is attained. More severe cases may require pralidoxime chloride (Protopam chloride) 25-50 mg/kg given slowly and intravenously as needed to reverse the symptoms and signs of intoxication.

595. The answer is A (1, 2, 3). *(Hoekelman, pp 1168, 1177, 1238.)* A mononucleosis syndrome may be caused by Epstein-Barr virus (EBV), cytomegalovirus (CMV), or *Toxoplasma*. The mononucleosis syndrome caused by cytomegalovirus is heterophile antibody negative. This syndrome sometimes occurs spontaneously, or it could be associated with prior fresh-blood perfusion carried out in conjuction with surgery. Echovirus infections are not associated with lymphadenopathy, hepatosplenomegaly, and atypical lymphocytes. EBV infections are usually heterophile positive in older children; CMV and *Toxoplasma* infections can be diagnosed by specific serological tests.

596. The answer is A (1, 2, 3). *(Hoekelman, p 1112. Schaller, J Pediatr 88:913-925, 1976.)* The HLA locus B27 is associated with ankylosing spondylitis, acute anterior uveitis, spondylitis associated with inflammatory bowel disease, Reiter's syndrome, and "reactive" arthritis that sometimes follows diseases caused by *Yersinia, Salmonella,* and *Shigella* organisms. Still's disease, which is not associated with B27, refers to the systemic type of juvenile rheumatoid arthritis (JRA) characterized by fever, toxicity, lymphadenopathy, splenohepatomegaly, and pericarditis. B27 is found on the 6th chromosome, within the HLA loci. It is present in greater than 90 percent of patients with ankylosing spondylitis compared with only seven to eight percent of the general population. Ankylosing spondylitis usually occurs in males between the ages of 15 and 30. The disease may begin in childhood with peripheral arthritis resembling JRA. Those children with JRA in whom spondylitis subsequently develops are usually boys in late childhood with a pauciarticular or lower limb arthropathy and negative rheumatoid factor assays.

597-599. The answers are: 597-A, 598-E, 599-D. *(Mausner, pp 127-128.)* Incidence and prevalence rates have been defined as follows: the incidence rate is the number of people who develop the disease (divided by the population at risk) in a given period. In the case of measles, only individuals who have neither been immunized nor had the disease would be included. Prevalence rates define the number of people who currently have a disease. The point prevalence rate is the number of people with the disease (divided by the total population) at a given time. The period prevalence rate is the number of people with the disease (divided by the total population) in a given period. This definition is not included in the question; therefore, "none of the above" is the answer. The point prevalence rate is used more commonly. Prevalence rates are particularly helpful for planning health services related to chronic illnesses, as they take into account the number of people with a disease rather than just the new cases. Incidence rates are of greater value for predicting risk of acute illnesses (i.e., those of short duration) among various groups and is therefore useful for predicting needed services.

600-603. The answers are: 600-D, 601-C, 602-A, 603-B. *(Hoekelman, pp 679-687. McGuigan, Pediatr Alert 3:67-68, 1978.)* Marihuana, along with alcohol, has become a common contributing factor in motor vehicle accidents in the adolescent and young adult population. This problem has been made worse by the increased potency of marihuana smoked by adolescents. Also of recent concern is the use of phencyclidine (PCP), termed "angel dust," a white crystalline powder that produces a variety of symptoms, including disorientation, excitability, slurred speech, a "staring" appearance, constricted pupils with horizontal nystagmus, increased deep tendon reflexes, and ataxic gait. Respiratory depression, cardiac arrhythmia, hypotension, and convulsions also have been reported with the use of angel dust. The abuse of opiates, such as heroin, frequently leads to hepatitis, often due to the use of contaminated needles. One of the most common causes of drug-related grand mal seizures in adolescents is the sudden withdrawal of phenobarbital from those abusing it or refusing to continue with therapeutic doses. Those with severe panic or psychotic reactions to LSD abuse may respond to the use of diazepam or haloperidol.

604-608. The answers are: 604-D, 605-B, 606-A, 607-D, 608-E. *(Hoekelman, pp 985, 1648, 1697, 1758, 1783.)* Because different organ systems develop differentially, environmental factors have effects that depend both on the age of the organism and the organ system involved. Thus, tetracycline can cause staining of those teeth in which enamel formation is still incomplete. Since enamel formation is complete (except for the third molars which are not visible in usual social interactions and are often removed) by age eight, tetracycline given after that age usually does not cause significant staining.

The normal vocalizing that occurs in the first eight months of life is not dependent upon hearing. If a patient less than that age is suspected of having a hearing impairment, formal audiology should be conducted regardless of the status of the vocalization.

The iron reserves in a full-term infant are usually adequate to prevent anemia in the first six months of life, even in the absence of significant amounts of dietary iron. Iron deficiency prior to six months is usually due to blood loss at or before birth (as from fetal blood loss into the maternal circulation, placenta previa, abruptio placentae, or twin-to-twin transfusions) or to inadequate iron stores at birth because of prematurity.

Occasional strabismus occurs in infants less than six months of age, but after that age, it should not be considered a normal variant. Because amblyopia ex anopsia is preventable, screening programs for strabismus in preschool children should be carried out by all people who give primary care. The earlier the diagnosis is made, the more likely the vision in the more severely affected eye can be restored to normal. After age eight the chance of restoring good vision is very small.

Because the skeletal system has its own sequence of growth and development, characteristic lesions may appear at specific ages. For example, most children who develop slipped femoral capital epiphysis are most likely to develop it between the ages of 11 and 16. Similarly, trauma, which to an adult would produce a ligamentous injury would, in a young adolescent, be more likely to produce a growth plate injury, since at that age ligaments are stronger than epiphyseal plates.

609-612. The answers are: 609-B, 610-C, 611-E, 612-A. *(Gellis, ed 9. pp 669-674.)* Methemoglobinuria, which can result from exposure to a variety of substances (including aniline dye, phenacetin, and sulfonamide), occurs when hemoglobin iron is oxidized from the ferrous to the ferric state, thus decreasing its oxygen-transport capacity. Methylene blue, which reverses this process usually is given as a one percent intravenous solution in a dose of 1 to 2 mg/kg over five to ten minutes, which may be repeated in three to four hours. Because of its toxic side effects, methylene blue is reserved for patients with methemoglobin levels above 30-40 percent or symptoms such as dyspnea, cyanosis, or an altered sensorium. Organophosphate poisoning is treated most effectively with a combination of atropine and pralidoxime (2-PAM). Naloxone hydrochloride (Narcan) is an effective antidote for propoxyphene, diphenoxylate (Lomotil), and most natural and synthetic narcotics. Deferoxamine mesylate (Desferal) is specific for iron intoxication. Dimercaprol (BAL) combines with arsenic and a variety of other metals, including bismuth, mercury, and lead.

613-615. The answers are: 613-E, 614-A, 615-B. *(Hoekelman, pp 679-686. Isselbacher, ed 9. p 987. Goodman, ed 5. pp 302-304.)* Although cocaine has been considered by many to be a safe way to experience euphoria, recent evidence indicates that this drug can cause high temperatures and even sudden death secondary to a cardiac arrhythmia. Death from respiratory failure can also result. The effects of cocaine and amphetamine abuse are often similar, but there is some question as to whether tolerance develops to cocaine; it does develop to amphetamines.

Hyperactivity, choreiform movements, tachypnea, tachycardia, and hypertension result from the use of amphetamines in ordinary doses, while excessive doses may also cause severe chest pain and unconsciousness. When administered intravenously, the effects of amphetamines may last for hours, as opposed to those of cocaine, which only last for minutes. Intracerebral hemorrhage and stroke have been noted with intravenous amphetamine use.

The phenothiazines are used therapeutically as tranquilizers, and some are used as antiemetics and antihistamines. Side effects are frequent and often serious; abuse of these drugs can bring on significant extrapyramidal side effects such as muscle spasms and dystonia, tremor, rigidity, and a shuffling gait. Phenothiazine usage is not usually associated with respiratory depression, nor are diazepam and chlordiazepoxide overdoses. Barbiturate abuse often results in an overdose with resultant dysarthria, ataxia, nystagmus, lethargy, and coma.

Lysergic acid diethylamide (LSD) is a hallucinogen that may induce fever, pupillary dilatation, increased deep tendon reflexes, and feelings so unpleasant that the individual is usually brought into the emergency facility in an acute panic reaction.

Appendix

Laboratory Values

Hematology

Table 1

Hematology

Age	Hemoglobin, g	% Hematocrit	WBC/mm³	% Polys	% Retics
1 day	16–22*	53–73*	18,000 (7000–35,000)	45–85	2.5–6.5
1 week	13–20*	43–66*	10,000 (4000–20,000)	30–50	0.1–4.5
1 month	16	53	10,000 (6000–18,000)	30–50	0.1–1.0
3 months	11.5	38	10,000 (6000–17,000)	30–50	0.7–3.0
6 months	12	40	10,000 (6000–16,000)	30–50	0.7–2.3
1 year	12	40	10,000 (6000–15,000)	30–50	0.6–1.7
2–6 years	13	43	9000 (7000–13,000)	35–55	0.5–1.0
7–12 years	14	46	8500 (5000–12,000)	40–60	0.5–1.0
			Absolute eosinophil count: 100–600/mm³; average, 250.		

* Under the age of 1 month, capillary hemoglobin and hematocrit exceed venous, the average difference being 3.6 g at 1 h, 2.2 g at 5 days, and 1.1 g at 3 weeks.

Table 2

Normal Blood Chemistry Values for Full-Term Infants

Determination	Cord	1–12 h	12–24 h	24–48 h	48–72 h
Sodium, meq/L*	147	143	145	148	149
(sample source: capillary)	(126–166)	(124–156)	(132–159)	(134–160)	(139–162)
Potassium, meq/L	7.8	6.4	6.3	6.0	5.9
	(5.6–12)	(5.3–7.3)	(5.3–8.9)	(5.2–7.3)	(5.0–7.7)
Chloride, meq/L	103	100.7	103	102	103
	(98–110)	(90–111)	(87–114)	(92–114)	(93–112)
Calcium, mg/100 mL	9.3	8.4	7.8	8.0	7.9
	(8.2–11.1)	(7.3–9.2)	(6.9–9.4)	(6.1–9.9)	(5.9–9.7)
Phosphorus, mg/100 mL	5.6	6.1	5.7	5.9	5.8
	(3.7–8.1)	(3.5–8.6)	(2.9–8.1)	(3.0–8.7)	(2.8–7.6)
Blood urea, mg/100 mL	29	27	33	32	31
	(21–40)	(8–34)	(9–63)	(13–77)	(13–68)
Total protein, g/100 mL	6.1	6.6	6.6	6.9	7.2
	(4.8–7.3)	(5.6–8.5)	(5.8–8.2)	(5.9–8.2)	(6.0–8.5)
Blood sugar, mg/100 mL	73	63	63	56	59
	(45–96)	(40–97)	(42–104)	(30–91)	(40–90)
Lactic acid, mg/100 mL	19.5	14.6	14.0	14.3	13.5
	(11–30)	(11–24)	(10–23)	(9–22)	(7–21)
Lactate, mm/L†	2.0–3.0	2.0			

* P. T. Acharya and W. W. Payne, *Arch. Dis. Child.,* **40**:430, 1965.

† S. S. Daniel, K. Adamsons, Jr., and L. S. James, *Pediatrics,* **37**:942, 1966.

Adapted from G. B. Avery: *Neonatology, Pathophysiology and Management in the Newborn,* Philadelphia: Lippincott, 1975, p. 1049, with permission.

CLINICAL CHEMISTRY

The normal values listed in Table 3 were primarily selected from the 1974 monograph *Normal Values for Pediatric Clinical Chemistry.*[1] This publication included several sets of normal values by different methods for each determination. Our purpose is to present guidelines for the interpretation of laboratory tests, not all-inclusive data. In keeping with the growing rise of the International System of Units (SI), Table 3 gives normal values in both standard and SI

units.[2] The multiplication factor necessary for conversion of standard to SI units is provided where applicable. In the SI system, grams per liter (g/L) designates measurement of mass concentration; mole (mol), the amount of a substance; mole per liter (mol/L), the substance concentration; and $\mu mol.s^{-1}/L$, used to report enzyme activity, the catalytic concentration.

Normal blood chemistry values for full-term newborns are given in Table 2.

[1] American Association of Clinical Chemists, *Normal Values for Pediatric Clinical Chemistry*, from the Special Committee on Pediatric Clinical Chemistry, August 1974.

[2] D. S. Young, Normal laboratory values (case records of the Massachusetts General Hospital) in SI units, *N. Engl. J. Med.*, **292:**795, 1975.

Table 3

Determination	Standard Units	Multiplication Factor	SI Units
Alkaline phosphatase:			
Newborn	73–226 m-IU/mL	NA*	NA
Child	46–111 m-IU/mL	NA	NA
Adolescent	57–258 m-IU/mL	NA	NA
Adult	6–61 m-IU/mL	NA	NA
Aldolase:			
Newborn	7.2–19.6 U/L (4 × adult)	1	7.2–19.6 mol.s⁻¹/L
Child	3.6–9.8 U/L (2 × adult)	1	3.6–9.8 mol.s⁻¹/L
Adult	1.8–4.9 U/L	1	1.8–4.9 mol.s⁻¹/L
Ammonia	<150 mg/100 mL	0.5872	<88.0 μmol/L
Amylase:			
Serum	<160 caraway u/100 mL	NA	
Urine	<30 caraway u/100 mL	NA	
Bicarbonate	18–25 meq/L	1.0	18–25 mmol/L
Bilirubin:			
>1 month	Total: <0.8 mg/100 mL	17.10	<13.6 μmol/L
	Direct: <0.4 mg/100 mL		<6.8 μmol/L
Calcium	9.0–11.5 mg/100 mL	0.2495	2.25–2.87 mmol/L
Carotene			
Birth to 6 months	0–0.4 μg/mL	1.863	0–0.74 μmol/L
6 months to adult	0.4–1.8 μg/mL		0.74–3.34 μmol/L
Chloride	95–105 meq/L	1.0	95–105 mmol/L
Cholesterol:			
0–1 year	65–120 mg/100 mL	0.02586	1.68–3.10 mmol/L
>1 year	95–195 mg/100 mL		2.46–5.04 mmol/L
Copper:			
0–6 months	<70 g/100 mL	0.1574	<11.02 μmol/L
6 months–5 years	27–153 μg/100 mL		4.2–24.0 μmol/L
5–17 years	94–234 μg/100 mL		14.8–36.8 μmol/L
Creatine phosphokinase	14–48 mU/mL	0.01667	0.23–0.8 μmol.s⁻¹/L
Creatinine:			
Newborn	0.8–1.4 mg/100 mL	88.40	70.7–123.8 μmol/L
Infant	0.7–1.7 mg /100 mL	88.40	61.9–150.3 μmol/L
Other	0.5–1.2 mg/100 mL	88.40	44.2–106.0 μmol/L
Glucose	55–100 mg/100 mL	0.05551	3.05–5.55 mmol/L
Haptoglobin	100–300 mg/100 mL	0.01	1.0–3.0 g/L
Iron:			
Serum Fe:			
Newborn	110–270 μg/100 mL	0.1791	19.7–48.4 μmol/L
4–10 months	30–70 μg/100 mL	0.1791	5.4–12.5 μmol/L
3–10 years	53–119 μg/100 mL	0.1791	9.5–21.3 μmol/L
>10 years	72–186 μg/100 mL	0.1791	12.9–33.3 μmol/L

* NA = not available.

Table 3 Continued

Determination	Standard Units	Multiplication Factor	SI Units
Total Fe Binding Capacity (TIBC):			
Newborn	262 (mean) μg/100 mL	0.1791	46.9 μmol/L
4–10 months	350 (mean) μg/100 mL	0.1791	62.7 μmol/L
3–10 years	386–522 μg/100 mL	0.1791	69.1–93.5 μmol/L
>10 years	280–360 μg/100 mL	0.1791	50.1–64.5 μmol/L
Lactate	1.0–1.8 meq/L	1.0	1.0–1.8 mmol/L
Lactic dehydrogenase:			
1 day–1 month	185–404 mU/mL	0.01667	3.1–6.7 μmol.s⁻¹/L
1 month–2 years	110–244mU/mL	0.01667	1.8–4.1 μmol.s⁻¹/L
3–17 years	86–165 mU/mL	0.01667	1.4–2.7 μmol.s⁻¹/L
Lead	<40 mg/100 mL	0.04826	4.93 μmol/L
Lipids:			
Total	400–1000 mg/100 mL	0.01	4.0–10.0 g/L
Phospholipids	166–300 mg/100 mL		
Triglycerides	30–150 mg/100 mL	0.01	0.3–1.5 g/L
Magnesium:			
Newborn	1.5–2.3 meq/L	0.5	0.7–1.15 mmol/L
Child	1.4–1.9 meq/L	0.5	0.7–0.9 mmol/L
Osmolarity	285–295 mosm/kg	1.0	285–295 mmol/kg
pH (arterial)	7.37–7.44	1.0	7.37–7.44
P_{CO_2}	35–45 mmHg	0.1333	4.7–6.0 kPa
P_{O_2}	80–100 mmHg	0.1333	10.7–13.3 kPa
Phosphorus (inorganic):			
Newborn	5.0–7.8 mg/100 mL	0.3229	1.6–2.5 mmol/L
1 month–1 year	3.8–6.2 mg/100 mL	0.3229	1.2–2.0 mmol/L
1–16 years	4.0–5.7 mg/100 mL	0.3229	1.3–1.8 mmol/L
Potassium	3.5–5.5 meq/L	1.0	3.5–5.5 mmol/L
Proteins:	g/100 mL	1.0	g/L

Age	Total	Albumin	Globulin
1–3 months	4.5–6.5	3.2–4.8	0.2–0.7
4–12 months	5.4–7.5	3.7–5.7	0.2–1.19
2–16 years	5.3–8.0	3.3–5.8	0.4–1.4

Determination	Standard Units	Multiplication Factor	SI Units
Sodium	136–145 meq/L	1.0	136–145 mmol/L
Transaminase:			
SGOT:			
Newborn	0–54 mU/mL	NA	NA
1 month–1 year	20–35 mU/mL	NA	NA
1–5 years	7–23 mU/mL	NA	NA
6–15 years	2–12 mU/mL	NA	NA
SGPT:			
Newborn	27–54 mU/mL	NA	NA
1 month–1 year	16–32 mU/mL	NA	NA
1–5 years	7–22 mU/mL	NA	NA
6–15 years	2–14 mU/mL	NA	NA
Urea nitrogen:			
Newborn	8–28 mg/100 mL	0.3569	2.9–10.0 mmol/L
1–16 years	10–20 mg/100 mL	0.3569	3.6–7.1 mmol/L
Uric acid	2.0–6.0 mg/100 mL	0.05948	0.12–0.36 mmol/L
Vitamin A	0.30–0.80 μg/mL	3.491	1.0–2.8 μmol/L
Vitamin E (tocopherol):			
Newborn	>0.3 mg/100 mL	NA	NA
Other	0.5–1.2 mg/100 mL	NA	NA

* NA = not available.

Bibliography

Aleck KA: Genetic-metabolic considerations in the sick neonate. *Pediatr Clin North Am* 25:431-451, 1978.

American Academy of Pediatrics, Committee on Drugs: Commentary on acetaminophen. *Pediatrics* 61:108-112, 1978.

Arnold EL (ed): *Helping Parents Help Their Children.* New York, Brunner/Mazel, 1978.

Avery GB (ed): *Neonatology: Pathophysiology and Management of the Newborn.* Philadelphia, JB Lippincott, 1975.

Beem MO, Saxon EM: Respiratory tract colonization and a distinctive pneumonia syndrome in infants infected with *Chlamydia trachomatis. N Engl J Med* 296:306-310, 1977.

Beem MO, Saxon EM, Tipple MA: Treatment of chlamydial pneumonia of infancy. *Pediatrics* 63:198-203, 1979.

Benirschke K: What pediatricians should know about the placenta. *Curr Probl Pediatr* II:10-11, 1971.

Brazleton TB: *Neonatal Behavioral Assessment Scale.* Philadelphia, International Ideas, 1974.

Buist NR: Metabolic screening of the newborn infant. *Clin Endocrinol Metab* 5:265-288, 1976.

Burton BK, Nadler HL: Clinical diagnosis of the inborn errors of metabolism in the neonatal period. *Pediatrics* 61:398-405, 1978.

Craig, W, Suh B: Theory and practical impact of binding of antimicrobials to serum proteins and tissue. *Scand J Infect Dis* 14:92-99, 1978.

Dallman PR, Siimes MA: Percentile curves for hemoglobin and red cell volume in infancy and childhood. *J Pediatr* 94:26-31, 1979.

Danforth DN (ed): *Obstetrics and Gynecology,* 3rd ed. Hagerstown, Md, Harper & Row, 1977.

Daniel WA: An approach to the adolescent patient. *Med Clin North Am* 59:1281-1282, 1975.

Department of Health, Education and Welfare/Public Health Service: Bacterial meningitis and meningococcemia—United States, 1978. *Morbidity and Mortality Weekly Report* 28:277-279, 1979.

Dewhurst CJ: Amenorrhea and the pediatrician. *Pediatr Clin North Am* 19:605, 1972.

Diem L, Lentor C (eds): *Scientific Tables,* 7th ed. Summit NJ, CIBA Pharmaceutical, 1970.

Drillien CM, Drummond M: *Neurodevelopmental Problems in Early Childhood: Assessment and Management.* Philadelphia, JB Lippincott, 1978.

Emans SJ, Goldstein DP: *Pediatric and Adolescent Gynecology.* Boston, Little Brown, 1977.

Esterly NB: Contact dermatitis. *Pediatr Rev* 1:85-90, 1979.

Farrell PM, Avery MD: Hyaline membrane disease. *Am Rev Respir Dis* 111:657-688, 1975.

Feldman WE: Bacterial etiology and mortality of purulent pericarditis in pediatric patients. Review of 162 cases. *Am J Dis Child* 133:641-644, 1979.

Fitzpatrick TB et al (eds): *Dermatology in General Medicine,* 2nd ed. New York, McGraw-Hill, 1979.

Fomon SJ: *Infant Nutrition,* 2nd ed. Philadelphia, WB Saunders, 1974.

Foung, S, Glader BE: Eosinophilia in children. *Pediatr Ann* 8:47, 1979.

Frasier SD: Growth disorders in children. *Pediatr Clin North Am* 26:1-14, 1979.

Friedman SB: Conversion symptoms in adolescents. *Pediatr Clin North Am* 20:873-882, 1973.

Fudenberg HH et al: *Basic and Clinical Immunology.* 2nd ed. Los Altos, Calif, Lange, 1978.

Fujiwara H, Hamashima Y: Pathology of the heart in Kawasaki disease. *Pediatrics* 61: 100-107, 1978.

Gardner H: *Developmental Psychology: An Introduction.* Boston, Little, Brown, 1978.

Gardner LI: *Endocrine and Genetic Diseases of Childhood and Adolescence,* 2nd ed. Philadelphia, WB Saunders, 1975.

Geiser CF: The histiocytosis syndromes. *Pediatr Ann* 8:54-64, 1979.

Gell PG, Coombs RR, Lachman PJ (eds): *Clinical Aspects of Immunology,* 3rd ed. Philadelphia, JB Lippincott, 1975.

Gellis SS, Kagan BM: *Current Pediatric Therapy 9.* Philadelphia, WB Saunders, 1980.

Golden GS: Tourette syndrome. The pediatric perspective. *Am J Dis Child* 131:531-534, 1977.

Goodman LS, Gilman A: *The Pharmacological Basis of Therapeutics,* 5th ed. New York Macmillan, 1975.

Granoff DM, Gilsdorf J, Gessert C et al: Haemophilus influenzae type B disease in a day care center: eradication of carrier state by rifampin. *Pediatrics* 63:397-401, 1979.

Green M, Haggerty RJ (eds): *Ambulatory Pediatrics Two: Personal Health Care of Children in the Office,* 2nd ed. Philadelphia, WB Saunders, 1977.

Greydanus DE, McAnarney ER: Contraception in the adolescent: current concepts for the pediatrician. *Pediatrics* 65:1-12, 1980.

Grodin JM: Secondary amenorrhea in the adolescent. *Pediatr Clin North Am* 19:619, 1972.

Grossman BJ, Mukhopadhay D: Juvenile rheumatoid arthritis. *Curr Probl Pediatr* 5:25-28, 1975.

Hambraeus L: Proprietary milk versus human breast milk in infant feeding. *Pediatr Clin North Am* 24:17-36, 1977.

Harley RD: *Pediatric Ophthalmology.* Philadelphia, WB Saunders, 1975.

Hoekelman RA et al (eds): *Principles of Pediatrics: Health Care of the Young.* New York, McGraw-Hill, 1978.

Hoeprich PD (ed): *Infectious Diseases,* 2nd ed. Hagerstown, Md, Harper & Row, 1977.

Hofmann AD: Adolescents in distress: suicide and out-of-control behaviors. *Med Clin North Am* 59:1429-1437, 1975.

Hofmann AD, Becker LD, Gabriel HP: *The Hospitalized Adolescent: A Guide to Managing the Ill and Injured Youth.* New York, Macmillan, 1976.

Hoppenfeld S: Back pain. *Pediatr Clin North Am* 24:884, 1977.

Hughes WT: *Pneumocystis carinii* pneumonia. *N Engl J Med* 297:1381-1383, 1977.

Isselbacher, KJ et al (eds): *Harrison's Principles of Internal Medicine,* 9th ed. New York, McGraw-Hill, 1980.

Jaffe FS: Sounding Board. The pill: a perspective for assessing risks and benefits. *N Engl J Med* 297:612-614, 1977.

Johnson RO, Clay SA, Arnon SS: Diagnosis and management of infant botulism. *Am J Dis Child* 133:586-593, 1979.

Johnston R, Magrab P: *Development Disorders: Assessment, Treatment, and Education.* Baltimore, University Park Press, 1976.

Journal of the American Medical Association: Standards for cardiopulmonary resuscitation (CPR) and emergency cardiac care (ECC). II. Basic life support. *JAMA* (suppl) 227: 841-851, 1974.

Kaplan BS, Thomson PD, de Chadarévian JP: The hemolytic uremic syndrome. *Pediatr Clin North Am* 23:761-777, 1976.

Kawabori I: Cyanotic congenital heart defects with increased pulmonary blood flow. *Pediatr Clin North Am* 25:777-795, 1978.

Kawasaki T, Kosaki F, Okawa S et al: A new infantile acute febrile mucocutaneous lymph node syndrome (MLNS) prevailing in Japan. *Pediatrics* 54:271-276, 1974.

Kempe CH et al: *Current Pediatric Diagnosis and Treatment.* 4th ed. Los Altos, Calif, Lange, 1976.

Kendig EL Jr, Chernick V (eds): *Disorders of the Respiratory Tract in Children,* 3rd ed. Philadelphia, WB Saunders, 1977.

Klein JO, Mortimer EA Jr: Use of pneumococcal vaccine in children. *Pediatrics* 61:321-322, 1978.

Koplan JP, Schoenbaum SC, Weinstein MC: Pertussis vaccine: an analysis of benefits, risks, and costs. *N Engl J Med* 301:906-911, 1979.

Kreisberg RA: Diabetic ketoacidosis: new concepts and trends in pathogenesis and treatment. *Ann Intern Med* 88:681-695, 1978.

Krugman S, Ward R, Katz SC: *Infectious Diseases of Children,* 6th ed. St. Louis, CV Mosby, 1977.

Kunin CM: Urinary tract infections in children. *Hosp Prac* II:91-98, 1976.

Lauder EC, Kanthor H, Myers G et al: Educational placement of children with spina bifida. *J Exceptional Child* 45:432-436, 1979.

Leichtman SR, Friedman SB: Social and psychological development of adolescents and the relationship to chronic illness. *Med Clin North Am* 59:1319-1328, 1975.

Levy G: Clinical pharmacokinetics of aspirin. *Pediatrics* 62:867-872, 1978.

Liebman WM: Recurrent abdominal pain in children: lactose and sucrose intolerance, a perspective study. *Pediatrics* 64:43-45, 1979.

Lockey RF, Bukantz SC: Allergic emergencies. *Med Clin North Am* 58:147-156, 1974.

Malmquist CP: Depression in childhood and adolescence. *N Engl J Med* 284:958-960, 1971.

Mamunes P: Newborn screening for metabolic disorders. *Clin Perinatol* 3:231-250, 1976.

Mann GV: The influence of obesity on health. Part II. *N Engl J Med* 291:226-232, 1974.

Mausner JS, Bahn AK: *Epidemiology: An Introductory Text.* Philadelphia, WB Saunders, 1974.

McAnarney ER: Adolescent pregnancy—a national priority. *Am J Dis Child* 132:125-126, 1978.

McAnarney ER, Greydanus DE: Adolescent pregnancy—a multi-faceted problem. *Pediatr Rev* 1:123-126, 1979.

McAnarney ER, Pless IB, Satterwhite B et al: Psychological problems of children with chronic juvenile arthritis. *Pediatrics* 53:523-528, 1974.

McGuigan M, Lovejoy FH: Recent developments in clinical toxicology. *Pediatr Alert* 3:67-68, 1978.

McMillan JA, Nieburg PI, Oski FA: *The Whole Pediatrician Catalog,* vol 1. Philadelphia, WB Saunders, 1977.

McMillan JA, Stockman JA, Oski FA: *The Whole Pediatrician Catalog,* vol 2. Philadelphia, WB Saunders, 1979.

Medical Letter: Drugs in breast milk. 21:21-24, March 1979.

Mendoza SA, Chan CM: Syndrome of inappropriate antidiuretic hormone secretion (SIADH). *Pediatr Clin North Am* 23:681, 1976.

Menkes JH: *Textbook of Child Neurology.* Philadelphia, Lea & Febiger, 1974.

Middleton E, Reed C, Ellis E (eds): *Allergy: Principles and Practice.* St. Louis, CV Mosby, 1978.

Miller D: *Ophthalmology: The Essentials.* Boston, Houghton Mifflin, 1979.

Miller HC, Merritt TA: *Fetal Growth in Humans.* Chicago, Year Book, 1979.

Miller M, Hall J: *Familial asymmetric crying facies. Am J Dis Child* 133:743-746, 1979.

Mishell DR: Contraception. *Am J Dis Child* 132:912-920, 1978.

Mokrohisky ST, Levine R, Blumhagen JD et al: Low positioning of umbilical-artery catheters increases associated complications in newborn infants. *N Engl J Med* 299:561-564, 1978.

Nadas AS, Fyler DC: *Pediatric Cardiology,* 3rd ed. Philadelphia, WB Saunders, 1972.

Nathan DG, Oski FA (eds): *Hematology of Infancy and Childhood.* Philadelphia, WB Saunders, 1974.

Nelhaus G: Brain tumors in children. *Pediatr Ann* 3:18-37, 1974.

Noonan JA: Association of congenital heart disease with syndromes of other defects. *Pediatr Clin North Am* 25:797-816, 1978.

Nyhan W: An approach to the diagnosis of overwhelming metabolic disease in early infancy. *Curr Probl Pediatr* VII:6-12, 1977.

Oski F, Naiman JL: *Hematologic Problems in the Newborn.* Philadelphia, WB Saunders, 1972.

Paradise JL: On tympanostomy tubes: rationale, results, reservations, and recommendations. *Pediatrics* 60:86-90, 1977.

Paradise JL, Smith CG, Bluestone CD: Tympanometric detection of middle ear effusion in infants and young children. *Pediatrics* 58:198-210, 1976.

Peterson B: Morbidity of childhood near-drowning. *Pediatrics* 59:364-370, 1978.

Pinkel D: Treatment of acute leukemia. *Pediatr Clin North Am* 23:117-130, 1976.

Pitts RF: *Physiology of the Kidney and Body Fluids,* 3rd ed. Chicago, Year Book, 1974.

Polgar G, Promadhat V: *Pulmonary Function Testing in Children.* Philadelphia, WB Saunders, 1971.

Rahal JJ Jr: Antibiotic combinations: the clinical relevance of synergy and antagonism. *Medicine* 57:179-195, 1978.

Reilly PP: What makes adolescent girls flee from their homes? An analysis of 50 such girls studied at Boston Juvenile Court. *Clin Pediatr* 17:886-893, 1978.

Rimoin DL, Horton WA: Short stature. Part I and II. *J Pediatr* 92:523-528, 697-704, 1978.

Rosenberg LE, Kidd KK: HLA and disease susceptibility: a primer (editorial). *N Engl J Med* 297:1060-1062, 1977.

Roy CC, Silverman A, Cozzetto FJ: *Pediatric Clinical Gastroenterology,* 2nd ed. St. Louis, CV Mosby, 1975.

Rudolph AM et al (eds): *Pediatrics,* 16th ed. New York, Appleton-Century-Crofts, 1977.

Safar P (ed): *Advances in Cardiopulmonary Resuscitation.* New York, Springer-Verlag, 1975.

Sahler OJ: *The Child and Death.* St. Louis, CV Mosby, 1978.

Schaffer AJ, Avery ME: *Diseases of the Newborn,* 4th ed. Philadelphia, WB Saunders, 1977.

Schaller JG, Omenn GS: The histocompatibility system and human disease. *J Pediatr* 86:913-925, 1976.

Scherzer AL, Gardner GG: Studies of the school age child with meningomyelocele: I. Physical and intellectual development. *Pediatrics* 47:424-430, 1971.

Schiff L: *Diseases of the Liver,* 4th ed. Philadelphia, JB Lippincott, 1975.

Schmitt BD: School phobia, the great imitator. *Pediatrics* 48:433-441, 1971.

Schmitt BD, Kempe CH: The pediatrician's role in child abuse and neglect. *Curr Probl Pediatr* 5:15-17, 1975.

Schuberth KC, Zittelli BJ: *The Harriet Lane Handbook,* 8th ed. Chicago, Year Book, 1978.

Scott MD, Crawford JD: Solitary thyroid nodules in childhood: is the incidence of thyroid carcinoma declining? *Pediatrics* 58:521-525, 1976.

Sell EJ, Harris TE: Association of premature rupture of membranes with idiopathic respiratory distress syndrome. *Obstet Gynecol* 49:167-169, 1977.

Settle GW: The anatomy of congenital talipes equinovarus. *J Bone Joint Surg* 45-A:1341-1354, 1963.

Shenker IR, Nussbaum M, Kaplan E: Delayed puberty and short stature in adolescents. *Pediatr Ann* 7:608-610, 1978.

Singer HS, Freeman JM: Head trauma for the pediatrician. *Pediatrics* 62:819-825, 1978.

Sleisenger MH, Fordtran JS: *Gastrointestinal Disease: Pathophysiology, Diagnosis, Management,* 2nd ed. Philadelphia, WB Saunders, 1978.

Smith AL: Management of animal and human bites. *Pediatr Alert* 4:45-48, 1979.

Smith CA (ed): *The Critically Ill Child: Diagnosis and Management,* 2nd ed. Philadelphia, WB Saunders, 1977.

Smith CK: Surgical procedures for correction of hypospadias. *J Urol* 40:239-247, 1938.

Smith DW: *Recognizable Patterns of Human Malformation: Genetic, Embryologic and Clinical Aspects,* 2nd ed, vol 7. Philadelphia, WB Saunders, 1976.

Smith DW, Klein AM, Henderson JR et al: Congenital hypothyroidism: signs and symptoms in the newborn period. *J Pediatr* 87:958-962, 1975.

Staheli LT, Smith JB: Knee problems in children. *Pediatr Clin North Am* 24:841, 1977.

Stiehm ER: Standard and special human immune serum globulins as therapeutic agents. *Pediatrics* 63:301-319, 1979.

Stiehm ER, Fulginiti VA: *Immunologic Disorders in Infants and Children.* Philadelphia, WB Saunders, 1973.

Tachdjian MO: *Pediatric Orthopedics.* Philadelphia, WB Saunders, 1972.

Thibeault DW, Gregor GA: *Neonatal Pulmonary Care.* Reading, Pa, Addison-Wesley, 1979.

Thomas A, Chess S, Birch HG: *Temperament and Behavior Disorders in Children.* New York, New York University Press, 1968.

Thompson RJ Jr, O'Quinn AN: *Developmental Disabilities: Etiology, Manifestation, Diagnosis and Treatment.* New York, Oxford University Press, 1979.

Touloukian RJ (ed): *Pediatric Trauma.* New York, John Wiley & Sons, 1978.

Vaughan VC III, McKay RJ, Behrman RE: *Nelson Textbook of Pediatrics,* 11th ed. Philadelphia, WB Saunders, 1979.

Verdain BH: Physical growth and development during puberty. *Med Clin North Am* 59: 1315-1316, 1975.

Ward JI: Haemophilus influenzae meningitis: a prospective national study of secondary spread in household contacts. *N Engl J Med* 301:122-126, 1979.

Weiner IB: Juvenile delinquency. *Pediatr Clin North Am* 22:673-684, 1975.

West CD: Asymptomatic hematuria and proteinuria in children: causes and appropriate diagnostic studies. *J Pediatr* 89:173-182, 1976.

Wettenhall HNB, Cahill C, Roche AF: Tall girls: a survey of 15 years of management and treatment. *J Pediatr* 86:602-610, 1975.

Wientzen RL, McCracken GH Jr: Pathogenesis and management of neonatal sepsis and meningitis. *Curr Probl Pediatr* VIII:3-54, 1977.

Wiese J, Osler M: Contraception in diabetic patients. *Acta Endocrinol* (suppl) 182:87-94, 1974.

Yow MD, Katz SL: *Red Book,* 18th ed. Evanston, Ill, American Academy of Pediatrics, Report of the Committee on Infectious Diseases, 1977.

Yunis A, Bloomberg G: Chloramphenicol toxicity: clinical features and pathogenesis. *Prog Hematol* 4:138, 1964.

Zelnick M, Kantner JF: Contraceptive patterns and premarital pregnancy among women aged 15-19. *Fam Plann Perspect* 10:135-142, 1978.

Ziai M, Janeway CA, Cooke R: *Pediatrics,* 2nd ed. Boston, Little Brown, 1975.